Case Studies in **Nursing Ethics**

Case Studies in
Nursing Ethics

Robert M. Veatch, Ph.D.

Professor of Medical Ethics
Joseph and Rose Kennedy
Institute of Ethics
Georgetown University
Washington, D.C.

Sara T. Fry, Ph.D., R.N.

Assistant Professor
School of Nursing
University of Virginia
Charlottesville, Virginia

Jones and Bartlett Publishers
Boston   London

Editorial, Sales, and Customer Service Offices

Jones and Bartlett Publishers
One Exeter Plaza
Boston, MA 02116
617-859-3900
1-800-832-0034

Jones and Bartlett Publishers International
7 Melrose Terrace
London W6 7RL
England

Library of Congress Cataloging-in-Publication Data

Veatch, Robert M.
  Case studies in nursing ethics.

  Includes bibliographies and index.
  1. Nursing ethics—Case studies.   I. Fry, Sara T.
II. Title.   [DNLM: 1. Ethics, Nursing. WY 85 V394c]
RT85.V4   1987   174'.2   86-27351
ISBN 0-87620-481-8

Printed in the United States of America
98 97 96 95   10 9 8 7 6 5

The authors and publisher have exerted every effort to ensure that
drug selection and dosage set forth in this text are in accord with
current recommendations and practice at the time of publication.
However, in view of ongoing research, changes in government
regulations, and the constant flow of information relating to drug
therapy and drug reactions, the reader is urged to check the
package insert for each drug for any change in indications and
dosage and for added warnings and precautions. This is particularly
important when the recommended agent is a new or infrequently
employed drug.

Preface

The biological revolution has brought about radical changes in health care. It has produced a set of problems in biomedical ethics that confront health care professionals as well as lay people making health care decisions. These developments have affected nursing dramatically. The nurse has long been the health care professional in closest contact with the patient, often perceiving ethical and other value differences among the patient, the physician, and other involved individuals. Increasingly nurses recognize that they have responsibility to be active, participating members of the health care team initiating actions when ethical questions emerge.

In the 1970s the use of case studies in medical ethics became an important way of helping health care professionals prepare for the increasing importance of ethical choices in health care. One of us prepared a collection published as *Case Studies in Medical Ethics* (Harvard University Press, 1977). That collection took medical ethics very broadly, emphasizing medical ethical decisions made by the entire range of health care professionals and lay people. While some of those cases involved nurses, it was clear that nurses face biomedical ethical problems in unique ways. They stand in special role relations with patients, families, physicians, and other members of the health care team. The two authors of this volume, having worked together for many years, realized that a special collection of cases focusing more specifically on the ethical problems facing nurses was needed. *Case Studies in Nursing Ethics* is the result of the collecting of those cases.

While the collection can be used as a source of ad hoc cases covering a wide range of topics, it can also be treated much more systematically. The authors were committed to organizing the cases in a format appropriate for the systematic study of applied ethics. The first part of the book deals with cases posing basic questions of the meaning and justification of ethical claims. It focuses on identifying ethical and other value problems and examining the role of codes and other sources of ethical reflection. The second part provides an opportunity to explore the basic principles of ethics as they have their impact on nursing. These principles are general and broad. As such they have impact on the ethical thinking of nurses in many different contexts. Part three provides an opportunity to apply these principles to more specific contexts in nursing practice and to examine some of the special frameworks for dealing with such topics as abortion, informed consent, and the care of the terminally ill. Taken together, the three parts of the book provide a text in basic ethics while at the same time showing how ethical theory is applied to the field of nursing. We hope that many readers will use this volume as an opportunity to confront systematically the full range of basic problems in ethics.

Almost all of the cases presented are based on real situations experienced by one of the authors or shared with us by one of the many nurses who helped develop this collection. Except in cases in the public domain as indicated with references to sources, the names and details have been changed to protect confidentiality and provide greater clarity of the ethical issues involved. Nevertheless, they grow out of real experiences faced by nurses who have been left ethically perplexed. A small number of cases, especially those, such as gene manipulation, involving future problems anticipated in nursing, have been constructed based on discussions with persons actively involved in clinical and policy-formulating settings.

A great number of people have helped us in preparing this collection. Our special appreciation is extended to Mrs. Eunice Kennedy Shriver for her long-term interest in the development of nursing ethics and to the Joseph P. Kennedy, Jr. Foundation for continued support of nurses in the study of ethics, from the early 1970s to the present. Their insights and influence are well represented throughout the entire volume.

Many individuals have helped us in the collection of case materials. Some have preferred to remain anonymous. Others have shared cases with us without wanting their names attached to specific cases. Among those to whom we are grateful are Jodie Lavin-Tompkins, Donna MacMillan-Scattergood, Deborah Marrington, Judith Melson, Lynn Noland, Carol Page, and Carolyn S. Rogers. Patricia Arford, Emilie Dolge, Manuel Fernandez, Caren Kieswetter, and Lynn Noland spent many hours in the preparation of the manuscript, and to them our appreciation is gratefully acknowledged. To the many nurses who have discussed preliminary versions of cases and commentaries, we are also grateful. Nurses face a tremendous challenge in formulating their own ethical positions and in dealing with those of patients and members of the health care team. We hope this collection of cases will help in meeting that challenge.

Robert M. Veatch
Sara T. Fry

Contents

List of Case Studies

indigent

Case Studies in **Nursing Ethics**

Four Questions
of Ethics

The term *nursing ethics* is controversial. Some insist that nursing ethics is a unique field posing issues that cannot be understood fully by adapting the professional ethics of physicians. They insist on the term *nursing ethics* because it connotes the uniqueness of the moral problems that nurses face in the health care setting.

On the other hand, others argue against the term. Some suggest that there is really very little that is morally unique to nursing. The same ethical principles and the same moral issues emerge in the health care setting whether one is a physician, nurse, or patient.

Case Studies in Nursing Ethics puts forth the view that nursing ethics is a legitimate term referring to a field that is a subcategory of biomedical ethics. Biomedical ethics is simply the ethics of judgments made within the biomedical sciences. The analysis of the ethical judgments made by physicians can be called physician ethics. Similarly, the analysis of ethical judgments made by nurses can be called nursing ethics. Like physician ethics, nursing ethics is a subsystem derived from a larger, general system of biomedical ethics.

Biomedical ethics as a field presents a fundamental problem. As a branch of applied ethics, biomedical ethics becomes interesting and relevant only when it abandons the ephemeral realm of theory and abstract speculation and gets down to practical questions raised by real, everyday problems of health and illness. Much of biomedical ethics, especially as practiced within the health professions, is indeed oriented to the practical questions of what should be done in a particular case. Nursing, like other health professions, is case oriented. Yet if those who must resolve the ever-increasing ethical dilemmas in health care treat every case as something entirely fresh, entirely novel, they will have lost perhaps the best way of reaching solutions: to understand the general principles of ethics and face each new situation from a systematic ethical stance.

This is a volume of case studies in nursing ethics. It begins by recognizing the fact that one cannot approach any ethics, especially nursing ethics, in the abstract. It is real-

Introduction adapted with permission of the publishers from *Case Studies in Medical Ethics* by Robert M. Veatch, Cambridge, Mass.: Harvard University Press, Copyright © 1977 by the President and Fellows of Harvard College.

life, flesh-and-blood cases that raise fundamental ethical questions. It also recognizes that a general framework is needed from which to resolve the dilemmas of nursing practice. The cases in this volume are therefore organized in a systematic way. The chapters and issues within the chapters are arranged in order to work systematically through the questions of ethics. Since the main purpose of the book is to provide a collection of case studies from which may be built a more comprehensive scheme for nursing ethics, the first few pages address more theoretical issues. The goal is to construct a framework of the basic questions in ethics that must be answered in any complete and systematic bioethical system.

Four fundamental questions must be answered in order to take a complete and systematic ethical position. Each question has several plausible answers, which have been developed over two thousand years of Western thought. For normal day-to-day decisions made by the nurse, it is not necessary to deal with each question. In fact, to do so would paralyze the nurse decision-maker. Most nursing decisions are quite ordinary—such as deciding when to ambulate a patient, when to flush an IV, or how often to check on a chronically ill patient—and do not always demand full ethical analysis. Other decisions, as in the case of emergency intervention, are not ordinary at all. Still, in both the ordinary and emergency situations it is possible to act without being immobilized by ethical and other value problems because some general rules or guidelines have emerged from previous experience and reflection. If ethical conflict is serious enough, it will be necessary to deal, at least implicitly, with all four of the fundamental questions of ethics.

WHAT MAKES RIGHT ACTS RIGHT?

At the most general level, which ethicists call the level of metaethics, the first question is: What makes right acts right? What are the meaning and justification of ethical statements?

At first, it may not be obvious what counts as an ethical problem in nursing. Nurses easily recognize the moral crisis in deciding to let an abnormal newborn die, choosing which of two needy patients will receive a heart transplant, participating in a late-term abortion for what, to the nurse, seems like trivial reasons, or helping a terminally ill patient in pain end his life. These situations clearly seem to involve ethical problems. Yet it is not immediately evident why we call these problems ethical while others faced more commonly in the routine practice of nursing are not so designated.

To make ethical problems obvious, several steps should be followed.

Distinguishing Between Evaluative Statements and Statements Presenting Nonevaluative Facts

Ethics involves making evaluations; therefore, it is a normative enterprise. Moving from the judgment that we can do something to the one that we ought to do something involves incorporating a set of norms—of judgments of value, rights, duties, responsibilities, and the like. Thus, in order to be ethically responsible in the practice of nursing, it is important to develop the ability to recognize evaluations as they are made in nursing practice.

To develop this ability, select an experience that, at first, seems to involve no particular value judgments. Begin describing what occurred and watch for evaluative words. Every time a word expressing value is encountered, note it. Among the words to watch for are verbs such as *want, desire, prefer, should,* or *ought.* Evaluations may also be expressed in nouns such as *benefit, harm, duty, responsibility, right,* or *obligation,* or in related adjectives such as *good* and *bad, right* and *wrong, responsible, fitting,* and the like.

Sometimes evaluations are expressed in terms that are not necessarily literal, direct expressions of evaluations but are clearly functioning as value judgments. The American Nurses' Association (ANA) *Code for Nurses,* for example, states that "the nurse provides services...unrestricted by considerations of social or economic status, personal attributes, or the nature of health problems."[1] By this statement, the ANA could be describing facts about the way all nurses behave. Obviously it is not, however. Rather, it is saying that the nurse ought to provide services without discrimination and that the good nurse does so provide them.

Distinguishing Between Moral and Nonmoral Evaluations

The process of distinguishing between moral and nonmoral evaluations can be much harder, since often the difference cannot be discerned from the language itself. If one says that the nurse did a good job of informing the patient about the reasons for instituting intravenous fluid therapy, the statement could express many kinds of evaluations. It could mean that the nurse did a good job legally—the nurse fulfilled the law. It could mean that the nurse did a good job psychologically—the job was done in a way that produced a good psychological impact on the patient. It could mean that the nurse did a good job technically—every relevant piece of information was conveyed accurately. Or it could mean the nurse did a good job ethically—the nurse did what was morally required. Conceivably, a good evaluation in one of these senses could simultaneously be a bad evaluation in some other sense.

Sometimes value judgments in nursing practice simply express nonmoral evaluations. Saying that the patient ate well does not express a moral evaluation of the way the patient consumed the food. Saying that another day's hospitalization will be good for the patient means only that the patient will be helped physically or psychologically, not morally. Even these apparently nonmoral judgments about benefits and harms, however, may quickly lead one into the sphere of ethics. When the client's judgment of what will be beneficial, for example, differs from the nurse's judgment, specific ethical dilemmas may emerge. A nurse who is committed morally to doing what will benefit the client will choose one course while the nurse who is committed to preserving client autonomy may reluctantly choose the other.

Ethical or moral evaluations are judgments of what is good or bad, right or wrong, having certain characteristics that separate them from other evaluations such as aesthetic judgments, personal preferences, beliefs, or matters of taste. The difference between the evaluations lies in the grounds on or the reasons for which the evaluations are being made.[2] Moral evaluations possess certain characteristics. They are evaluations of human actions, institutions, or character traits, rather than inanimate objects such as paintings or architectural structures. Not all evaluations of human actions are moral evaluations, however. We may say that the nurse is a good administrator or a good teacher without making a moral evaluation. To be considered moral, an evaluation must have additional characteristics. Three characteristics are often mentioned as the distinctive characteristics of moral evaluations. First, the evaluations must be ultimate. They must have a certain preemptive quality, meaning that other values or human ends cannot, as a rule, override them.[3] Second, they must possess universality. Moral evaluations are thought of as reflecting a standpoint that applies to everyone. They are evaluations that everyone, in principle, ought to be able to make and understand (even if some, in fact, do not do so).[4] Finally, many add a third, more material, condition: that moral evaluations must treat the good of everyone alike. They must be general in the sense that they avoid giving a special place to one's own welfare. They must have an other-regarding focus or, at least, must consider one's own welfare on a par with that of others.[3,5,6]

Moral judgments possessing these characteristics can sometimes conflict with one another. Conflicts over whether the nurse ought to care for a client in the way thought to be most beneficial or that would preserve the client's autonomy (even though harm may result) can involve conflicts between moral characteristics. If that is the case, any clinical decision in nursing practice that involves a conflict over values, potentially involves a moral conflict. The nurse may be faced with the choice between preserving the client's welfare or that of someone else. The nurse may have to choose whether to keep a promise of confidentiality or provide needed assistance for a client even though a confidence would have to be broken. The nurse may have to decide whether to protect the interests of colleagues or of the institution, whether to serve future patients by striking for better conditions or serve present patients by refusing to strike. These are moral conflicts in nursing. Chapter 1 presents a series of cases in which both moral and nonmoral evaluations are made in what appear to be quite ordinary nursing situations. The main task is to discern the value dimensions and to separate them from the physiological, psychological, and other facts.

Determining Who Ought to Decide

A closely related problem that depends on the question of what makes right acts right is that of who ought to decide. This is the focus of Chapter 2. Having learned to recognize the difference between the factual and evaluative dimensions of a case in nursing ethics, one will constantly encounter the problem of who ought to decide or where the locus of decision-making ought to rest. Chapter 2 presents cases with a wide range of sources of moral authority, from institutions, patients, families, physicians, and administrators to professional committees and the general public.

The choice among these decision-makers depends, at least in part, on what it is that ethical terms mean, or more generally, what it is that makes right acts right. Several answers to this question have been offered. One answer is rooted in the fact that different societies seem to reach different conclusions about whether a given act is right or wrong. Holders of this view go on to say that an act is morally right means nothing more than that it is in accord with the values of the speaker's society or simply that it is approved by the speaker's society. This position, called social relativism, explains rightness or wrongness on the basis of whether the act fits with social customs, mores, and folkways. One problem with this view is that it seems to make sense to say that some act is morally wrong even though it is approved by the society of the speaker. That would be impossible if moral judgments were based simply on the values of the speaker's society.

A second answer to the question of what makes right acts right attempts to correct this problem. According to this position, to say that an act is right means that it is approved by the speaker. This position, called personal relativism, reduces ethical meaning to personal preference. This means that behavior thought to be immoral by some is approved by others. Some say that the reason this can happen is that moral judgments are merely expressions of the speaker's preference.

Such differences in judgment, however, may have another explanation than that ethical terms refer to the speaker's own preferences. Those disagreeing might simply not be working with the same facts. To claim that two people are in moral disagreement simply because the same act is seen as right by one person or society and wrong by another requires proof that both see the facts in the same way. Differences of circumstances or belief about the facts could easily account for many moral differences.

In contrast with social and personal relativism, there is a third, more universal group of answers to the question of what makes right acts right. These positions, collectively called universalism or sometimes absolutism, hold that, in principle, acts that are called morally right or wrong are right or wrong independent of social or personal biases. Certainly some choices merely involve personal taste: flavors of ice cream or hair lengths vary from time to time, place to place, and person to person. But these are matters of preference, not morality. No one considers the choice of vanilla morally right and chocolate morally wrong. Other evaluations appeal beyond the standards of social and personal taste to a more universal frame of reference. When these are concerned with acts or character traits—as opposed to, say, paintings or music—they are thought of as moral evaluations.

However, the nature of the universal standard is often disputed. For the theologically oriented, it may be a divine standard. According to this view, calling it right to disconnect a respirator keeping alive a terminally ill, comatose patient is to say that God would approve of the act. This position is sometimes called theological absolutism or theological universalism.

Still another view among universalists takes empirical observation as the model. The standard in this case is nature or external reality. The problem of knowing whether an act is right or wrong is then the problem of knowing what is in nature. Empirical absolutism, as the view is sometimes called, sees the problem of knowing right and wrong as analogous to knowing scientific facts.[7,8] Whereas astronomy is the attempt to discern the real nature of the universe of stars and chemistry the real nature of atoms as ordered in nature, ethics is an effort to discern rightness and wrongness as ordered in nature. The position sometimes takes the form of a natural law position. As with the physicist's law of gravity, moral laws are thought to be inexplicably rooted in nature. Natural law positions may be secular or may have a theological foundation such as in the ethics of Thomas Aquinas and traditional Catholic moral theology.

Still another form of universalism or absolutism rejects both the theological and empirical models. It supposes that right and wrong are not empirically knowable, but are nonnatural properties known only by intuition. Thus, the position is sometimes called intuitionism or nonnaturalism.[9] Although, for the intuitionist or nonnaturalist, right and wrong are not empirically knowable, they are still universal. All persons should, in principle, have the same intuitions about a particular act, provided they are intuiting properly. Still others, sometimes called rationalists, hold that reason can determine what is ethically required.[10]

There are other answers to the question of what makes right acts right. One view—in various forms called noncognitivism, emotivism, or prescriptivism—which ascended to popularity during the mid-twentieth century, saw ethical utterances as evincing feelings about a particular act.[11–13] A full exploration of the answers to this most abstract of ethical questions is not possible here.* Ultimately, however, if an ethical dispute growing out of a case is serious enough and cannot be resolved at any other level, this question must be faced. If one says that it is wrong to tell the truth to a dying patient because it will produce anxiety, and another says that it is right to do so because consent to treatment is a moral imperative, some way must be found of adjudicating the dispute between the two principles. Then one must ask what it is that makes right acts right, how conflicts can be resolved, and what the final authority is for morality.

WHAT KINDS OF ACTS ARE RIGHT?

A second fundamental question of ethics moves beyond determining what makes right acts right to ask: What kinds of acts are right? This is the realm of normative ethics. It questions whether there are any general principles or norms describing the characteristics that make actions right or wrong.

Consequentialism

Two major schools of thought dominate Western normative ethics. One position looks at the consequences of acts, the other at what are taken to be inherent rights and wrongs. The first position claims that acts are right to the extent that they produce good consequences and wrong to the extent that they produce bad consequences. The key evaluative terms for this position, known as utilitarianism or consequentialism, are *good* and

*For basic surveys of ethical theory see Frankena W: Ethics, 2nd ed. Englewood Cliffs, NJ, Prentice-Hall, 1973; and Warnock GJ: Contemporary Moral Philosophy. New York, St Martin's Press, 1967. For more detailed introductions see Brandt RB: Ethical Theory: The Problems of Normative and Critical Ethics. Englewood Cliffs, NJ, Prentice-Hall, 1959; Beauchamp TL: Philosophical Ethics: An Introduction to Moral Philosophy. New York, McGraw-Hill, 1982; Feldman F: Introductory Ethics. Englewood Cliffs, NJ, Prentice-Hall, 1978; and Taylor PW: Principles of Ethics: An Introduction. Encino, CA, Dickenson, 1975. For readings containing classical sources see Brandt RB: Value and Obligation: Systematic Readings in Ethics. New York, Harcourt, Brace & World, 1961; and Melden AI (ed): Ethical Theories: A Book of Readings, 2nd ed. Englewood Cliffs, NJ, Prentice-Hall, 1967.

bad. This is the position of John Stuart Mill and Jeremy Bentham, as well as of Epicurus, Thomas Aquinas, and capitalist economics. Aquinas, for example, argued that the first principle of the natural law is that "good is to be done and promoted and evil is to be avoided."[14]

Aquinas stands at the center of the Roman Catholic natural law tradition. He illustrates that natural law thinking (which is one answer to the first question of what makes right acts right) is not incompatible with consequentialism. The two positions are answers to two different questions. While natural law thinkers are not always consequentialists, they can be.

Classical utilitarianism determines what kinds of acts are right by figuring the net of good consequences minus bad ones for each person affected and then adding up to find the total net good.[15] The certainty and duration of the benefits and harms are taken into account. Unfortunately, this form of consequentialism is indifferent to who obtains the benefits and harms. Thus, if the total net benefits of providing nursing care to a relatively healthy but powerful figure are thought to be greater than those of providing it to a sicker Medicare recipient, the healthy and powerful ought to be given the care without further ethical debate.

Traditional nursing ethics, like physician ethics, is oriented to benefiting patients. This tradition combines the utilitarian answer to the question of what kinds of acts are right with a particular answer to the question of to whom is moral duty owed. Loyalty is to the patient, and the goal is to what will produce the most benefit and avoid the most harm to the patient.

Nursing ethics traditionally holds that the nurse's primary commitment is to the client's care and safety. Some interpret this as emphasizing protecting the client from harm as being prior to benefiting the client. Like the principle of physician ethics, *primum non nocere* or "first of all do no harm," it gives special weight to avoiding harm over and above the weight given to goods that can be produced.

Among physicians the principle of doing no harm is often interpreted conservatively so that harm is avoided by nonaction. Nurses may be more active in avoiding harm, especially when they take an advocacy role to attempt to prevent a harm to the client. In either case, however, when nursing ethics gives special weight to certain kinds of consequences (*i.e.,* avoiding harm), it is still further distinguished from classical utilitarianism.

These problems of the relation between classical utilitarianism (which counts benefits to all in society equally) and traditional nursing ethics (which focuses on the individual patient and sometimes gives special weight to avoiding harms through the prescriptive duty of advocacy) are raised in the cases in Chapter 3.

Nonconsequentialism

In contrast to these positions that are oriented to consequences, the other major group of answers to the question of what kinds of acts are right asserts that rightness and wrongness are inherent in the act itself independent of the consequences. These positions are collectively known as nonconseqentialism. They are sometimes called formalism or deontologism. They hold that right- and wrong-making characteristics may be independent of consequences. Kant stated the position most starkly.[10]

Chapter 4 takes up problems of health care delivery and in doing so poses probably the most significant challenge to the consequentialist ethic. The dominant ethical principle of health care delivery is that of justice. Taken in the sense of fairness in distributing goods and harms, justice is held by many to be a right-making ethical characteristic even if the consequences are not the best. The problem is whether it is morally preferable to have a higher net total of benefits in society even if unevenly distributed, or to have a somewhat lower total good but to have that good more equally distributed. Utilitarians would argue that net benefits tend to be greater when benefits are distributed more evenly (because of decreasing marginal utility). They claim that the only reason to distribute goods, such as health care, evenly is to maximize the total good. On the other hand, the formalist who holds that justice is a right-making characteristic independent of utility does not require an item-by-item calculation of benefits and harms before concluding that the unequal distribution of goods is *prima facie* wrong, that is, wrong with regard to fairness.

Another major challenge to consequentialism comes from the principle of autonomy. Where classic utilitarianism leads to a moral principle of demanding noninterference with the autonomy of others in society because this produces greater net benefits, Kantian formalism leads to the moral demand that persons and their beliefs be respected per se. The problems of conflict between the nurse's nonconsequentialist duties to respect autonomy or self-determination of individual clients and consequentialist duties to produce benefit are discussed in Chapter 5.

Another ethical principle that many formalists hold to be independent of consequences is that of truth-telling or veracity. As with the other principles, utilitarians argue that truth-telling is an operational principle designed to guarantee maximum benefit. When truth-telling does more harm than good, according to the utilitarians, there is no obligation to tell the truth. To them, telling the dying patient of his condition can be cruel and therefore wrong. In contrast, to one who holds that truth-telling is a right-making ethical principle in itself, the problem of what the dying patient should be told is much more complex. This problem of what the patient should be told is the subject of Chapter 6.

Another characteristic that formalists may believe to be right-making independent of consequences is the duty of fidelity, especially the keeping of promises. Kant and others have held that breaking a promise will at least tend to be wrong independent of the consequences. If it were to become a usual practice, the act of promising itself would become useless. The formalist, although granting this danger, argues that there is something basically wrong in breaking a promise and that to know this one need not even go on to look at the consequences. The formalist might, with the utilitarian, grant that to look at consequences may reveal even more reasons to oppose promise-breaking, but this is not necessary to know that promise-breaking is *prima facie* wrong.

The nurse–patient relationship can be viewed essentially as one involving promises, contracts, or, to use a term with fewer legalistic implications, covenants. The relationship is founded on implied and sometimes explicit promises. One of these promises is that information disclosed in the nurse–patient relationship is confidential, that it will not be disclosed by the nurse without the patient's permission. The principle of confidentiality in ethics is really a specification of the principle of promise-keeping in ethics in general. In Chapter 7, cases present the various problems growing out of the ethical principle of fidelity.

The cases in Chapter 8 introduce a final principle that can be included in a general ethical system: the principle of avoiding killing. All societies have some kind of prohibition on killing. The Buddhists make it one of their five basic precepts. Those in the Judeo-Christian tradition recognize it as one of the Ten Commandments. The moral foundation of the prohibition on killing is not always clear, however. For some people, who base their ethic on doing good and avoiding evil, prohibiting killing is simply a rule summarizing the obvious conclusion that it usually does a person harm to kill him. If that is the full foundation of the prohibition on killing, then killing is just an example of a way that one can do harm.

This presents a problem, however. Many people believe that they are aware of special cases in which killing someone may actually, on balance, do good. It will stop a greater evil that the one killed would otherwise have committed, or it will, in health care, possibly relieve a terminally ill patient of otherwise intractable pain. Is killing a human being always a characteristic of actions that tends to make them morally wrong, or is it wrong only when more harm than good results from the killing? For those who hold that killing is always a wrong-making characteristic, avoiding killing takes on a life as an independent principle much like veracity, autonomy, or fidelity. The cases in Chapter 8 explore these questions.

HOW DO RULES APPLY TO SPECIFIC SITUATIONS?

There is a third question in a general ethical stance. It stems from the fact that each case raising an ethical problem is in at least some ways situationally unique. The ethical principles of benefiting, justice, autonomy, truth-telling, fidelity, and avoiding killing are extremely general. They are a small set of the most general right-making characteristics. Applications to specific cases require a great leap. The question is, how do the general principles apply to specific situations? As a bridge to specific cases, an intermediate, more specific set of rules is often used. These intermediate rules probably cause more problems in ethics than any other component of ethical theory. At the same time, they are probably more helpful as guides to day-to-day behavior than anything else.

The problems arise, in part, because of a misunderstanding of the nature and function of these rules. Rules may have two functions. They may simply serve as guidelines summarizing conclusions we tend to reach in moral problems of a certain class. When rules have this function of simply summarizing experience in similar situations of the past, they are called rules-of-thumb, guiding rules, or summary rules.

In contrast, rules may function to specify behavior that is required independent of individual judgment about a specific situation. The rules against abortion of a viable fetus or against killing a dying patient are examples of rules that are often directly linked to right-making characteristics. Sometimes this kind of rule is called a rule of practice.

The rule specifies a practice that, in turn, is justified by the general principles. According to this rules-of-practice view, it is unacceptable to overturn a general practice simply because to do so in a particular case would produce a better outcome.

The conflict between those who take the rules more seriously and those who consider the situation to be the more critical determinant of moral rightness has become one of the major ethical controversies in the mid-twentieth century. It is sometimes called the rules–situation debate.[16–19] At one extreme is the rigorist, who insists that rules should never be violated. At the other is the situationalist, who claims that rules never apply because every situation is unique. Probably both positions in the extreme lead to absurdity. The rigorist is immobilized when two of his rules conflict. The situationalist is immobilized when he treats a situation as literally new with no help from past experience in similar if not identical situations.

The rules–situation debate does not lend itself to special cases grouped together. The problem arises continually throughout the cases in this volume. The final question, however, requires special chapters with cases selected to examine the problems raised.

WHAT OUGHT TO BE DONE IN SPECIFIC CASES?

After the determination of what makes right acts right, what kinds of actions are right, and how rules apply to specific situations, there still remain a large number of specific situations that make up the bulk of problems in nursing ethics. The question remains, what ought to be done in a specific case or kind of case? Nursing, being particularly oriented to case problems, is given to organizing ethical problems around specific kinds of cases. Ethics, too, is sometimes divided into the problems of birth, life, and death.

The first two parts of this volume emphasize the overarching problems of how to relate facts to values, who ought to decide ethical questions, and matters of justice, autonomy, truth-telling, fidelity, and avoiding killing. These are among the larger questions of biomedical ethics. Part Three shifts to cases involving specific problem areas. Cases in Chapter 9 raise the problems of abortion, sterilization, and conception control. Chapter 10 moves to the related problems of genetic counseling and engineering and of intervention in the prenatal period. The next chapters take up, in turn, the problems of psychiatry and the control of human behavior; human experimentation, consent, and the right to refuse medical treatment; and, finally, death and dying.

The answer to the question of what ought to be done in a specific case requires the integration of the answers to all of the other questions if a thorough analysis and justification is to be given. The first line of moral defense will probably be a set of moral rules and rights thought to apply to the case. In abortion, the right to control one's body and the right to practice nursing as one sees fit are pitted against the right to life. In human experimentation, the rules of informed consent pertain. Among the dying, rules about euthanasia conflict with the right to pursue happiness; and the right to refuse med-

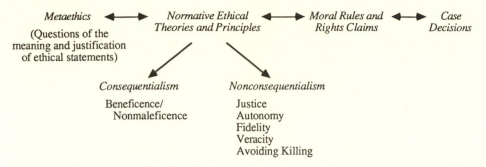

Figure 1.   The stages of ethical analysis.

ical treatment conflicts with the rules that the nurse ought to do everything possible to preserve life.

In many cases the conflict escalates from an issue of moral rules and rights to the more abstract stage of ethical principle. It must be determined, for example, whether informed consent is designed to maximize benefits to the experimental subject or to facilitate the subject's freedom of self-determination. It must also be explored whether harm to the patient justifies withholding information from the patient or whether the formalist truth-telling principle justifies disclosure.

The problem of what ought to be done in a specific case also requires a great deal of information other than moral judgments. It requires considerable empirical data. Value-relevant biological and psychological facts have developed around many case problems in biomedical ethics. The predictive capacity of a flat electroencephalogram may be important for the definition of death. The legal facts are relevant for the refusal of treatment. Basic religious and philosophical beliefs of the patient may be critical for resolving some cases in nursing ethics. It is impossible to present all of the relevant medical, genetic, legal, and psychological facts that are necessary for a complete analysis of any case, but it is possible to present the major facts required for understanding. Readers will have to supplement these facts for a fuller understanding of the cases, just as they will have to supplement their reading in ethical theory for a fuller understanding of the basic questions of ethics.

These four basic questions in ethics can be thought of as four different stages of ethical analysis. If the answer to the specific case is not apparent, one might see if some rules or rights claims are relevant. At that point one would have to know how rules apply to specific situations. If the rules do not give a clear answer, then one will have to move to the next stage, the stage of deciding what ethical principles are morally relevant. Finally, if one questions the basic principles, he or she is forced to consider the most fundamental questions, those of metaethics. An ethical analysis can start at the most specific stage, that of cases, and move to other stages, or one might try to be more systematic by starting with the most fundamental questions and moving to more and more specific stages. These movements are illustrated in Figure 1.

References

1. American Nurses' Association: Code for Nurses with Interpretive Statements, p 1. Kansas City, American Nurses' Association, 1985
2. Frankena W: Ethics, 2nd ed, p 62. Englewood Cliffs, NJ, Prentice-Hall, 1973
3. Beauchamp TL, Childress JF (eds): Principles of Biomedical Ethics. 2nd ed, pp15–17. New York, Oxford University Press, 1983
4. Fried C: Right and Wrong, p 12. Cambridge, MA, Harvard University Press, 1978
5. Rawls J: A Theory of Justice, pp 131–136. Cambridge, MA, Harvard University Press, 1971
6. Baier K: The Moral Point of View: A Rational Basis of Ethics, pp 106–109. New York, Random House, 1965
7. Firth R: Ethical absolutism and the ideal observer theory. Philosophy and Phenomonological Research 12:317-345, 1952
8. Broad CD: Some reflections on moral-sense theories in ethics. Proceedings, The Aristotelian Society 1944-45, pp 131–166
9. Ross WD: The Right and the Good. Oxford, Oxford University Press, 1939
10. Kant I: Groundwork of the Metaphysic of Morals, trans Paton HJ. New York, Harper & Row, 1964
11. Ayer AJ: Language, Truth, and Logic. London, Victor Gollancz, 1948
12. Stevenson CL: Ethics and Language. New Haven, Yale Univeristy Press, 1944
13. Hare RM: The Language of Morals. Oxford: Clarendon Press, 1952
14. Thomas Aquinas: Summa Theologica, I-II, A. 94, Art. 2. Fathers of the English Dominican Province (ed): London, R & T Washbourne, 1915
15. Bentham J: An introduction to the principles of morals and legislation. In Melden AI (ed): Ethical Theories: A Book of Readings, pp 367–390. Englewood Cliffs, NJ, Prentice-Hall, 1967
16. Rawls J: Two concepts of rules. The Philosophical Review 44:3-32, 1955
17. Fletcher J: Situation Ethics: The New Morality. Philadelphia, Westminster Press, 1966
18. Ramsey P: Deeds and Rules in Christian Ethics. New York, Charles Scribner's Sons, 1967
19. Bayles MD (ed): Contemporary Utilitarianism. Garden City, NY, Doubleday, 1968

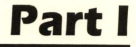
Part I

Ethics and Values in Nursing

Chapter 1

Values in Health and Illness

Nursing is a clinical profession that includes systematic problem-solving (the nursing process) through assessment and nursing management of identified patient needs. Throughout this process, the nurse makes countless decisions concerning nursing diagnoses, construction and implementation of the nursing care plan, and evaluation of the patient's progress toward health. Each decision requires the nurse to combine a wide range of facts (or data) with a set of values to determine what ought to be done to help the patient fulfill his or her health needs. The facts assessed are drawn from many different areas: medical and psychosocial histories, physiological status, economic status, and aesthetic and religious orientations. The collection and analysis of the facts alone, however, can never lead to a conclusion that a particular nursing intervention is morally justified. To reach a conclusion about what is morally justified in nursing practice, the nurse must combine relevant facts with a set of values. Thus, the first task of the study of cases in nursing ethics is to identify the many evaluations that take place in nursing practice and separate the moral from the nonmoral components in these evaluations.

IDENTIFYING EVALUATIONS IN NURSING

The first two cases demonstrate the various kinds of values in clinical decisions made by nurses in quite ordinary, routine nursing practice. Neither case raises traditional, dramatic ethical issues, but both clearly force the nurse to make ethical decisions. Moreover, they both involve many other kinds of evaluations that are not ethical at all. The evaluations include matters of taste (whether physical or psychological risks are more weighty), matters of aesthetics (which of two environments is more pleasant), matters of law (whether it is legally acceptable to risk a baby's life to conform to the wishes of its parents), and matters of what are sometimes called "value orientations" (fundamental stances about such basic issues as whether a nurse ought to try to dominate nature or let nature take its course). However, questions of moral evaluation become central to the cases as they develop. Basic questions are raised about what the nurse *ought* to do in the moral sense. In analyzing these cases, notice the evaluations that occur and determine which of the evaluations are moral.

Case 1: The Patient Who Objected to a Posey Belt

Isaac Livingston had led a good life. He had worked as a pharmaceutical sales-man for 45 years before retiring 6 years before his most critical medical problems began. Now, at 72, he was hospitalized for what the nursing staff suspected might be his last time. He was suffering from carcinoma of the prostate that had metastasized to the bone and sapped his strength. His current hospital admission was triggered by an episode of blacking out undoubtedly related to a serious drop in blood pressure. The pain of the tumor, the side effects of the medication (meperidine, 100 mg q 3–4 hours as necessary, and chlorpromazine, 10 mg qid as needed for nausea from the chemotherapy), and his lethargy combined to make him somewhat groggy. Moreover, Mr. Livingston often desired to get up and out of his room "to get some air," as he put it.

To make matters worse, Mr. Livingston suffered from a partial paralysis of the left leg of some 15 years' duration, apparently caused by spinal cord damage related to pressure from a spinal disk. All of these led the nursing team to be concerned about potential injury should Mr. Livingston fall while getting out of bed, as he often did. Margaret Howard, the evening charge nurse, felt that the problem had reached a crisis when she found Mr. Livingston on the floor at 10 PM one evening. Apparently, he had fallen trying to get out of his bed. Ms. Howard decided to restrain Mr. Livingston with a Posey belt. His admission orders included the use of this method of restraint at the nurse's discretion.

To Ms. Howard's surprise, Mr. Livingston, in spite of his rather incoherent state, vociferously protested the use of the belt. Although he understood that the belt was intended for his own good and that the nurses thought it was dangerous for him not to have it, Mr. Livingston intensely disliked the use of this restraint.

The next evening, Ms. Howard learned by reading the nursing notes that he had objected to the restraint many times during the day. She was approached at the nurses' station by Mr. Livingston's son during visiting hours that same evening. The son explained that Mr. Livingston had been trapped in a burning building when he was a child and since then had been extremely afraid of being trapped, of suffocating, or of being confined in small rooms.

This explained some of Mr. Livingston's behavior, but Ms. Howard was still seriously concerned about the danger to a 72-year-old man, groggy with medication and partially paralyzed, of falling as he wandered from his bed. It was her judgment that continued use of the restraint was indicated for good nursing practice.

She explored her options: She could follow his urgent request that the Posey belt be removed. She could insist that in her clinical judgment good care required continued restraint. She could ask for guidance from the resident on call or ask that Mr. Livingston's physician be consulted in the morning.

Commentary

The problem faced by Ms. Howard and her colleagues at first seems rather mundane. The Posey belt decision hardly falls into the same class of moral controversy as the more exotic ethical issues of genetic manipulation, defining death, or even discussing a terminal diagnosis with a patient. Yet, upon reflection, it is clear that evaluations took place throughout Ms. Howard's interaction with Mr. Livingston. Even the brief case report presented here is full of value judgments. Mr. Livingston's life was a *good* life. He was *suffering* from carcinoma of the prostate and from partial paralysis. *Suffering* is necessarily an evaluation. One cannot suffer and judge the sensation to be good in this respect.

The evaluations continue in the account of the immediate problem facing Ms. Howard. Mr. Livingston found it *desirable* to get up and out of his room, whereas the nursing team was worried about *injury,* something that necessarily has a bad connotation. Moreover, Mr. Livingston *protested* vociferously and *objected* many times. On the other hand, Ms. Howard was concerned about the *danger* to Mr. Livingston's health if he were unrestrained.

Three different levels of evaluations are taking place: choices about mental and physical health, choices about more fundamental value orientations, and choices about what is ethically acceptable behavior. At the first level, evaluations related to physical and mental outcomes seem to be in conflict. The nurse was naturally concerned about the real and significant physical risk to Mr. Livingston if he were free to get up at will in his sedated and disoriented state. Mr. Livingston, on the other hand, seemed to have a rather different agenda. He was relatively unconcerned about risks of physical injury from a fall, but extraordinarily concerned about the psychological sense of well-being that came from being free to move about and "get some air." That concern was, in part, derived from a unique experience in Mr. Livingston's past.

When Ms. Howard learned from Mr. Livingston's son of this unique history, she was able to include in her considerations the unique psychological trauma of restraint for her patient. She still, however, did not reach what was apparently Mr. Livingston's conclusion—that, on balance, greater benefit would come from avoiding the restraint. It could well be that the two simply compared avoiding physical injury and experiencing psychological distress differently. If avoiding a broken hip is a good worthy of substantial psychic trauma, then Ms. Howard's evaluation of the relation of the two kinds of benefits makes sense. If, on the other hand, one places more emphasis on the potential psychological harm involved, then Mr. Livingston's behavior is understandable.

So far, this only suggests that differences are possible in essentially nonmoral evaluations. It does not yet get us to the level of ethics. However, there may be other levels of evaluations going on in this case. Underlying the specific evaluations of physical and mental outcomes may be a second level of evaluation involving deeper, more fundamental beliefs and values. These more basic evaluations are sometimes called "value orientations" or, taken together, a world view.[1] They deal with the human's relationship with nature, whether one ought to be active and aggressive or more passive in letting nature take its course, whether it is better to be oriented to goals in the future or focus more on the present or past, whether people are to be regarded as tending toward good or evil, and how individuals relate to other individuals and groups. Individuals, as well as cultures, tend to take stands on these basic value orientations. Moreover, they sometimes regard them as moral obligations rather than simply matters of preference. People sometimes believe they have a duty to plan for the future or to avoid intervening aggressively in natural processes.

It is possible that differences in basic value orientations will, in part, account for disagreements over what counts as good nursing care of patients. In Mr. Livingston's case, physicians and nurses have made judgments about proper medication levels that are not the only possible courses of medication. For example, if Mr. Livingston remains in pain, the nurse would have the option of increasing the administration of meperidine up to the prescribed amount. Since the narcotic has been authorized for use "as necessary," certain judgments must be made balancing pain relief and the side effects of the medication. In this case, since the sedating effect of the medication is adding significantly to Mr. Livingston's risk, the nurse has several options. If the nurse takes the view that the role of the health professional is to make full use of pharmacologic and other medical means to control the natural processes, the nurse could take steps to increase the narcotic to the limits of the prescribed amount. The nurse could go beyond that, asking the physician to increase the dosage. More frequent administration, higher dosage levels, and shifting to a more potent narcotic (such as morphine) are all available options. Their choice would reveal a take-charge value orientation leading to increased pain relief and even more sedation, perhaps decreasing the tendency for Mr. Livingston to want to get out of bed.

On the other hand, if the nurse took the attitude that the health professional should use great caution in tampering with the natural processes, the toxic and addictive potential of the drugs might be feared to the point that blood levels would be lightened as much as possible. The nurse could, for example, extend the times between the administration of both the narcotic and the antinausea medication. This attitude of respect for natural processes in its extreme form could lead to abandoning narcotics altogether in favor of propoxyphene hydrochloride or other analgesics presumed by many to be nonaddictive. One of the effects of working from this value orientation might be the reduction of sedation to the point where Mr. Livingston's risk of falling would be lessened.

These basic differences in value orientation begin to sound like differences in what may be called ethical values. They are often perceived as differences in obligation rather than mere personal preferences. A nurse might argue that it is wrong, even morally wrong, to sedate a patient to avoid the Posey belt problem. The nurse might also argue that it is morally wrong to eliminate the problem by lightening a patient's medication to the point that he is in excruciating pain or nauseated from his chemotherapy.

Beyond these value orientations, there is still a third level of evaluation going on in Mr. Livingston's case. It is at this level that true moral judgments are involved. The true moral problems are likely to arise if Ms. Howard remains convinced of her conclusion that use of the Posey belt is in Mr. Livingston's interest, on balance, after she learns of the uniquely discomforting psychological impacts on him. If, under those circumstances, Mr. Livingston continues to insist that the belt be removed, we have before us one of the classic ethical problems in health care ethics. If the nurse acts on the traditional, rather paternalistic principle that she should do what she thinks is in Mr. Livingston's interest, the belt will be left in place, morally violating his autonomy (not to mention any legal questions raised). If, on the other hand, she acts out of the principle of respect for the autonomy of persons and removes the restraint, she temporarily abandons her commitment to the health, welfare, and safety of the patient. Good nursing care will be directly dependent on whether the nurse should act to promote autonomy or should act to do what she thinks is in the interest of the patient's health, welfare, and safety. Which ought to be done is a matter of ethical principle.

Even if the nurse decides to abandon her conception of patient welfare in order to promote Mr. Livingston's autonomy, she may consider the impact of the decision on other patients, co-workers, or herself. In removing the restraint, Ms. Howard may feel compelled morally to spend more time checking on Mr. Livingston, thus providing less adequate care for other patients. If the patient falls again, as anticipated, she and the other hospital staff will have additional burdens. Even if the hospital is so well-staffed that other patients are not put at additional risk, Ms. Howard and her co-workers will still suffer the inconvenience of extra work and worry in the form of an incident report. On the one hand, it is ethically questionable that a nurse should restrain a patient simply to lighten her work load and avoid a potentially troublesome situation. On the other hand, however, part of nursing ethics will inevitably have to include the question of the limits of the burden a patient should be permitted to put on a nurse or her co-workers. It seems that there should be some moral limit on how much extra work a nurse should have to do in order to cater to the idiosyncratic preferences of a single patient.

In dealing with both of these concerns about the interests of other parties—the interests of the other patients and of the nurse—a full analysis of the ethics of nursing practice will have to consider the legitimate moral role of various social interests. Is the welfare of others totally irrelevant morally, as some traditional ethics would have us believe? If not, is it the aggregate total of benefits and harms of an action that count? Or do certain kinds of benefits and harms take precedence—benefits to the neediest, for example?

Finally, when Ms. Howard explores her options, she will have to take some stand on the ethics of the relationships she has with other professionals and with the patient. In deciding among her options, she must decide whether she stands in a relationship of obligation to the patient, her nursing colleagues, the hospital administration, the resident on call, and Mr. Livingston's attending physician, as well as others in her personal life. Morality is, in part, a matter of loyalty and fulfillment of commitments. If Ms. Howard feels bound morally to the profession of nursing as a source of moral insight, she may well turn to sources within the profession for help in resolving her problem. She may consult a code of ethics, standards of nursing practice, or the advice of her nurse–colleagues. If she feels bound in loyalty to the hospital as an institution, she may consider legal liability of the institution, as well as standards for appropriate care established by the hospital administration. If she feels obligated to the medical personnel involved in the case as her sources of authority, she will insist on turning to them for advice or even for "orders." If she sees the patient as the center of moral authority regarding his own care, she may yield to the patient not only on the question of the Posey belt, but also on what moral norms ought to be used for resolving the problem. Finally, since she has other centers of moral loyalty in her personal life—her church, her family, her own personal system of beliefs and values—she will have to decide how these are appropriately integrated into the decision.

What starts out as a simple problem of patient management ends by introducing us to virtually the entire range of ethical problems in nursing. In the case that follows, we shall see in another context how ethical and other types of evaluations raise issues, sometimes in unexpected ways.

Case 2: The Nurse–Midwife and Crisis in a Home Delivery

Twenty-seven-year-old Melissa Owens was eagerly awaiting the birth of her first child. Married for 3 years, she and her husband Roger had recently opened a small business in a growing suburban community. When it became apparent that Mrs. Owens was pregnant, she and her husband visited Nurse–Midwives, Inc., a home birth service available in their community. The emphasis on pre-natal nutrition, childbirth preparation classes, and the opportunity to give birth to their firstborn in their own home appealed to the Owens' belief in birth as a natural body process. They were also strongly attracted to the relaxed approach of the four certified nurse–midwife partners and their agreement that Mr. Owens could participate in the birth as much as he and his wife desired.

During the months of pregnancy, Mr. and Mrs. Owens attended the bi-weekly childbirth preparation classes given by their nurse–midwife, Ms. Lisa Bennington, and her partner, Mrs. Betty Thornton. A friendly and supportive re-lationship developed between the couple and the nurses, based on their mutual beliefs about the birth process and the value of early infant–maternal bonding in the family setting. Since Mrs. Owens had enjoyed a healthy, uneventful preg-nancy, Ms. Bennington anticipated no problems during labor and delivery.

Now, in her 41st week of pregnancy, Mrs. Owens began to feel the long-awaited contractions signaling labor. Called to the Owens' home, Ms. Benning-ton found her patient in the early phase of labor, 4 cm dilated and 70% effaced. Her amniotic membranes were intact, and Mrs. Owens seemed in good health and spirits. The baby's presentation (head, or vertex) and position (left occipi-toanterior, or LOA) were considered favorable for both mother and baby. In min-imal pain, Mrs. Owens was encouraged to walk around the house to stimulate labor.

Mrs. Thornton soon joined her partner at the home. She confirmed Ms. Bennington's findings, which were discussed by telephone with the nurse–mid-wives' obstetrical "back-up," Dr. Lester Holmes. A strong believer in the overall safety of hospital delivery but supportive of the nurse–midwives' practice, he en-couraged them to call him if any unexpected problems developed during Mrs. Owens' labor.

Within an hour, Mrs. Owens' amniotic membranes ruptured, and the labor contractions became stronger. As the time passed, everything seemed to be pro-gressing normally until Ms. Bennington noted a marked decrease in the fetal heart rate during contractions. After each contraction, however, the fetus seemed to regain its normal heart rate. Both nurse–midwives noted this pattern over several strong contractions. Changing Mrs. Owens' position did not seem to alter the pattern. They realized that an unexpected problem (*i.e.*, cord compression) could be developing. Since Mrs. Owens was now almost fully dilated, birth of the baby could occur within a short time. Their concern about the fetal heart rate thus required prompt attention. According to their contractual agreement with Mr. and Mrs. Owens, the nurse–midwives explained the decelerations of the fetal heart rate during contractions, its possible meanings, and the various choices that might have to be made.

Mrs. Thornton thought that Dr. Holmes should be contacted to arrange immediate transport to the hospital. She considered any change in the status of the fetus during labor at home a good reason to change to a hospital delivery. Ms. Bennington, however, did not think that the situation warranted hospital delivery. She thought home delivery was of such value to parents and child that some minimal risk to the fetus was tolerable. She also knew that her patient had very strong feelings about bearing her child at home with her husband's participation. Ms. Bennington strongly supported these wishes. Her own belief in home rather than hospital delivery encouraged her to avoid transporting any patient to the hospital unless a dramatic change occurred in the fetal heart rate or other problems became evident. At this point, Mr. and Mrs. Owens voiced their own insistence on home delivery unless some definite danger to the life of their child was evident.

Ms. Bennington considered the possible choices she might make: She could yield to the Owens' wishes to stay at home unless definite risk to the fetus was evident. She could observe the fetal heart for another 30 minutes, which was as much risk as she personally thought acceptable. She could defer to her partner's judgment that the technological advantages of a hospital delivery room were immediately warranted by the situation. She could even choose not to make a decision by calling Dr. Holmes to ask for his guidance. She felt sure, however, that he would recommend immediate hospitalization.

Commentary

The safety of home versus hospital delivery is an important issue in contemporary approaches to childbirth. Believing that hospital services have been the most important factor in the improved outcomes of pregnancy in the past two decades, some health professionals, especially physicians, emphasize the unpredictability of events during childbirth, which can increase risk to the life of the fetus or mother during a home delivery.[2-4] On the other hand, advocates of home delivery cite statistics demonstrating decreased rates of infant mortality and of premature and cesarean births, as well as increased psychological benefits from home childbirth.[5-10] Wedged between the two extremes of high technology, physician-managed, in-hospital births and the lay–midwife approach of the home birth movement, the certified nurse–midwife is faced with an array of competing values.

In choosing to become a certified nurse–midwife, Ms. Bennington has made a significant value judgment. She has demonstrated her preference to use nursing knowledge in the bearing and birth of children rather than in the care of adults or even in nursing specialties such as oncology nursing. In choosing to join with Mrs. Betty Thornton and her other partners in Nurse–Midwives, Inc., she has also demonstrated a value preference for independent practice over that of institution-based practice. Nearly 90% of all nurse–midwives are employed by hospitals, public health agencies, physicians in private practice, or the military services. Only 10% of all nurse–midwives practice in either a maternity service operated predominately by nurse–midwives (7.6%) or in a private nurse–midwifery practice (2.4%) such as Nurse–Midwives, Inc.[11] Ms. Bennington and her partners have decided to choose a style of practice based on values emphasizing independent practice within nurse–midwifery itself.

Ms. Bennington has also chosen to attend births in the home rather than in the hospital. This choice is based on a set of values that are apparently rather unusual for nurse–midwives. Only 3% of practicing certified nurse–midwives attend home deliveries.[12] Assuming that she and her partner, Mrs. Betty Thornton, have hospital privileges by which they can admit patients for in-hospital care, choosing to deliver Mrs. Owens' baby at home indicates that they consider home birth to be of considerable physical or psychological benefit to the parents and the expected child.

In several studies that compared nurse–midwife–managed prenatal care and delivery with physician-managed care and delivery, improved birth statistics in nurse–midwife–managed deliveries were demonstrated for both low-risk and high-risk obstetrical patients.[13,14] These statistics are, of course, open to debate. Some have argued that the samples are not really comparable, that fetal monitoring in modern obstetrics affects the data, or that certain critical effects (such as those stemming from anoxia) are not measurable for many years. Ms. Bennington has chosen to interpret the data available to her in such a way that they support her conclusion that home delivery is, physically, a safe childbirth alternative. Those interpreting the data with other values might be more skeptical. She has made her judgment despite other studies demonstrating that up to one third of women who go into labor at home must be transported to the hospital for some complication of delivery.[3,6] Thus, for women who choose home delivery over hospital delivery, Ms. Bennington is ready to provide a service based on mutual judgments of benefits, both psychological and physical, judgments that will not necessarily be shared by other nurses, physicians, or lay people.

Even Melissa and Roger Owens have made a value judgment in deciding to consult Nurse–Midwives, Inc. for the birth of their child. To them, a home delivery signifies the naturalness of birth. Rather than the technological or unnatural setting of a hospital, they prefer childbirth in their own home, where they and close friends can share in the event. But even the preference of home delivery for these reasons may not be the most significant value judgment for Mr. and Mrs. Owens. It may be the choice itself, the freedom to choose how one wants to give birth, that is also important.

In the past, the bearing and birth of a child was considered an illness-related event under little control of the consumer. While midwife services have always been available to the rural poor or to those residing in economically depressed areas, most American women, particularly those in the middle class, have had little choice except to visit an obstetrician for prenatal care and hospital delivery. Advocates of home birth are now urging women to reclaim responsibility for childbirth by requesting birth alternatives from which to choose. Influenced by the women's health movement, many women like Mrs. Owens feel that decisions about birth are too important to be left solely to the obstetrician. What emerges as an important value judgment in maternity services is being able to choose the mode of birth for one's child.

Up to this point, the many value judgments in this case are nonmoral and demonstrate nonmoral conflict. Ms. Bennington's judgments in selecting nurse–midwifery, independent practice, and home birth over hospital delivery all indicate nonmoral evaluations made on the basis of personal preference or tastes. The judgments of Mr. and Mrs. Owens are based on similar nonmoral evaluations. Even the conflict between physical and psychological benefits and harms posed by the choice of home delivery versus hospital delivery is nonmoral. Neither judgment possesses any of the characteristics of moral evaluations. But as we have already demonstrated, nonmoral conflict can easily lead one into the realm of ethics and ethical conflict.

Influenced by the many nonmoral value judgments that have led her to practice certified nurse–midwifery, Ms. Bennington must make additional judgments, particularly concerning the rightness or wrongness of allowing Mrs. Owens to continue in labor at home with marked decelerations of the fetal heart rate during contractions. She must decide whether she has a duty to the fetus that would lead to hospitalization—perhaps a duty to preserve life or a duty to protect the health and welfare of the fetus—and, if so, whether that would lead to more immediate hospitalization than the Owens would desire. She must relate her obligation to respect the values of the parents to her own values and those of her colleagues and others involved in the case. If she decides that the situation does not pose a serious enough threat to the fetus' health and that Mrs. Owens' choice of home birth is to be respected, Ms. Bennington may decide to wait and see if birth occurs within a short period of time. In deciding to wait, she would be acting on the basis of the ethical principle of autonomy or respect for self-determination of persons. If increased decelerations of the fetal heart rate during contractions should occur, Ms. Bennington might then decide to act on the basis of her duty to the health and life of the fetus. Although the autonomy of the parents would be overridden by this decision, Ms. Bennington would still be acting on the basis of a moral principle: preserve life, preserve health, or serve the welfare of the fetus.

Mrs. Thornton has already made a moral evaluation by insisting that the change in fetal status warrants hospital delivery and its available technology. This evaluation is based on the moral wrongness of allowing labor to continue without medical assistance once fetal distress, no matter how slight, is demonstrated. While Mrs. Owens has a value preference for respecting parental choice for home delivery, Mrs. Thornton is claiming that she has a moral obligation to act in the fetus' best interest when any change in fetal status occurs in a home-managed labor. Her evaluation automatically places her in the position of acting on paternalistic grounds: Mr. and Mrs. Owens' autonomous choice to deliver at home will be set aside for what Mrs. Thornton judges to be in the fetus' best interest and perhaps in the interest of the parents as well.

At this point, it is very difficult to determine where the conflict exists. It may be that the nurse–midwives simply disagree on the empirical facts of the physical risk to the fetus from the change in heart rate. They may also disagree over the relative importance of the physical risk and the psychosocial advantages of the home birth. However, there may be a moral conflict between their obligation to the fetus—to preserve life, promote health, or serve the interests of the fetus—and what is called for by their obligations of loyalty to the parents, the profession of nursing, or the back-up physician. There may be, finally, a conflict over whether the autonomy of the parents should take moral precedence over the duty of the nurse to serve the fetus' welfare. Thus, both moral and nonmoral evaluations permeate the practice of nursing even in apparently routine decisions such as restraining a patient or arranging in-hospital care when a patient's labor at home takes an unexpected turn.

IDENTIFYING ETHICAL CONFLICTS

Once it is apparent that value choices are made constantly in nursing and other health professional practice, it will not be surprising that many of the choices involve an ethical component. They may involve conflict between the duty to the patient and the duty to society. These conflicts may involve the clash between two ethical duties (such as the duty to respect and promote autonomy and the duty to benefit the patient). They may involve tension between the ethical positions of professional and religious groups to which the nurse is loyal. They may involve tension between the rights of patients and the nurse's self-interest and welfare. The following cases illustrate, in turn, each of these problems.

Benefit to the Patient vs. Benefit to Others

One of the most common and straightforward ethical conflicts the nurse faces is conflict between an obligation to benefit the client and an obligation to benefit others. The dilemma is signaled in the third point of the *Code for Nurses* of the American Nurses' Association (ANA). If a nurse were to take the ANA code as definitive moral guidance, the nurse would act, according to the *Code for Nurses*, "to safeguard the client and the public when health care and safety are affected by incompetent, unethical, or illegal practice of any person."[15(p 6)] Both the client and public welfare are on the nurse's agenda. The first type of moral dilemma faced by the nurse is what should be done when the two come into conflict.

Traditionally, the obligation to serve the interests of the client takes precedence, but the realities of modern, complicated health care delivery systems exert pressures on the nurse to compromise the client's welfare, especially when substantial benefits will accrue to others and very little is lost by the patient. The current movement to involve the nurse in responsible cost containment in order to reduce rapidly expanding growth of health care costs illustrates the problem of the conflict between the welfare of the individual and society.

Case 3: The Nurse and Cost Containment: The Duty to Society

Ramon Ortega, a 42-year-old farm laborer with a history of hypertension, had been experiencing headaches on an almost daily basis for 2 to 3 weeks. Disturbed by the persistent and severe nature of the headaches, he visited the state-supported health clinic serving his rural community. Ms. Tracey Anderson, the family nurse–practitioner and sole staff member of the clinic, listened as Mr. Ortega described his headaches. She then performed an initial examination, which revealed good general health with the exception of an elevated blood pressure of 190/100. Since Mr. Ortega had described some dizziness and visual disturbances during his headaches, Ms. Anderson also completed a neurologic assessment. Everything seemed within normal limits except for Mr. Ortega's peripheral vision. Ms. Anderson's assessment demonstrated that he had some difficulty seeing objects in the visual field on his left side. Ms. Anderson realized that this disturbance was probably a manifestation of his present headache in combination with his known visual deficit. Since no other abnormalities were demonstrated, the possibility of a more serious problem seemed remote according to Ms. Anderson's judgment. Yet Mr. Ortega was very distressed by his headaches. He asked the nurse what he could do to prevent the headaches or, at least, what could be done to lessen the pain he was experiencing. Could she be sure that no other problem was causing the headaches?

Several months previously, Ms. Anderson would not have hesitated to refer Mr. Ortega to University Medical Center, 110 miles away, for physician examination and a neurologic evaluation of his headaches. She would have done this for no other reason than to relieve the patient of his worry and to confirm the absence of a more serious problem. She still believed that, on balance, the referral would be of some help. In recent weeks, however, the state agency that funds the rural health clinics had urged all health clinic personnel to be careful in referring patients for costly laboratory or evaluative testing with the added expense of clinic-sponsored transportation. The agency had decreased monies to support the personnel and services in rural health clinics since the agency-supported health care services bill had been defeated in the state legislature. In fact, the continued operation of the rural health clinics depended on how well individual clinics contained costs, even though they provided greatly needed services to populations such as the low-income farm community in which Mr. Ortega lived.

Ms. Anderson had been cutting operating costs of her clinic in every way she could, particularly in her judicious referral of patients to University Medical Center. However, she could not overlook the fact that Mr. Ortega was distressed by his headaches and that there was the possibility, albeit remote, that he was presenting with early signs of impending cerebrovascular disease, the effects of which could seriously affect him and his family. She was uncertain about what choice to make.

Commentary

The health cost containment effort has generated pressures on health professionals such as Tracey Anderson to be conscious of the socioeconomic impact of their decisions. Some cost containment decisions by these professionals can be made without moral dilemma. Some procedures may turn out to be useless or even detrimental, on balance, to the patient. If the procedure under consideration is going to hurt the patient more than it helps, it is simply good nursing practice to eliminate it. If money is saved in the process, that is a fortuitous side effect.

If the procedure is one in which the benefits and harms for the patient are just about equally balanced and the patient has no strong preferences for the procedure, then the fact that it would be costly for a health clinic to do the procedure might plausibly be good reason to avoid doing it. In such a case there is no good reason to go ahead.

However, Ms. Anderson's dilemma is more complicated. She has concluded that, on balance, Mr. Ortega will be helped by a referral for a neurologic work-up. It will at least provide psychological comfort, and there is a slim chance that therapeutically critical information will be revealed.

The moral traditions have almost all included within their lists of ethical principles some sense of a moral obligation to do good for other people or "to promote beneficence," as contemporary philosophy calls it. Ms. Anderson senses that beneficence is what is at stake here. She wants, in the words of the ANA *Code for Nurses*, "to safeguard the client and the public." She has correctly perceived, however, that in this particular situation the two standards may well be in direct conflict with one another. To make matters worse, the members of the public who are most likely to benefit directly from Ms. Anderson's cost consciousness are other patients in her rural health clinic area. The funds conserved by judicious compromise of Mr. Ortega's interests will be of benefit to other clients whose welfare she is also obliged to serve.

Two major options seem to be open to her. First, she could take the ANA *Code for Nurses* conclusion that "the nurse's primary commitment is to the health, welfare, and safety of the client"[15(p 6)] and apply it rigorously from the perspective of the client standing before her. If the client's welfare is primary and she has concluded that, on balance, he would benefit from a referral, then her moral dilemma is solved. Being concerned about the welfare of others is morally subordinate to the welfare of the individual. If that moral priority is chosen, following the state agency's directive to be cost conscious in such situations would be morally unacceptable. Of course, from the standpoint of the state agency, someone will have to be concerned about the society's welfare. Therefore, it would impose constraints on Ms. Anderson for the kind and amount of referrals she could make. In certain special, marginal cases she would not be permitted to make a referral even if she thought it was in her client's (marginal) interest.

Ms. Anderson's other option is to abandon the notion that the welfare of the client always takes priority over public welfare. That would permit her to take into account the social welfare impact on others—the state agency, taxpayers, and her other clients. She might, from this perspective, try to produce the greatest good, taking the welfare of all into account. She could strive for the greatest good for the greatest number, to use the classic utilitarian phrase.

There may be other options open to Ms. Anderson, options that would permit her to take into account certain benefits to society, but not others, when she decides whether, morally, she should put the care of her client above all other considerations. The balancing of the two kinds of interests might depend, for instance, on whether promises have been made to her client or to the state agency. It might depend on how she, her profession, and the society see the role of the nurse. It might depend on whether her

client's needs or the needs of others who might be helped with the funds are more urgent. Any of these factors might be seen by the nurse, the profession, clients, or others
in society as morally relevant, in addition to the amount of benefit and harm involved.
The problem of how benefits to the client relate to benefits to others will be the first major moral issue confronted in many cases in nursing ethics. These alternatives will be explored further in the cases in Chapter 3.

The Rights of the Patient vs. the Welfare of the Patient

Not all ethical problems faced by the nurse involve conflict between the welfare of the
patient and the welfare of others. Often the consequences to other parties are not really
an issue. Rather, the problem is that the nurse sees several courses of action open in
which different interests, claims, or rights of the patient seem to be in conflict. Sometimes these are merely matters of kinds of benefit to the patient. As in the Posey belt and
home childbirth cases, physical welfare of the patient may conflict with psychological
welfare. Long-term health concerns may conflict with short-term concerns.

In other cases, however, it does not seem to be a simple matter of different kinds of
benefits. Rather, other moral dimensions seem to be added. One course of action may
produce the most benefit for the patient, whereas another course protects some right or
corresponds to some moral obligation. Nurses, as well as anyone, may feel that certain
kinds of actions—telling the truth, keeping promises, avoiding killing, and so forth—
are simply morally required even if they do not necessarily produce good consequences.
Sometimes an action can be seen as having several different morally relevant components; the production of good and bad consequences, the breaking of a promise, the violation of autonomy of another might all be parts of the same action contemplated by the
nurse. If so, it is sometimes said that the acton is *prima facie* wrong insofar as it is an
act, for example, of lying, but simultaneously that it is *prima facie* right insofar as it produces good consequences. *Prima facie* rightness or wrongness is thus a characterization
of a component of an action, not necessarily of the action as a whole. The morality of
the action as a whole—one's duty proper as it is sometimes called—will depend on how
the various elements are taken into account.

Often the *prima facie* moral dimensions of an action are expressed not as duties,
but as rights; that is, they are expressed not in terms of the one bearing the obligation to
act, but from the perspective of the one who might make a moral claim. A *right* is a justified claim that one may make on another. A *moral right* is a morally justified claim, a
claim justified on the basis of moral principles or moral rules.[16(pp 143–155),17] As a justified
moral claim, a right, at least as the term is normally used, cannot be defeated or overridden by pointing out that an action required by the right will have bad consequences.

Many situations faced by the nurse pose the problem of a right of the patient conflicting with benefit to the patient; that is, one course seems to protect the patient's right,
whereas another course would produce more good for the patient. The tension between
rights and benefits is illustrated in the next case.

Case 4: Allowing Self-Care or Acting in the Interests of the Patient

Racheal Peterson, a 14 year old with childhood diabetes, visited the outpatient clinic of a large urban hospital every 3 months. On this particular visit, the new clinic nurse, Meredith Walker, noticed that Racheal's injection sites on her thighs contained many hard, reddened areas. Miss Walker asked Racheal to demonstrate how she administers her daily insulin. It became obvious to Miss Walker that Racheal was not following aseptic technique in the preparation of the injections and was not adopting a systematic pattern of rotating injection sites. Since Racheal had been a diagnosed diabetic for 3 years and no problems had been documented prior to this visit, Miss Walker wondered why Racheal was seemingly becoming careless in her self-care. In addition, Racheal related "snacking binges" and the difficulty of being diabetic when other teenage friends could eat whatever they want. Since Racheal's urine specimen showed a 3+ glucose, Miss Walker was also concerned about the long-term effects of high glucose levels on Racheal's health. She decided to be firm with this young patient and point out exactly what risks to her health Racheal was creating by not following her diet, by being careless about her insulin administration, leading to possible injection site infections, and by having a general lack of concern for her medical problems. Miss Walker also told Racheal that she might need to be admitted to the hospital for stabilization of her diet and insulin therapy for her "own best interests" if Racheal continued with her lack of self-care and concern.

Racheal was angered by the nurse's strong warnings and the threat of future hospitalization. She also objected to Miss Walker's decisions about how she should administer her daily insulin, rotating injection sites. Since Racheal had never liked giving her injections in her abdomen or arms, she had decided to give most injections in her thighs, claiming that it is "her choice" and that she could decide what she wanted to do with her own body.

After Racheal left the clinic angrily, Miss Walker discussed the visit with a more experienced nurse. This nurse explained that Racheal's attitude is common among diabetics in early adolescence and is reflective of the anger they feel about being different or not being able to participate in activities to the same extent as teenage friends. She brushed away Miss Walker's plan to initiate hospitalization by stating, "Wait until she puts herself into a diabetic crisis and is hospitalized; then she will be willing to assume more self-responsibility for her care."

Miss Walker strongly disagreed with this attitude. She believed that Racheal's long-term interests as a diabetic would be best served by reeducation and hospitalization to stabilize her condition. Although she recognized and supported Racheal's right to determine how she would care for herself, she also thought that she should act in Racheal's best interests by doing whatever she could do to prevent a future diabetic crisis, which could have long-term effects on Racheal's health. Yet, Miss Walker was uncertain what she should do: allow Racheal to determine her health care herself, or act in her perceived best interests by calling her mother and making arrangements for in-hospital care.

Commentary

This case, like the Posey belt case, poses in stark form the conflict between benefit to a patient and the rights of a patient. Unlike the Posey belt case, however, there seems to be good reason to believe that the patient really would benefit from improved care in administering her insulin. In the Posey belt case, the course that would benefit Mr. Livingston seems open to substantial controversy, especially after the psychological dimensions and the patient's history of a fear of enclosures are taken into account. In Racheal Peterson's case, however, it is harder to claim that, on balance, she really is better off following her care plan rather than the nurse's. It might be argued that Miss Walker's plan is so upsetting to her that, on grounds of benefit to the patient, the nurse should concede. Yet, if there were ever a case where the nurse knows best, this would certainly appear to be it.

This case is ethically interesting because Miss Walker recognizes and supports what she calls "Racheal's right to determine how she will care for herself." Ethical standards for the nursing profession indicate that minors have moral rights "to determine what will be done with his/her person; . . .; and to accept, refuse, or terminate treatment." The nurse is to respect these rights to "the fullest degree permissible under the law."[15(p 4)] That makes it a case in which, from Miss Walker's perspective, the rights of the patient and the professional mandate to protect these rights conflict with the nurse's felt duty to benefit the patient.

The first line of debate might focus on the nature of the rights claim being made. Does anyone really have a right to determine to take such risks with his or her own body? In short, is the rights claim being considered a justified one? Does this right include taking risks that place one's health at serious risks? Libertarian rights theorists and holders of more paternalistic perspectives differ. Even if competent adults have such a right, does that right extend to adolescents? Does it include adolescents whose disease patterns may contribute to their apparently inappropriate preferences?

A rights claim, if it exists at all, must be exercised by an individual who is a substantially autonomous, independent decision maker. It is widely recognized that age is a relevant factor in deciding whether someone is autonomous. As a general rule, minors are not presumed autonomous for purposes of making many critical decisions. However, the mere fact that one is a minor or that one has a chronic illness cannot, in itself, be taken as definitive evidence of incompetency for purposes of making such choices. Minors are, on occasion, found capable of making autonomous judgments, even on serious, life-and-death issues. We also recognize the minor's right to make decisions in the case of abortion and treatment for venereal disease. The critical question for one who accepts a general right to determine self-care based on the general principle of autonomy will be whether this young woman, a 14-year-old diabetic, is capable of autonomous actions.

For others who reject the principle of autonomy and the right of self-determination on such matters that might derive from that right, the moral problem is rather different. The overriding moral principle is likely to remain the principle of beneficence, a commitment to do what is in the patient's interests. Several critical features must be present to justify a paternalistic intervention such as the one Miss Walker is contemplating. There must be good reason to believe that the intervention really will be beneficial.

There must be good reason to believe that the person intervening, in this case, Miss Walker, is qualified to know that the action will be beneficial.[18–22] Some analysts of paternalism and its justifications also insist that there must be some due process to make sure that Racheal Peterson's rights are not violated. This might, for example, include court review to determine whether she is competent to decide for herself—whether she really comprehends the consequences—and also to determine whether the proposed intervention really is the most beneficial course.

The case poses the conflict between the right of the patient to decide about self-care based on the principle of autonomy and the duty of the nurse to benefit the patient. This tension and the general problem of autonomy will be explored further in the cases in Chapter 4.

Moral Rules and the Nurse's Conscience

The last two cases presented classic problems of ethics: first, where benefits to the patient conflict with benefits to others, and, second, where benefits to the patient conflict with the rights of the patient. Sometimes, however, the nurse may experience ethical conflict even though there is little apparent disagreement or doubt over these basic questions of principle. People may agree on the ethical principle at stake and still disagree on the application of the principle to a specific case problem. The gap between the very abstract principle and the specific case can be large. Nurses and others reflecting on moral problems often find it helpful to turn to moral precepts that are intermediate in their specificity between principles and cases. Moral rules often fulfill this role.* The rule, "always get consent before surgery," bridges the gap between an abstract principle such as the principle of autonomy or respect for persons and the health care professional's decision at the bedside. For example, the nurse in a triage unit knows the moral rules of triage that bridge between abstract principles of justice and nursing care decisions in specific disaster situations.

Instead of stating as a moral rule that the health professional has a duty to get consent before surgery, one might say much the same thing by claiming that the candidate for surgery has a right to consent to the surgery. Moral rules and rights are often correlative in this way. Whether the language of rules or rights is used, however, both normally provide guidelines for action or description of moral practices at an intermediate level of generality. (For this reason, they are, together, sometimes called "middle axioms" of morality.[16, 23–25]) The various moral rules pertaining to abortion are all examples of these middle level moral rules expressing in different traditions what various abstract principles such as the principles of beneficence, autonomy, avoiding killing, or the sacredness of life might imply for the abortion situation.

Different social groups are likely to hold somewhat different and sometimes conflicting rules on a particular problem area. These disagreements about moral rules may take place even among people who do not disagree on the most general principles.

---

*Moral rules state, at a middle level of generality, what action is required of someone who has a duty to act. If one wanted to state what action is required of some other individual or group from the point of view of the one acted upon, the language of rights might be used to the same end.

The nurse stands in relationship to many groups at any one time. The nurse may be a member of various religious, ethnic, socioeconomic, political, and familial groups, as well as being a member of one or more professional groups. Each group is likely to come to a different conclusion about any particular issue. The nurse's religious group may come to a moral conclusion (expressed in rules of conduct) on an issue such as abortion that may not be precisely the same as that reached by one's professional group. The nurse thus experiences ethical conflict at the level of moral rules when a rule of one's religious group prohibits one from participating in specific aspects of patient care, whereas the rules of some other social or professional group offer no such prohibition or even consider such participation morally required. This conflict is especially acute if one accepts as binding the claim of the ANA *Code for Nurses* that "the provision of quality nursing care is not limited by personal attitudes or beliefs."[15(p 3)] The disagreement may or may not include differences on the more abstract ethical principle. It clearly involves, however, disagreement at the level of moral rules. The following case illustrates this problem.

Case 5: The Nurse Asked to Assist in an Abortion

Mrs. Betty Phelps worked part-time in a small suburban hospital. Since she was familiar with the hospital's routines and the staff, she was often asked by the nursing supervisor to work in those patient care areas short on nursing staff for that particular shift. Today, she was asked to work in the recovery room. Within an hour, however, the nursing supervisor called and asked her to report to A-4, the suite of rooms where elective abortions were usually performed. Hesitating, Mrs. Phelps told the supervisor that she did not believe in abortion. A devout Roman Catholic, she considered abortion the killing of human life and a mortal sin. Would it be possible for the supervisor to find someone else to help out at A-4? The supervisor said that she understood and would try to find another nurse. In the meantime, however, Dr. Graham needed someone to prep his patient and set up the room for the abortion. Since Mrs. Phelps was not busy at the moment, could she go to A-4 and at least prep Dr. Graham's patient? Mrs. Phelps reluctantly agreed to this arrangement as long as the supervisor would send another nurse to replace her. The supervisor assured her that she would do this.

In A-4, after preparing the equipment and room, Mrs. Phelps prepped Dr. Graham's patient, an unmarried 16 year old approximately 8 weeks pregnant. She then told the physician that his patient was ready but that she would not participate in the proceedings. Another nurse would arrive shortly who would assist him. Dr. Graham protested, saying in an annoyed tone of voice to Mrs. Phelps, "Do you think I have all day to wait while the nursing staff puts its moralism and emotions in order? Everyone—the patient, the fetus, and the community—will be better off not having to deal with one more illegitimate child requiring public support."

When Mrs. Phelps stated that her religious and moral beliefs did not allow her to participate in an abortion, Dr. Graham pointed out that the fetus was just "a piece of tissue" and not really human life. Thus, there was nothing morally

wrong with performing abortions early in pregnancy. Now, would Mrs. Phelps please come into the room and assist him? When Mrs. Phelps declined, Dr. Graham stalked angrily down the hallway, claiming that it was a sad day for patients when nurses decided that they would not provide needed care.

Commentary

The question of participation in an abortion inevitably raises questions about the morality of abortion itself, including the surrounding issues of when life begins and the supposed right to life. These are the issues usually contained in any conflict over abortion. They are certainly present in this case, but there are other components as well.

It may seem, at first, that the ethical conflict in this case exists between the nurse and the physician—whether or not the nurse should "obey" the physician's request to assist in the abortion. However, the issue is really one of conflicting moral rules that direct professional acts. Although it is not obvious, Dr. Graham is responding to his patient's request for abortion out of a Hippocratic emphasis on benefiting the patient and, in this case, a calculation of what is the greatest benefit, on balance, to everyone concerned with this pregnancy. The unmarried teenager will be benefited by not having an unwanted child at this stage of her life. Society will be benefited by not having to support another person at public expense. On balance, the benefits of aborting the teenager's unwanted pregnancy are greater than any perceived harms to the patient, according to Dr. Graham.

Mrs. Phelps, however, is not responding to the situation solely out of a benefit-producing principle. She is responding out of a personal value structure influenced by religious belief, which claims that life begins at conception, the fetus is human life, and the destruction of human life is murder and therefore a sin; thus direct abortion where the life of the mother is not in question is an unspeakable crime, which the practicing Roman Catholic cannot participate in or support.[26] She may, in fact, agree that Dr. Graham is correct in the amount of benefit to be produced by aborting this patient. However, the mere production of benefit does not make abortion right according to her religious beliefs and personal values. She may even feel that, as a professional, she *should* act in the interests of a patient's welfare in all circumstances. Yet she cannot do so, in good conscience, in the case of abortion. Her religious group has come to a conclusion on the issue of abortion that prohibits her participation in professional acts involving abortion.

Even when Dr. Graham counters the nurse's objections by pointing out that, yes, we do respect human life, but the fetus in this case is not human life, and therefore it is morally acceptable to abort the products of conception in this pregnancy, the act is still not right for Mrs. Phelps. In fact, it is irrelevant to Mrs. Phelps whether the fetus' age is 8 weeks or 30 weeks. Fetal age is simply not important in the face of a personal belief that all fetal life is of value and should not be aborted.

We can well imagine how fervently Mrs. Phelps hopes that the nursing supervisor will soon send another nurse to assist Dr. Graham. Even though she agrees with the physician and the professional patient-benefiting ethic for all other aspects of health care, deciding not to assist Dr. Graham in this procedure on the basis of religious-group–directed moral rules has placed her in a very uncomfortable position. The difference between her choice of nonparticipation in the act of abortion and participation in other

health acts for the benefit of the patient lies within the strength of the moral rule generated and supported by religious beliefs. Whether or not the abortion will or should be performed, with or without Mrs. Phelps' assistance, is not the important question. What is important is on what basis and to what extent do personal values and beliefs influence professional acts in routine nursing care?

Limits on Rights and Rules

The fact that a nurse may be a member of a religious group favoring one moral rule on abortion and simultaneously be a member of some other social or professional group favoring some other moral rule suggests that there must be some limit on these moral rules. At least, when two different moral rules come into conflict, the nurse will have to decide how each is limited in order to resolve the conflict.

Sometimes the nurse may discover limits on certain moral rules or rights related to nursing care even when they do not come into direct conflict with other rules or rights. One kind of limit may be encountered when the nurse has been released from an obligation. If a nurse promises to keep confidential some information about the patient's sexual history, the nurse would normally be obliged to act on the moral rule requiring that the confidence be kept. The moral rule might be seen as being derived from the general principle of promise-keeping. What, however, if the nurse decides it would be very important to disclose the information to the consulting psychiatrist? If the nurse asked the patient for permission to disclose and the patient granted that permission, we would probably conclude that the nurse has been released from the rule of confidentiality.

The release might come, according to some interpretations, from the behavior of one of the parties rather than from a verbal release. If one of the parties to a contract fails to fulfill the specified part of the bargain, the other might thereby be released, at least, in some circumstances.

A second kind of limit on a moral rule or a moral right may be built into the rule or right itself. Even if there has been no "release," most moral rules, if stated carefully, include within them exceptions. The confidentiality rule, for example, often carries with it the exception "unless breaking confidence is required by law." The rule that the nurse should provide nursing care that will benefit the patient probably includes some implied limits. The nurse may be expected to provide care "up to a reasonable level" or "within the nurse's competence."

The following case is one in which the nurse must determine what limits, if any, are placed on the duty to provide patient care.

Case 6: The Visiting Nurse and the Obstinate Patient: Limits on the Right to Nursing Care

Mr. Jeff Williams, team leader in Home Care Services at the county health department, was preparing to visit Mr. Rufus Chisholm, a 59-year-old patient diagnosed as having emphysema during a recent hospitalization. Well known to the health department, Mr. Chisholm was unemployed as a result of a farming accident several years ago. Hypertensive as well as overweight, he was also a heavy cigarette smoker of long duration despite his decreased lung function. Mr. Williams' reason for visiting him today was to find out why Mr. Chisholm had missed his second scheduled chest clinic appointment. He also wanted to find out if this patient was continuing his medications as ordered.

As Mr. Williams parked his car in front of his patient's house, he could see Mr. Chisholm sitting on the front porch smoking a cigarette. A flash of anger made him wonder why he continually tried to teach Mr. Chisholm reasons for not smoking and why he took the time out from his busy home care schedule to follow up on Mr. Chisholm's missed clinic appointments. This patient certainly did not seem to care about his own health, at least so far as giving up smoking was concerned.

During the home visit, it was determined that Mr. Chisholm had discontinued the use of his prophylactic antibiotic and was not taking his expectorant and bronchodilator medication on a regular basis. In addition, his blood pressure was 210/114, and he coughed almost continuously. Although he politely listened to Mr. Williams' concerns about his respiratory function and the continued use of his medications, Mr. Chisholm simply made no efforts to take responsibility for his health care. Even so, another clinic appointment was made, and Mr. Williams encouraged the patient to attend.

As he drove to his next appointment, Mr. Williams wondered to what extent he was obligated as a nurse to spend time on patients who took no personal responsibility for their health. He also wondered if there was a limit to the amount of nursing care an uncooperative patient could expect from a community health service.

Commentary

Employed within a health care system whose goal is to provide nursing care services at public expense for those who need and desire this service, the nurse is confronted with the occasional patient who fails to follow the recommended health care plan. When this happens, the nurse may experience moral conflict. The nurse who personally values health and the provision of quality nursing care may view the patient who continually engages in health-risking behaviors as a waste of personal time, professional skill, and public monies. Yet the nurse may also feel professionally obligated to provide nursing care in response to the patient's right to health care services.

One approach to this issue is to regard patients like Mr. Chisholm as having a limited claim on nursing care services. His claim may be limited because other clients have a claim on Mr. Williams' time and nursing services. In this case, benefits to others must be balanced against the benefit of nurse attention and care to Mr. Chisholm.

His claim may also be limited because he has failed to fulfill his part of the contract relationship between client and nurse. Failure on his part thus releases the nurse from the duty to provide care that would normally be required.

However, there is one other reason why the client's rights claim to care may be limited. It may be that personal interests of the nurse—to finish up paperwork in the office, go out for dinner with one's spouse, or even party with friends—may take precedence once certain levels of health care services have been provided. This may be true even when no failure in the contract relationship on the part of the client exists. But who sets the limit on how much nursing care one is entitled to receive, and who is to say when the nurse has fulfilled obligations to the client? It is the question of who has ethical authority in defining the moral requirements and moral limits of the practice of nursing to which we turn in Chapter 2.

References

1. Kluckhohn FR, Strodtbeck DL: Variations in Value Orientations. Evanston, IL, Row, Peterson, 1961
2. Home or hospital confinement? (editorial) Br Med J 2:845, 1977
3. Adamson GD, Gare DJ: Home or hospital births? JAMA 243:1732–1736, 1980
4. Moawad AH: Some problems of professionally attended home births. J Reprod Med 19:298, 1977
5. Montgomery T: A case for nurse-midwives. Am J Obstet Gynecol 105:309–313, 1969
6. Mehl LE, Peterson GH, Shaw NS et al: Complications of home birth: An analysis of a series of 287 home births from Santa Cruz County, California. Birth Family J 2:123–135 1975
7. Arms S: Immaculate Deception. Boston, Houghton Mifflin, 1975
8. Mehl GH, Peterson GH, Whitt M et al: Outcomes of elective home births: A series of 1,146 cases. J Reprod Med 19:281–290, 1977
9. Melson J: Testimony presented to the New Jersey Board of Medical Examiners, April 2, 1980
10. Burneet JA, Jones JA, Rooks J et al: Home delivery and neonatal mortality in North Carolina. JAMA 244:2741–2745, 1980
11. Research and Statistics Committee of the American College of Nurse Midwives: Nurse Midwifery in the United States: 1976–1977, p 18. Washington, DC, American College of Nurse Midwives
12. Nurse midwifery to be used at Stanford Hospital. Health Care Horizons, March 1, 1981, pp 6A–B
13. Leny BS, Wilkinson FS, Marine WM: Reducing neonatal mortality rate with nurse-midwives. Am J Obstet Gynecol 109:50–58, 1971
14. Haire D: Improving the outcome of pregnancy through the increased utilization of midwives during labor and delivery. Public hearing sponsored by the Mayor's Blue Ribbon Commission of Infant Mortality, Washington, DC, February 14, 1980
15. American Nurses' Association: Code for Nurses With Interpretive Statements. Kansas City, MO, The Association, 1985
16. Feinberg J: Rights, Justice, and the Bounds of Liberty: Essays in Social Philosophy. Princeton, Princeton University Press, 1980
17. Beauchamp TL, Childress JF: Principles of Biomedical Ethics, 2nd ed, pp 49–55. New York, Oxford University Press, 1983
18. Dworkin G: Paternalism. Monist 56:64–84, 1972
19. Paternalism. In Wasserstrom R (ed): Morality and the Law, pp 107–126. Belmont, CA, Wadsworth, 1971
20. Gert B, Culver CM: Paternalistic behavior. Philosophy and Public Affairs 6(Fall):45–67, 1976
21. Gert B, Culver CM: The justification of paternalism. In Robison WL, Pritchard MS (eds):

Medical Responsibility: Paternalism, Informed Consent and Euthanasia, pp 1–14. Clifton, NJ, The Humana Press, 1979

22. Gert B, Culver CM: The justification of paternalism. Ethics 89(Jan):199–210, 1979
23. Gert B: The moral rules: A new rational foundation for morality. New York, Harper & Row, 1970
24. Lyons D: Rights. Belmont, CA, Wadsworth, 1979
25. Bennett JC: Principles and the context. In Bennett JC et al: Storm Over Ethics, pp 1–25. Philadelphia, United Church Press, 1967
26. Connery JR: Abortion: Roman Catholic perspectives. In Reich WT (ed): The Encyclopedia of Bioethics, pp 9–13. New York, The Free Press, 1978

Chapter 2

The Nurse and Moral Authority

Introduction

The nurse's ability to identify ethical and other evaluative judgments in clinical or policy-making situations is a skill that may be sufficient to resolve many ethical problems. Some tensions may be resolved simply by recognizing that a dispute or a feeling of uneasiness arises because ethical or other value choices are at issue. In more difficult cases, however, the nurse may still not know which of two or more options is the best or the most morally right one to choose. At this point, the nurse may turn to traditional sources for help. She or he may seek the opinions of colleagues, consult other health professionals, or turn to a code of ethics such as the American Nurses' Association (ANA) *Code for Nurses*. Other possible sources of guidance for making these difficult judgments include the institutional rules, the law, the broader mores of society, the nurse's religious tradition, or the client's value system.

Whereas merely consulting with one of these potential authorities may sometimes resolve tensions or reveal to the nurse what appears to be the right course of action, at other times, the nurse may still be perplexed. On these occasions the question will inevitably arise: "By which of these authorities, if any, ought I to be influenced?" Which should be viewed as a legitimate source for clarifying and justifying ethical positions?

The problem is a classic one in ethics. Before we proceed to determining what principles or rules for behavior are the right ones, we need to have some basis for assessing the alternative sources of such principles or rules. This is the problem philosophers often refer to as the problem of metaethics, or understanding the meaning and justification of our moral judgments.[1-4] Some have held, for example, that an action, a rule, or a principle is right only when it is approved by God or by one's religious tradition. That would be a religious basis for answering the question of moral authority. One of the advantages of such a religious system is that moral judgments are usually thought of as universal in the sense that everyone has some common ultimate frame of reference.

Everyone looking at the same problem ought to come to the same conclusion. There really is, for one working in this kind of religious world view, a right answer to each of our ethical questions.

Others, working in a more secular framework, also believe that there are really right answers to our moral questions. They might be rationalists, like Immanuel Kant, who believe that reason will ultimately be the foundation of right judgments.[5] Still others think that there is a single right or wrong answer, but that it must be known intuitively.[6]

By contrast, some people have given up the idea that there is a single ultimate source of moral authority. They may believe that expressions of moral judgments are merely expressions of the speaker's personal feelings or the judgments of one's society.[7,8] Medical professional groups have for many years written codes sometimes implying that either they themselves were the source of their moral rules or that they were, at least, the ones in the best position to identify the morally correct course.[9]

Nurses have often been caught in a tension among many groups who claim to be the correct or legitimate sources of moral authority. This chapter presents some cases designed to help one think through these competing claims. For example, is it right to turn off a respirator because a physician says to do so? Because the hospital lawyer says to turn it off? Should the question of the approval of society as a whole be a consideration? What if the nurse is a member of a professional association that specifies in its code of ethics that a particular behavior is called for or is categorically unethical? Does the fact that the code approves of the nurse's participation in research on children who cannot consent necessarily make that participation ethical? What if the nurse is a member of a religious group? Does that provide a source of moral authority for decisions in nursing? What if the religious group's judgment conflicts with some other judgments the nurse obtains when he or she seeks advice? What if it conflicts with the physician's judgment, with the judgment of the state licensing board, the consensus of the nurse's colleagues, or the ANA's code of ethics? It is the tension between the professional code and a religious tradition that provides the problem raised in the case of the nurse who thought that the ANA *Code for Nurses* was wrong.

THE AUTHORITY OF THE PROFESSION

Case 7: The Nurse Who Thought the ANA Code for Nurses Wrong

Martha Levy, staff nurse in a small nursing home in a Midwest community, has just reviewed the physician's orders for Mr. Carson, an 84-year-old man who is being readmitted to the nursing home after a 6-week stay at the county medical center. Suffering from diabetes, chronic brain syndrome, frequent urinary tract infections, and heart disease, Mr. Carson had been admitted to the medical center for treatment of his gangrenous left foot. He was largely unaware of his surroundings but did move his extremities and moan loudly when the nursing staff tried to talk to him or move him. There was no expectation that his condition would improve significantly. An amputation had been recommended to prevent additional deterioration of his condition and possible death, but the operation had been refused by Mr. Carson's niece, his only surviving relative and legal guardian. The niece, Mrs. Myers, refused to consent to the surgery on the basis that Mr. Carson would not have consented to the procedure if he were competent and able to state his wishes. The surgery was not performed, and over a period of several weeks, Mr. Carson's condition improved to the point that he could be discharged to the nursing home, his residence for the past 6 years.

While he was in the medical center, a nasogastric tube had been inserted to facilitate Mr. Carson's feeding and nutritional intake. The physician's orders stated that he was to be fed a high-protein, low-sodium, tube-feeding preparation every 4 hours. This order would not pose any problem in the nursing home, because several of the home's residents were on regular tube feedings per nasogastric tube. During the first 24 hours after his return, nursing staff noted that he apparently did not like his tube feedings; Mr. Carson moaned, turned his head, and waved his arms when the tube feedings were administered. The nurses restrained his arms and held his head tightly while the tube feeding was given. Once it was given, he apparently tolerated the tube feeding well.

The following day, Mrs. Myers visited her uncle and was visably upset by his general condition, the presence of the nasogastric tube, the feeding routine, and what she considered was his obvious dislike of the procedure. She told the nurse that the feeding tube had been removed during the last few days of his stay at the medical center with her whole-hearted consent. She had not been aware that it had been reinserted the day of discharge to the nursing home. Mrs. Myers called her uncle's physician from the nursing home and asked that the feeding tube be removed. Even though it was doubtful that Mr. Carson would be able to take sufficient nutrition by mouth, the physician agreed to removal of the nasogastric tube. He then called Mrs. Levy and asked that she remove Mr. Carson's nasogastric tube.

Mrs. Levy objected to the decision to remove the tube and refused to remove the tube herself. She felt that Mr. Carson would be unable to receive adequate nutrition without the tube and that removing the tube would contribute to a deterioration of the patient's condition. Despite his reactions to the tube feedings, she did not want to participate in what, in her opinion, might contribute to Mr. Carson's death. Her reasons, in part, stemmed from the fact that she was a strictly observant Orthodox Jew. She had learned that the Talmudic tradition places the highest emphasis on the duty to do what is necessary to preserve an identifiable, individual human life. She had, in discussions with her rabbi, debated on several occasions the ethics of maintaining terminally ill patients, especially those who were near death. She had gradually become convinced of the wisdom of her religious tradition, which had consistently taught that even moments of life should be preserved. Her religious commitment required her to do what she could to ensure that risk of death be avoided, or at least minimized.

However, other nursing staff and Mr. Carson's physician sharply disagreed with Mrs. Levy. They cited the right of the patient to refuse treatment, as exercised by his legal guardian, and the obligation of the nurse to refrain from prolonging the dying process. When Mrs. Levy consulted the ANA *Code for Nurses* for direction, she discovered that the obligation of the nurse to "provide services with respect for human dignity and the uniqueness of the client..." had recently been interpreted by the profession in the following manner: "Nursing care is directed toward the prevention and relief of the suffering commonly associated with the dying process. The nurse may provide interventions to relieve symptoms in the dying client even when the interventions entail substantial risks of hastening death."[10(p 4)] She interpreted this statement to mean that nurses may remove nasogastric tubes from comatose individuals, even though their removal would reduce adequate nutrition and hydration in the patient and might hasten death. The professional ethic would apparently agree with the niece's and the physician's decisions to remove the feeding tube.

Clearly, Mrs. Levy was facing a difficult moral dilemma: The ethics of her nurses' association pulled her in one direction while her religious heritage pulled her in another. Her problem was which, if either, should take precedence.

Commentary

Mrs. Levy is faced with a conflict between two potential sources of moral help in resolving her dilemma, and, as she understands them, they are in conflict. The ANA *Code for Nurses* places great emphasis on the autonomy of the patient and the nurse's duty to respect the integrity of the choices made. True, in this case, Mr. Carson's wishes are being transmitted by his niece, but his wishes appear to be clear. In fact, the ANA code specifically endorses the use of a surrogate decision-maker.

On the other hand, Mrs. Levy's religious tradition, as she understands it with the help of her rabbi, is one that insists on the moral obligation to preserve life, even for a terminally ill patient such as Mr. Carson.[11] In some cases, the nurse might be able to resolve the conflict by appealing to the "conscience clause" in the interpretations of the ANA code. The code says, "If ethically opposed to interventions in a particular case because of the procedures to be used, the nurse is justified in refusing to participate."[10(pp 3–4)] In this case, however, the moral conflict is more difficult. Mrs. Levy is asked to remove a nasogastric feeding tube, with the realization that Mr. Carson's life will be shortened. Simply withdrawing from the case so that some other nurse will remove the tube would not satisfy her religiously rooted obligation to preserve life. Mr. Carson would still die.

A similar problem might occur if a decision not to attempt resuscitation were made by Mr. Carson or his niece and placed in the medical record. In such a case, it might be awkward for Mrs. Levy to withdraw from the case. She, for example, might be the only nurse on the floor for her shift. On the other hand, if she were to honor the decision not to resuscitate if he needed resuscitation during her shift, she would be violating her religiously based duty.

The underlying issue raised by Mrs. Levy's dilemma is the question of what the status of various codes and ethical interpretations should be in helping the nurse formulate her own conscience. On balance, the two kinds of authority Mrs. Levy is considering seem to be quite different. One makes claims about what is ethically correct for the whole of life and will be accepted to the extent that one accepts the particular religious tradition. The other makes claims about a particular sphere of one's life, in this case, nursing. It will be accepted to the extent that one believes that professional groups actually invent the morality of their members, or to the extent that one believes that the collective wisdom of the professional group is the best way of knowing what is right for its members.

Technically, the codes of ethics of various professional associations are binding on the members of those associations, but only to the extent that the association can censure its members for violations. The ultimate penalty, presumably, would be expulsion from the association. But should Mrs. Levy consider that her professional association has special ethical authority in determining what is ethical for nurses? Historically, some health professionals have claimed that the professional group actually creates the ethical duties for its members. Insofar as one wants to be a member in good standing, one would consider the profession's judgment definitive. Others have argued, however, that ethics is a matter that cannot simply be invented by any group of human beings, that what is ethically required must be grounded in some source beyond mere convention— in reason, universal moral law, or divine authority.

If that is the case, the issue would become one of whether the professional group is authoritative in understanding and articulating the moral obligations of professionals. It might be argued that clinical experience or socialization into the meaning and goals of the profession is essential before one can understand what a nurse ought to do.

There are also critics of this position, however. Surely health care professionals have special duties, duties that would not apply to people in other roles. Being uniquely dedicated to the client is only the most apparent of these duties. Just as police or military officials or parents have special ethical responsibilities, so do health care professionals. Yet the question is whether one has to be a member of one of these groups in order to understand what the group members' duties are. Presumably both parents and nonparents understand why the role of parent includes a bias in favor of the welfare of one's own children. Both police and nonpolice recognize that police behave in special ways, that they use violence in ways not authorized for others, for example.

A similar question arises for the ethics of the professions. Do members of the professions have a special authority in deciding what the professional's duty is? If so, the pronouncements of professional associations should be given special weight by Mrs. Levy and others wanting to know their professional obligations. If they do not, then Mrs. Levy might listen to what they say, but not consider them definitive or authoritative. They are more the opinion of one group about the special duties of that group.

How should Mrs. Levy view the authority of her religious tradition and her rabbi as teacher in deciding what she ought to do in the face of a decsision not to provide nutrition, hydration, or resuscitation? It is the nature of religious institutions that they claim to have authoritative ways of knowing. They know through revelation, reason, tradition, or inspired prophecy. They claim moral authority. Of course, not everyone accepts that authority as definitive, but its members do, at least to some extent.

If Mrs. Levy considers herself a member of the Orthodox Jewish community, she presumably accepts the moral authority of her tradition. It is not that she will necessarily automatically accept what her rabbi says as definitive, but she should at least consider carefully the wisdom of her religious tradition, and, to the extent she considers herself a part of that tradition, she should consider its sources of moral knowledge authoritative. Mrs. Levy's question should be whether she feels that her professional group ought to be given the same status. If it should, she may be in the terrible situation of having two sources of moral insight she considers authoritative that are in conflict. Does a professional group have claims to moral authority the way a religious tradition does?

THE AUTHORITY OF THE PHYSICIAN

In other cases, the tension the nurse faces over the source of moral authority is not between the professional code and and some other source of authority to which she is committed, such as her religion. It is between her own sense of what is right and the viewpoint of other people involved in the case: the physician, the institutional authorities, the society at large, or the client. The next group of cases examines in turn each of these kinds of conflict. In each case, the nurse's problem is deciding whether she should compromise her own ethical commitments and substitute the ethical framework of someone else.

Case 8: Following the Physician's Orders: The Nurse as Moral Spectator

Gretchen Sears, a 20 year old in midpregnancy, was admitted to a small community hospital early one evening when she developed signs of premature labor and delivery. Although Mrs. Sears had undergone two prenatal checkups, both she and her obstetrician, an elderly but well-respected practitioner in the community, were uncertain about her stage of pregnancy. Alerted by the labor room staff, the nurse in the special care nursery, Roger Simmons, prepared for the possible admission of an infant of unknown gestation. Mr. Simmons was a neonatology nurse specialist and had recently been employed by the hospital. He quickly alerted the pediatric associate, Dr. Frank Barnes, on call for the evening.

In the labor room, the obstetrician explained to Mrs. Sears that it was very unlikely that her infant would be alive when delivered. Both she and her husband were urged to reconcile themselves to the loss of the pregnancy. Within an hour, Mrs. Sears delivered the product of her first pregnancy, a very small female infant, in the labor room bed. The infant breathed spontaneously, however, and was quickly rushed to the special care nursery. Nurse Roger Simmons examined the tiny infant. Weighing 680 grams, she was pink and had a heart rate of 140. No physical abnormalities were noted. From the infant's physical development, the nurse estimated its gestational age at 27 to 28 weeks. Based on this information, Mr. Simmons anticipated that the infant would be placed on respiratory support and transported to the nearest tertiary care faculty . He quickly called Dr. Barnes and began supporting the infant's respiratory efforts. After examining the infant, however, Dr. Barnes told Mr. Simmons, "I'm not sure we ought to be too aggressive with this infant. I'm going to talk with the obstetrician before we go any further." Mr. Simmons was surprised, since he was accustomed to instituting treatment for infants of this size (and even smaller

infants) in his previous position in a large medical center. He knew how important early treatment and quick transport to another facility might be to this infant's survival.

Within a few minutes, the obstetrician arrived to consult with Dr. Barnes.
After some discussion, Dr. Barnes discontinued the ventilation support, telling
Mr. Simmons that they would not be giving the infant any further treatment. In
his opinion, the infant was too small to survive. Mr. Simmons disagreed with Dr.
Barnes. He then asked if Mr. and Mrs. Sears were aware of their child's condition
and her chances for survival if transported. Dr. Barnes stated that both he and the
obstetrician were going out to talk with the parents. The obstetrician added,
"Look, these parents are just young kids getting started with their lives. They
don't have the resources or know-how to take care of the kind of problems this
child will create. They'll have more babies." As the physicians left the nursery to
inform the parents, Dr. Barnes told Mr. Simmons to keep the infant comfortable
and call him "when its heart stops beating."

Commentary

As in the previous case, the nurse may feel the moral tension between two different
kinds of moral authority. In this case, however, Mr. Simmons does not feel moral am-
bivalence within himself because of having to choose between religious and professional authority. He seems to be convinced of what is morally required. His problem is
rather that someone else—a physician in a traditional position of authority—has made
a choice apparently based on some other set of moral principles.

Mr. Simmons presumably formed his own conclusion, drawing on sources of
moral authority of importance: his religious and philosophical convictions, his sense of
the commitments he has made as a professional nurse, and other sources of significance
to him. On the other hand, Dr. Barnes has apparently concluded that it is ethically appropriate, or at least ethically permissible, for him to decide on his own to let the Sears'
baby die. Dr. Barnes may have had several reasons for his decision. He may have
thought that the baby would be sufficiently handicapped if it survived to justify his letting her die. He may have thought that the Sears were not capable of being adequate parents. He may have thought that the costs to society would not justify doing what was
necessary to give the child a chance to live. For whatever reason, Dr. Barnes was making a moral judgment just as was Mr. Simmons. The critical question is whether there
is any reason to assume that Dr. Barnes' judgment should automatically take
precedence.

Were the choice one based on medical knowledge, many would hold that Dr.
Barnes' judgment has a special authority. After all, he is the one with the medical skill.
By the same token, were the decision one requiring nursing expertise, Mr. Simmons'
judgment might be given special weight. Yet, there was no evidence in the case presented that Dr. Barnes and Mr. Simmons disagreed over anything requiring either a physician's or nurse's expertise. They appeared to disagree over the morality of letting a
baby die who might live if saved, but who might live with some degree of debilitation.
Is it acceptable for a physician to let such a baby die? is the first ethical question. If so,
is it acceptable to do so without the knowledge and permission of the parents?

Dr. Barnes has presumably drawn on his religious or philosophical belief system in deciding that it was acceptable to let the baby die. He may have been informed by the physician's Hippocratic tradition, which urges the physician to use his own judgment to do what will benefit the patient.[12] Is there any reason, however, why either the personal religious and philosophical views of the physician should be definitive? Presumably, some other physician, had he been on call that evening, would have brought to the case some other set of beliefs and values. It is hard to see why the fate of the patient should be decided by the luck of the draw as it determines who happens to be on call on a given evening. By the same token, it is hard to imagine why a professional code or professional consensus, should one exist among physicians, should be definitive in deciding the baby's fate. On the other hand, it is hard to see why Mr. Simmons' own beliefs and values or the code of his profession is definitive either.

A number of avenues of response have been proposed for the nurse caught in the situation wherein the physician or some other *de facto* decision maker may have inappropriately claimed moral authority in situations such as this. What is your assessment of each of the following?

1. Discussing with nursing colleagues the wisdom of the treatment plan of the physician
2. Discussing with the physician directly concerned whether the course he is following is ethically appropripate
3. Appealing through nursing channels, for example, through the nursing supervisor
4. Taking the issue to a hospital ethics committee
5. Going directly to Mr. and Mrs. Sears
6. Reporting the situation to local child abuse authorities for review

In considering each of these courses and any others that can be added to the list, ask yourself whether the persons to whom Mr. Simmons might appeal have any authority—either moral or legal—to override the decision made by Dr. Barnes.

THE AUTHORITY OF THE INSTITUTION

The profession, the nurse's religious tradition, and the physician are not the only ones proposing interpretations of moral duties for the nurse. At times the nurse's hospital or other health care institution may have moral commitments of its own from which it attempts to structure the nurse's obligations. This raises the question of whether the nurse's moral duty and that of the health care institution are always compatible.

Case 9: The Nurse Covering the Maternity Unit

Herma Gonzales was a nurse for a medical–surgical nursing unit of a small county hospital in the Midwest. She was a recent graduate of an undergraduate program in nursing and had worked on her unit for approximately 2 months.

During this time, she had become familiar with most of the unit's routines and felt confident of her nursing abilities. One Saturday evening, the nursing supervisor came to her unit right at the beginning of the shift and stated that someone would need to be pulled to cover the 10-bed maternity unit temporarily. The regular evening nurse had experienced car trouble on the way to work and would be approximately 1 1/2 hours late getting to the hospital. Since the medical–surgical unit was relatively quiet, the supervisor thought that the LPN working with Mrs. Gonzales could handle the unit. The supervisor wanted Mrs. Gonzales to cover the maternity unit, because the emergency room nurse had just notified her of an impending admission to the maternity unit.

Mrs. Gonzales quickly went to the maternity unit, where she received report from the waiting day shift nurse. The report revealed nothing extraordinary except the new admission that the emergency room had just called about. They would be transporting the new admission to the maternity unit in a few minutes. The patient was a 24-year-old woman in her last trimester of pregnancy. She had two living children and a history of precipitous labor. She was apparently in the early stages of labor. Because of her labor and delivery history and the fact that she lived 25 miles from the hospital, she was being admitted for close observation.

As soon as she checked her patients, Mrs. Gonzales called the nursing supervisor to let her know that she would need assistance with this particular patient. She was not competent in maternity nursing and was concerned about the potential needs of the patient. Did the supervisor have a more experienced RN who could cover the maternity ward? The supervisor said that she did not and told Mrs. Gonzales not to worry. An RN was needed on the ward to admit the patient, but the supervisor knew that the regular nurse would be arriving soon. As soon as she arrived, Mrs. Gonzales could go back to her regular unit.

Within minutes, the patient arrived from the emergency room. Mrs. Gonzales checked her vital signs and put the patient into bed. The patient was having regular and strong uterine contractions; her blood pressure was 176/118, pulse, 98 and faint, and respirations, 24. The patient seemed very anxious and restless. The fetal heart rate (FHR) was 146 and faint but regular. Mrs. Gonzales again called her supervisor. She wanted the supervisor to come to the floor immediately and relieve her of the responsibility for this patient. She simply did not feel competent to handle the situation, and it would be another 30 minutes, at least, before the regular nurse could be expected. How could hospital policy calling for the presence of an RN on the floor during the admission override Mrs. Gonzales' obligation to not take on responsibilities for which she did not feel competent?

Commentary

Much like the physician in the previous case, Mrs. Gonzales' hospital had a moral position from which it was acting. The administrators felt obligated to make sure that their nursing skills, which were in short supply because another nurse was delayed, would be used as efficiently as possible. To them, this meant letting the LPN cover the medical-surgical floor and shifting Mrs. Gonzales temporarily to the maternity unit. They argued, probably correctly, that this staffing would do more good for patients than any other arrangement, given the emergency that had developed. The hospital administrators necessarily adopt a social ethic, one that is committed to moral treatment of all the persons within their institution. As such, they would appear to have the right and the responsibility to use their personnel in accord with their ethical obligation.

Mrs. Gonzales and other nurses in clinical settings are not administrators. They should be open to the possibility that they have an ethical obligation that differs from that of administrators. The nurse's obligation is normally thought to be more directly to the health, welfare, and safety of the individual client. The ANA, the most well-recognized interpretor of the nurse's ethical obligation, warns against incompetent practice. Many nurses would hold that they have a duty not to practice where they are not appropriately educated and competent and therefore might feel obliged to refuse to practice on a unit where they believe they cannot do an adequate job.

Some nurses might make an exception in an emergency, when their refusal means that patients in need will not receive any nursing attention at all. Others might feel obliged, even in an emergency situation, to refuse to practice nursing under circumstances in which they are convinced they would not practice competently. Nurses should be open to the possibility that the administrators' ethical mandate and that of the nurses are quite different. This will be an issue in many of the cases in Chapters 3 and 4.

THE AUTHORITY OF SOCIETY

There are times when it is not the physician or the hospital, but society that places moral pressure on the nurse. The following two cases examine the authority of society in articulating moral duties for the nurse and how the nurse should respond to those pressures.

Case 10: Medications by Unlicensed Technicians*

Rose McGovern, Director of Nursing of an 80-bed nursing home facility in an urban setting, has just learned that a bill has been introduced in the state legislature to allow medications to be given by unlicensed technicians in nursing homes throughout the state.

Mrs. McGovern is outraged. As a long-standing advocate of skilled nursing home care, she knows that the administration of medications to elderly clients is much more than the mere giving of ordered dosages of chemical substances. Medication administration provides the best opportunity for the qualified nurse to assess the total health state of the elderly person. Although medication technicians have been allowed by law to give medications in state owned and psychiatric hospitals within her state for many years, the practice has never been

*Adapted from Fry ST: Ethical issues: Politics, power, and change. In Talbott S, Mason D (eds): Political Action: A Handbook for Nurses, pp 133-140. Reading, MA, Addison-Wesley, 1985. Used with permission

legislated for general hospitals or for nursing homes. In fact, the state nurses' association and the state association of nursing homes have always agreed that the administration of medicines in nursing homes is a nursing function and must be performed by licensed personnel (RNs and LPNs). Mrs. McGovern maintains that the ANA *Code for Nurses* makes clear that the health, welfare, and safety of the patient will be the nurse's primary consideration. She is convinced that the state has no business authorizing nonlicensed technicians to perform nursing functions and that such a proposal could easily compromise the welfare and safety of patients. Now, that position is being directly challenged in the legislature.

After a few hurried telephone calls, Mrs. McGovern and her colleagues in the state nursing home association learn that the bill has been referred to committee. They also learn that the bill was introduced by a representative in support of a group of businessmen who are building a large nursing care facility for the elderly in his rural district. The businessmen have argued that employing medication technicians in nursing homes is more cost effective than using licensed personnel, and, if the technicians are properly trained and supervised, their use presents no additional risk to nursing home residents. Since the number of elderly needing nursing home care and the cost of employing licensed nursing personnel have risen dramatically in the last few years, the bill is viewed as a means to help provide low-cost nursing care for the state's elderly citizens. The bill has the support of the state medical association and the state pharmaceutical association.

Within 36 hours, the bill comes out of committee, is passed, and is sent to the governor for signing. Mrs. McGovern, other directors of nursing homes, and officials of the state nursing home association send an urgent message to the governor opposing the potential legislation. They also request time to study the use of medication technicians in nursing homes. Mrs. McGovern wonders whether the state has the authority to risk patients' welfare in this way.

Commentary

This case raises the problem of the relationship of the nursing profession to society and what role society and the profession ought to have in articulating norms of nursing conduct. The proposed legislation authorizing the use of medication technicians might, at first, appear to trigger an empirical disagreement. The supporters of the legislation claim that the unlicensed technicians would be cheaper and would pose "no risk" to patients. Mrs. McGovern is apparently convinced that patients would be in at least some risk if unlicensed technicians administered medication.

The case would become more interesting ethically if both sides were to agree that there is probably some increased risk for patients, although that risk may be small. If this is admitted, then the dispute may really be one over moral principles. Mrs. McGovern appeals to the ANA code to identify what she takes to be the most important ethical principle: working for the health, welfare, and safety of patients. Presumably, the state, if it accepts the arguments of the supporters of the bill, is operating on a somewhat

different norm, something like the notion that small risks are worth taking if they will save significant amounts of money.

If this is not a simple dispute over the factual matter of whether the use of unlicensed medical technicians would lead to increased risks for patients, then it is a dispute over the relative authority of the nursing profession and the state in deciding which norm should apply.

Some might argue that the nursing profession has legitimate authority for articulating the moral norms for nurses, but that the state has taken the task of administering medication in nursing homes out of the nurses' purview. In that case, the nursing profession could continue to articulate norms for nurses, but not for those working outside nursing.

That argument might simply shift the issue to that of whether the profession or the society as a whole has the authority to determine what is within the purview of nursing. In any case, the critical problem remaining is what the relation should be between the profession and the broader society.

Some would hold that when it comes to articulating moral norms for a professional group such as nurses, the profession is the only group with the experience, skill, and sensitivity to make the decision. They would ask, "Why should state legislators tell nurses what the norms should be for the practice of their profession?"

The defenders of the involvement of the broader society in picking the norms for professionals reject this position. They may well concede that when it comes to matters requiring technical competence, only the members of the profession are adequately experienced to speak authoritatively. Only physicians can speak authoritatively about the prognosis of a particular patient or the predicted effects of a treatment. Only nurses can determine the diagnosis and treatment of human responses to actual or potential health problems.

However, there may not be disagreement over the technical, empirical question of whether patients are at risk (a question over which nurses might claim special expertise). The dispute may be over which of two moral norms is appropriate for institutionalizing policy regarding administration of medication. If the dispute is really one over moral norms, it is not clear that being a professional in a particular field gives one expertise in choosing moral norms for social practices. The dispute might, in effect, be over how much risk is worth taking in order to save money.

If that is the nature of the argument, then it could be concluded that the authority of the broader society is substantial. Different groups within society are likely to have different preferences for moral norms and different views about how much risk is worth taking. Nurses may be more inclined against taking risks with patients than is the general public. However, some other professional group, such as accountants, may be much more supportive of risk-taking than the general public. The issue for debate is whether the expertise that one gains when one becomes a member of a profession has anything to do with the kinds of judgments required in choosing moral norms governing the conduct of the profession as it interacts with the public. Society as a whole may well have authority to articulate moral norms of conduct—such as deciding that marginal risks are justified.

The position of society as the group articulating the norms for nursing is not ex-

actly parallel to the position of some other profession such as that of physicians. It seems clear that one professional group cannot claim the authority to determine what the norms shall be for the conduct of another profession. It is more difficult to determine the extent to which society as a whole should be able to play an active role in determining what the norms of conduct are for the professions.

THE AUTHORITY OF THE CLIENT

Thus far in this chapter we have explored the moral authority of a number of agents. The question being addressed is who might the nurse appropriately turn to as an authority for deciding what morality requires. We have examined the authority of religious tradition, professional groups, physicians, and society. One more possible source of authority that a nurse might consider is the client. Every client comes to the nurse with a set of beliefs and moral values. Clients have some sense of what is required of them ethically. They draw on their own religious or philosophical systems. They are influenced by others in the society. In any case, they are capable of reaching moral conclusions about the kind of health care they desire and how the nurse, physician, and other health care professionals ought to act. Sometimes those convictions may be at odds with the nurse's own judgments. In the following case, the relation of the nurse's own moral convictions to those of the client will be explored.

Case 11: The Patient Who Wanted the Bedrails Down

Mr. Clinton Hightower, a 79-year-old man afflicted with Parkinson's disease, had been a patient at Sweet Pines Convalescent Home for less than 18 hours. Within that time, however, he had made himself known to every staff member and to most of the patients in the facility. His particular manner of doing this consisted in loudly calling, "Nurse! Nurse! Is anybody there?" whenever he wanted to get out of bed and go to the bathroom (which was frequently) or wanted his glasses (which he often lost in the folds of the bedding).

As Doris Franklin, the night nurse, quietly made her rounds of the patients, she could hear his loud, insistent voice. It had not been more than 20 minutes since she had been in Mr. Hightower's room. Now he was calling for her again. What could he need now? As she walked the last steps to the door of his room, he was rattling the bedrails. "Please don't keep me trapped in my bed like this," he bellowed. "I'm not an invalid. I want to be able to get out of bed and go to the bathroom whenever I want. Why are these things on my bed?" As Mrs. Franklin helped him out of bed and watched him shakily proceed with his walker to the bathroom, she again explained that siderails were used on all the patients' beds at night. While Sweet Pines was a facility that offered a home-like atmosphere for its residents, the night nurse insisted that siderails be placed on all the beds during hours when patients were sleeping. Since Mrs. Franklin and a nursing aide were the only night staff for the 45 elderly residents of the facility, the bedrails helped ensure that no one would attempt to get out of bed for routine visits to the bathroom without assistance from Mrs. Franklin or the aide. The low incidence of patient falls at night was proof that the practice helped protect the patients from injury as a result of falling.

Unfortunately, Mr. Hightower was not satisfied with Mrs. Franklin's explanation. He insisted that he would take responsibility for himself and for any injuries that he might incur as a result of falling. The bedrails were a great annoyance to him and were keeping him from resting at night. Mrs. Franklin would not change her mind. Although, in general, she respected any patient's requests for self-care, she was adamant about the use of bedrails at night, particularly for any patient with Parkinson's disease. In her professional judgment, to fail to use siderails at night on the bed of an elderly client, no matter how competent and oriented he or she might be, was to put the patient at risk of injury. Mr. Hightower was very displeased, and his frequent trips to the bathroom made it a very difficult and unpleasant night for both him and Mrs. Franklin.

When she arrived for work the next night, Mrs. Franklin was surprised to see a note in the Kardex that Mr. Hightower was not to have siderails put on his bed at night. He had signed a statement for the facility's administrator releasing Sweet Pines and the staff of all responsibility for any injuries that he might incur as a result of falling while getting out of bed. This certainly relieved Mrs. Franklin of any legal responsibility for injuries that Mr. Hightower might incur. But did it relieve her of her moral responsibility to protect him from harm? Mrs. Franklin did not think that it did! Yet Mr. Hightower seemed to think that *he* was the best judge of professional responsibility where his risk of injury from falling out of bed was concerned.

Commentary

Once again, the initial issue is whether there is a moral dispute or merely one involving professional judgment. Mrs. Franklin and Mr. Hightower may be arguing about who is the better judge of whether Mr. Hightower is at risk if he has the bedrails down. Surely, Mrs. Franklin has had much more experience than Mr. Hightower in caring for elderly patients with Parkinson's disease who are new residents in convalescent homes. Although she probably does not know as well as Mr. Hightower how mobile he is (since he had been at Sweet Pines for only a day), she does have experience with patients falling while getting out of bed.

A more sophisticated assessment of the risks and benefits of the bedrails would, of course, have to include not only the risk of falls, but also the risks of psychological stress from Mr. Hightower's feelings of confinement. Mr. Hightower might well be better able to assess the overall risks and benefits than Mrs. Franklin.

It is not clear, however, that the dispute is merely one of assessing risks and benefits. It may well be that Mrs. Franklin and Mr. Hightower are operating with different ethical principles. Mrs. Franklin's principle seems to be one of a duty to protect her patients from harm, of placing the client's care and safety as the first consideration. Mr. Hightower's principle is probably not as narrow. He may, if pressed, say that his goal is not his safety but rather his overall well-being, including his happiness and other psychological considerations. He may even, if pressed further, make another claim. He may say, that he wants the freedom to live his own life, even if it puts him at risk and even if it turns out not to make him as well off as he might otherwise be. The dispute may be over which of two principles—patient safety or patient autonomy—ought to govern Mrs. Franklin's actions.

If that is the case, then the nurse needs to know how to relate her own instincts about the right principle of action to Mr. Hightower's judgment. When religious authority was a possible source of the norms for nursing conduct, we saw that there was good reason for the nurse who was committed to a particular religious tradition to treat the religious tradition as authoritative. Likewise, in case 10, we saw that arguments could be made leading to the conclusion that the society as a whole might be able to articulate moral norms governing nursing conduct.

In contrast, the moral authority of the individual physician and of professional groups was more complex. We examined arguments that led to the conclusion that neither individual physicians nor professional groups should be viewed as having any special expertise in articulating moral norms.

The problem posed by Mr. Hightower is more complex. Surely, there is no particular reason to assume that the 79-year-old Parkinson's disease patient is an expert in determining moral norms. He might, in fact, be a wise and respected citizen of the community who has traditionally provided its moral leadership, but nothing in the case scenario suggests that. There seems to be no reason to assume Mr. Hightower is any more of an authority in choosing moral norms than was Dr. Barnes in the case in which he decided to let a prematurely born infant die.

Mr. Hightower may not be claiming to be an authority in choosing moral norms for the nursing profession, however. He is probably making a much more simple claim: that in deciding about his own care, within certain limits , the care ought to be governed by his own values and ethical commitments. Mr. Hightower is probably not making the same claim that the society seemed to be making through its legislature in the case involving the use of unlicensed medical technicians. He is not claiming that all of nursing should be governed by some moral norms articulated from outside nursing. Rather, he is merely asking for the freedom to have his own personal care governed by his norms. If Mrs. Franklin ought to yield to Mr. Hightower with regard to the bedrails, it is not because Mr. Hightower has general moral authority. It is rather because he is the primary client and claims that his care should be provided on his terms.

At the same time, the limits of client authority need to be assessed. What should happen, for example, if the nurse cannot participate in the client's care on the client's terms without violating her own conscience? What do we make of Mrs. Franklin's continuing reservations after Mr. Hightower signs a release? It seems unlikely that Mrs. Franklin's objections to Mr. Hightower's moral position are so great that she would choose this issue to take a stand on conscience. However, there might be some moral positions of clients that so violate Mrs. Franklin's ethical framework that she ought not to cooperate. What, for example, if Mr. Hightower's condition deteriorated, and he said that the moral framework he wanted for his care was one that accepted active mercy killing? At some point, the authority that comes from clients must have its limits.

References

1. Brandt RB: Ethical Theory: The Problems of Normative and Critical Ethics, pp 151–294. Englewood Cliffs, NJ, Prentice-Hall, 1959
2. Frankena W: Ethics, 2nd ed, pp 95–116. Englewood Cliffs, NJ, Prentice-Hall, 1973
3. Feldman F: Introductory Ethics, pp 160–247. Englewood Cliffs, NJ, Prentice-Hall, 1978
4. Taylor PW: Principles of Ethics: An Introduction, pp 175–227. Encino, CA, Dickenson Publishing Co, 1975
5. Kant I: Groundwork of the Metaphysic of Morals, Paton HJ (trans). New York, Harper & Row, 1964
6. Ross WD: The Right and the Good. Oxford, Oxford University Press, 1939
7. Sumner WG: Folkways. Boston, Ginn, 1906
8. Westermarck EA: Ethical Relativity. Paterson, NJ, Littlefield, Adams, 1960
9. Veatch RM: A Theory of Medical Ethics, pp 79–107. New York, Basic Books, 1981
10. American Nurses' Association. Code for Nurses with Interpretive Statements. Kansas City, American Nurses' Association, 1985
11. Bleich JD: The obligation to heal in the Judaic tradition: A comparative analysis. In Rosner F, Bleich JD (eds): Jewish Bioethics, pp 1–44. New York, Sanhedrin Press, 1979
12. Edelstein L: The Hippocratic oath: Text, translation and interpretation. In Temkin O, Temkin CL (eds): Ancient Medicine: Selected Papers of Ludwig Edelstein, pp 3–64. Baltimore, The Johns Hopkins Press, 1967

Part II

Ethical Principles in Nursing

The ability to recognize ethical and other value issues in nursing care situations and the understanding of proper sources of moral authority in nursing are foundational to the analysis of ethical dilemmas in nursing. When used in conjunction with codes of ethics for nurses these skills help build a framework for analyzing specific case problems in nursing care. A framework—an ethical theory for nursing, if you like—can be built up in several stages. At the level of specific case problems, intuitions often provide perfectly adequate solutions to ethical problems. In fact, most of the ethical decisions that a nurse must make during the course of the day are made on the basis of intuitive knowledge.

However, many patient care problems are more serious and require more than intuitive knowledge of its ethical dimensions. Our common sense intuitions often do not provide a clear answer. Sometimes what seems to be the ethically obvious course to us is opposed by a colleague, a physician, an administrator, or a patient. In these situations, it is often helpful to appeal to other levels of the framework for help in thinking through the alternatives and reasons for making various choices.

Above the level of specific case decisions is a second level of rules or guidelines that, depending on one's view about how rigidly they should be adhered to, provide either guidelines or firm answers to the problem being faced. These rules are specific enough to apply to concrete situations but general enough to be used widely. "Always get informed consent before surgery" is an example. So are rules such as, "It is wrong to kill a patient actively even for mercy." Many of the provisions in the American Nurses' Association (ANA) *Code for Nurses* contain rules of this nature.

Sometimes rules are stated from the point of view of the person who has a claim rather than that of the one upon whom the claim is made. In these cases, the language of rights is often used. The claim that the patient always has the right to give an informed consent before surgery is directly parallel to the rule that one must always obtain the patient's informed consent before surgery. When the language of rights is used in this way, the rights are often thought to be derived from the rules.

At some point it may become necessary to call into question one of the rules—to debate whether the rule is justified or properly formulated. For example, if we are really not sure whether it is always wrong to kill for mercy, we may feel a need to appeal to still a higher level. It is widely accepted in ethics that the moral rules reflect another level of our framework for ethical reasoning. This level is the level of ethical principles—principles such as doing good and avoiding evil, promoting justice, respecting autonomy, telling the truth, keeping promises, and avoiding killing. These principles are often given the names, respectively, of the principles of justice, beneficence, nonmaleficence, autonomy, veracity, and fidelity. Avoiding killing is sometimes referred to as the principle of the sacredness of life. There are, according to some ethical theories, more ethical principles than the seven already mentioned. Other theorists, however, claim that all of ethics can be reduced to an even shorter list of principles, perhaps even one principle, such as beneficence.

Regardless of the number of principles ascribed to, ethical principles make up the third level of a framework for analyzing ethical problems. Yet, we might want to ask if one ethical principle is of greater authority than another. To ask which principle ought to be accepted over another principle one would have to deal with the very basics of an ethical theory. There are two dominant normative theories available. One holds that the issue of right and wrong is fundamentally a matter of producing good consequences and avoiding evil consequences. This approach—often called consequentialism—is illustrated by the ethical position referred to as utilitarianism, the idea that the ethically correct course is the one that produces the greatest good on balance. The alternative is to insist that right and wrong cannot be reduced totally to producing good consequences. These positions—of which there are many different varieties—all agree that there are inherent right or wrong characteristics of certain actions or rules. For example, acts or rules that involve lying, breaking a promise, or distributing resources unfairly are often considered to be acts with wrong-making characteristics. Theories that espouse this view, are called nonconsequentialistic. (Sometimes these positions are also called formalist or deontological.) Consequentialist theories and nonconsequentialist theories, together with their variations, constitute what can be called normative ethics.

Finally, we may have to ask the most basic questions of ethics as a way of attempting to understand and justify our theory. This level, called metaethics, deals with the source of ethics and the ways we know and justify ethical positions. These levels are illustrated in Figure 1 in the Introduction.

The cases in Part II have all been selected because they raise some problem related to one or more general ethical principles. Chapter 3 looks first at the two principles directly related to the consequences of ethical actions: the principles of producing good and avoiding evil or, as they sometimes called, the principles of beneficence and nonmaleficence. The remaining chapters in Part II analyze cases involving the principles of justice, autonomy, truth-telling, keeping promises, and avoiding killing.

Chapter 3

Benefiting the Client and Others: The Duty to Produce Good and Avoid Harm

Virtually everyone agrees that producing good and avoiding harm are relevant to ethics in some way. The ethics of health care professionals have given special emphasis to the consequences of actions. The Hippocratic Oath states this twice. At one point in the oath, the physician pledges to work "for the benefit of the sick according to my ability and judgment; I will keep them from harm and injustice." At a later point in the oath, the physician pledges, "whatever houses I may visit, I will come for the benefit of the sick."[1]

Nursing ethics has a similar emphasis. The Florence Nightingale Pledge includes the promise, "I will abstain from whatever is deleterious and mischievous...and devote myself to the welfare of those committed to my care."[2] The American Nurses' Association (ANA) *Code for Nurses* has language that is similar in its moral impact. The explanation of the third point of the code begins, "The nurse's primary commitment is to the health, welfare, and safety of the client."[3(p 6)]

These code statements sound so benign that they appear uncontroversial, almost platitudinous. Yet we begin to encounter some problems as we probe more deeply into some of the cases in this volume. Sometimes the duty to benefit the client will come into direct conflict with some other ethical requirements, such as respecting the autonomy of the client or distributing resources fairly. These conflicts between producing good consequences for the client and fulfilling the requirements implicit in other ethical principles will be explored in later chapters.

Even when we focus exclusively on the consequences of nursing actions, there are unexpectedly difficult problems in trying to decide exactly what it means to have a primary commitment to the client's care and safety. There are also problems in trying to decide whether we really ought to protect the client if, when the impact on others in the society is taken into account, less good is done on balance.

One problem frequently encountered by the nurse is whether the nurse's responsibility is to benefit the client, taking into account *all* the ways that he or she might be ben-

57

efited. That is what the Hippocratic Oath seems to ask of physicians. An account of *all* benefits to the patient can, however, lead the health professional into areas where he or she has little or no competence. It might include producing social, psychological, economic, and religious benefits for the client—forcing the health care professional to overstep the limits of his or her ability. The ANA *Code for Nurses* seems to ask this of the nurse. Point three of the code states that the nurse's primary commitment is to the client's health, welfare, *and* safety.

A second problem that often occurs in deciding how to produce benefit and avoid harm concerns whether avoiding harm to the patient has a higher priority than benefiting the patient. Some ethical analysts have claimed that the duty to avoid harming the client is more stringent than that of benefiting.[4-6] That may explain why a nurse would feel more responsible if she has injured a patient by giving a wrong medication than if she simply fails to benefit a patient (say, because she is busy helping other clients). On the other hand, if it is more important to avoid harm than to benefit, the implications can be very conservative. The nurse could perfectly fulfill the ethical requirement of avoiding harm to clients by simply never doing anything for them. In the cases that follow, watch to see if the consequences involved are those of having the nurse produce benefit or avoid harm.

A third problem often revolves around the two very different approaches to doing good and avoiding harm. Traditionally, the utilitarians simply counted the net amount of good and harm for each person affected by an individual action and added to find the total amount of good (minus harm) produced.[7] Each action would be considered separately, with an implicit calculation of harms and benefits produced each time. Within the past 20 years, many philosophers who are committed to an ethic of consequences have adopted a different strategy. They have proposed calculations of benefits and harms as a way of evaluating alternative rules of conduct. The rule (or set of rules) that will produce the best consequences would then be adopted. When decisions must be made about individual actions, no direct calculation of consequences is made. One simply applies the rule that has previously been determined to produce the best consequences. For example, the rule, "always get informed consent before surgery," might be adopted because it has better consequences than any alternative rule. (We shall see later that that is not the only reason to adopt it or necessarily even the best reason to do so.) Thus when it comes to specific cases at the bedside, one would simply apply the rule rather than try to calculate *in the individual case* whether consequences are better if consent is obtained. This position, referred to as rule utilitarianism or rule consequentialism, has recently gained great favor among sophisticated consequentialists.[8,9]

Finally, there is a major tension between the consequences of nursing and other health professional ethics and more general ethical theories devoted to the principles of beneficence and nonmaleficence. Most consequentialist theories hold that the goal of ethics is to do as much good as possible, considering the benefits to all people affected by one's actions. Yet many health care ethics put limits on the consequences that are to be considered. They limit the nurse or other health professional to consideration of benefits and harms for the client. Remember, it is the client's health, welfare, and safety that are the nurse's chief concerns according to the ANA *Code for Nurses*.

On what basis are such limits placed, and how is the welfare of the client traded off against the welfare of various other people about whom the nurse might be concerned? The ANA *Code for Nurses*, for example, also talks about the nurse being concerned about the common good and of participating in research that is not for the benefit of the client. It speaks of the nurse's responsibility to the public. Does not the nurse also have an obligation to benefit the institution, society at large, the profession of which she is a member, and, especially, specific, identified persons who are not her clients, but who could be helped greatly by her efforts? Finally, are there ever times when the nurse can compromise the client's care and safety in order to serve the nurse's own interests or those of the nurse's family? These are the issues of the cases in this chapter.

BENEFIT TO THE CLIENT

Because it is widely accepted that the health professional's duty is to benefit the client and protect the client from harm, it is best to begin with a series of cases that help clarify exactly what this means and what problems arise in trying to benefit clients and protect them from harm. We shall address later in the chapter the more complex cases involving conflicts between benefit to the client and benefit to others, such as the institution, the society, the profession, identified nonclients, and oneself or one's family.

In trying to decide how to benefit one's clients and protect them from harm, three separate problems arise:

1. Should the nurse strive to produce the greatest possible general benefit for the client, or should the nurse focus only on health benefits?
2. Should the nurse give special weight to protecting the client from harm, or do benefits and harms get the same weight in calculating net benefits?
3. Should the nurse try to do what is most beneficial in each individual case or should the nurse think in broader terms, say, by acting on a set of rules that will produce more good on balance than any other set of rules?

Health Benefits vs. Overall Benefits

Case 12: The Patient Who Did Not Want To Be Clean*

Marion Downs, a community health nurse, must decide whether to refer her patient, 72-two-year-old Sadie Jenkins, to the community fiduciary for consideration of conservatorship and guardianship. Miss Jenkins has no living relatives and lives alone in a one-room apartment furnished with a bed, refrigerator, table, chair, lamp, and small sink. Since she does not have a stove, two meals per day are supplied by her landlord. With the support of her Social Security check and food stamps, she has adequate money for her needs and has lived for over 10 years in these arrangements. She is also in good physical health.

Ms. Downs has made four home visits to Miss Jenkins to check her vital signs and medication routine following recent treatment in the Health Center's

*Adapted from Cross L: The right to be wrong. Am J Nurs 83:1338, 1983

Hypertension Clinic. Although Miss Jenkins has made excellent progress and no longer requires visits from the community health nurse, her landlord, the other residents of her small apartment building, and her immediate neighbors are urging the nurse to "do something" about Miss Jenkins. Admittedly, Miss Jenkins' apartment has a strong odor from the long-term accumulation of dust, dirt, and mold. Cockroaches can be seen in the apartment, and an unemptied bedpan is often sitting next to Miss Jenkins' bed (it is "too much trouble" to walk down the hallway to the bathroom shared by Miss Jenkins and two other tenants). Ms. Downs has noticed that Miss Jenkins has worn the same soiled clothes every time she has been to her apartment. It is also obvious that Miss Jenkins has not bathed for a long time, her hair is unwashed, and she apparently does not clean her fingernails and dentures. In addition, her toenails are so long that they have perforated the canvas of her tennis shoes, apparently the only shoes that she likes to wear.

Yet, Miss Jenkins is comfortable with her life-style and does not want to change her living arrangements. Although Ms. Downs has offered to contact agencies to help Miss Jenkins—homemaker service, counseling, and senior citizen's group—Miss Jenkins says that she is comfortable and does not want (or need) help from anyone. Moreover, Ms. Downs is aware that she has several other patients who have severe needs for nursing care in the most traditional sense. She knows that if she interrupts her schedule of visits for the day to help place Miss Jenkins, she will not be able to use her skills as a nurse for these other patients as well as she might. Should Ms. Downs use her role of community health nurse to create an arrangement whereby Miss Jenkins would lose the right to control her person, her financial resources, and her environment? Can an individual in the community be forced to be clean and to live in a clean environment? How far should a nurse go in providing "good" for a patient, and who determines what is "good" for Miss Jenkins?

Case 13: Is Leaving the Nursing Home Beneficial?

Mrs. Gertrude Swensen was 86 years old. She had been a resident of St. Luke's Village for slightly over a year. St. Luke's is a self-contained lifetime care community near Miami. She decided to move in after the death of her husband and after surgery for a tumor behind her right ear. In the community she has her own apartment, receives one hot meal a day in a common dining room, and has access to a full range of services, including a church, a library, a beauty shop, and many recreational activities. She is very happy in the community, which she considers an ideal environment for someone who has difficulty caring for herself. Because she has no immediate family, the large one-time fee she paid in exchange for the commitment to lifetime support was no problem for her. Her mind was put at ease knowing that there was a nursing home right within the community that would be available should she ever need it.

Her medical problems were not severe. She had adult-onset diabetes requiring regular oral medication. Her main problem, however, was that the wound from her ear surgery had never healed properly. Two weeks ago she began feeling weaker and had difficulty coming down to the dining room for dinner. She was having difficulty walking and often forgot to change the dressing on her surgical wound. Mrs. Lillian Feldman, the nurse from the community who was visiting her in her apartment, felt that she should move to the nursing home, until she regained her strength.

Mrs. Swensen had gone reluctantly. Now, 2 weeks later, she was beginning to feel a little stronger. She still had trouble walking and was forgetful, but she desperately wanted to be back in her own apartment. She wanted to be near her friends and to eat dinner with them instead of in her nursing home room.

She complained to Mrs. Feldman that she was getting restless and wanted to go back to her apartment. Mrs. Feldman was concerned. She had seen Mrs. Swensen try to walk and nearly fall. She knew she would have difficulty remembering to take her medication and would not be able to change the dressing on her ear by herself. The relationship that had developed between Mrs. Swensen and Mrs. Feldman was a close one. Mrs. Feldman knew that her patient would do whatever she recommended. Mrs. Feldman was convinced that Mrs. Swensen's health required a longer stay in the nursing facility.

Commentary

Marion Downs and Lillian Feldman are two nurses facing a similar problem. They both are committed to the health and welfare of their clients but are having difficulty determining exactly what that means. The ethic of the health professions is traditionally one committed to benefiting the patient, but one of the problems is trying to determine how health benefits relate to other goods that may be on the clients' agendas.

In the first case, that of Sadie Jenkins, the nurse (Ms. Downs) appears to believe that Miss Jenkins would be better off in a nursing care facility. She might be better off medically, but she would certainly be better off in other ways. She would at least be in a clean environment. She would have good meals and would have her clothes and grooming taken care of.

Miss Jenkins might argue with Ms. Downs about whether, taking everything into account, she would be better off. Miss Jenkins might concede that medically she would be better off, but that does not appear to be Miss Jenkins' chief concern. She appears to prefer her familiar home environment and the control that she can exercise, even if it leads to a less-than-ideal living situation.

Moreover, Ms. Downs is aware that other patients need her services, and those services are ones that only she, as a skilled nurse, can provide. The problem is one of whether Ms. Downs should take as her responsibility the total welfare of the patient, including problems such as house cleaning, grooming, and maintenance of clothing that are not traditionally nursing problems, or whether she should remain committed to nursing skills in the narrower sense.

The ANA *Code for Nurses* commits her to the health, welfare, and safety of her patients. Does that limit her to traditional nursing care and medical safety? If so, she would have to justify working to institutionalize Miss Jenkins on health grounds narrowly conceived. Moreover, she would have to give special attention to the health needs of her other patients rather than the non-health needs of Miss Jenkins.

On the other hand, if the ethical mandate of nurses is to benefit the client (without restriction to whether the benefits are health benefits), Miss Jenkins may receive very different treatment. On the one hand, her house cleaning, grooming, and clothing needs are legitimately included in the nurse's agenda. On the other, Miss Jenkins' psychological well-being also must receive full consideration; and Miss Jenkins does not appear to believe that she will be better off on balance if she moves to a nursing care facility.

A similar problem faces Mrs. Feldman. If the medical and health needs of Mrs. Swensen are the nurse's first consideration (if that is what commitment to her health, welfare, and safety means), then surely Mrs. Feldman should recommend that she stay longer in the nursing home of the community. On the other hand, if Mrs. Swensen's total well-being is Mrs. Feldman's objective, then her care and safety might well have to be compromised.

When Mrs. Feldman takes on the role of advisor to Mrs. Swensen, this presents an interesting problem. If Mrs. Feldman makes her judgment while focusing only on Mrs. Swensen's medical needs, health, and safety, then it would appear that health concerns would be a strong consideration. However, no rational person would make such choices solely on the basis of what maximizes his or her health. People have their general welfare in mind, including many dimensions that could lead to decisions that are risky to health.

If Mrs. Feldman tries to take into account not only her health but the other dimensions of Mrs. Swensen's welfare (the way that Ms. Downs appeared to be doing), another problem arises. As a nurse, Mrs. Feldman has no particular skill in making decisions that promote the welfare of patients outside the health sphere. In fact, in comparing the health and nonhealth dimensions of the choice, she might reveal an overcommitment to the health aspect. She has, after all, committed herself to a health profession.

Thus, if by the principle of doing good (beneficence) the nurses limit their attention to the health aspects of their clients' welfare, they are omitting what may be the most important concerns of their clients. On the other hand, if they expand their horizon to attempt to promote the overall welfare of their clients, they venture into areas in which they have no special skill, they dilute their energies so that they can spend relatively less time doing those things for which they are specially educated, and they run the risk of overlooking the unique ways in which their clients assess their overall welfare.

One thing should be clear from these cases. Striving to maximize the health or medical well-being of clients cannot be the same thing as striving to maximize their overall well-being. Which agenda should Ms. Downs and Mrs. Feldman adopt?

Benefiting vs. Avoiding Harm

Case 14: When "Doing Good" May Harm the Patient

The nurses in a critical care unit had been under a great deal of stress from very ill patients, a high census, and frequent staff illnesses during a 2-week period. On one particular evening, two nurses recognized that they were developing the symptoms of an upper respiratory infection that had been affecting other members of the staff. Since they had three postoperative patients needing one-to-one care and were receiving another admission from the emergency room, the nurses solicited medication from the house staff in order to suppress their symptoms and "keep going." While they were able to remain working on the unit and *not* contribute to an already critical staffing situation, they recognized that they might be causing more harm by communicating their illnesses to already vulnerable patients and by the mistakes they made while under the influence of medications (antihistamines).

The two nurses contemplated the alternatives. They were convinced that the additional risk to the patients was quite small, and they believed that the patients were in real need of the one-to-one care that could only be provided if they remained on duty. They concluded that, on balance, the good they could do would exceed the risk of harm, but they wondered: Is there a special obligation for health professionals to avoid harm?

Commentary

Although this seems to be a very simple, routine problem for two nurses, the ethical question the case raises is a fascinating one. In thinking about the ethics of nursing based on benefits and harms to patients, sometimes the formula is used that is derived from the Hippocratic Oath. The health professional's duty is to benefit the patient and protect the patient from harm. In this form, the benefits and harms are on a par. One standard way of approaching health care decisions is to anticipate the expected benefits and the expected harms of alternative courses (taking into account the probabilities in each case).[7] In this situation, the nurses would reflect on the good they could do if they care for patients and on the harm that they could cause (the possible transmission of an infection or the mistakes they could make under the influence of their own medication). They would also reflect on the benefits the patients would forego if the nurses were to go out sick. If benefits and harms are on a par, the nurses would simply compare the net benefits (the benefits minus the harms). As long as the benefits from their nursing care exceeded the projected harms, they would be morally justified in covering up their illnesses in order to serve their patients.

There is an alternative way for health professionals to compare benefits and harms. It is expressed in the slogan *"primum non nocere"*—"first of all do no harm."[10,11] Many believe that it is also from the Hippocratic Oath, but it is not. In fact, it is no where to be found in any Hippocratic writings or in any ancient medical ethics writings. It appears to have emerged in about the middle of the nineteenth century.

Its meaning is as obscure as its origin. It may be just a careless way of saying that health professionals should maximize net benefits for their patients, but it may also have a very different meaning.

Some people hold that it is worse ethically to hurt someone than to fail to help him or her.[4-6] They would hold, for example, that it would be worse to take food away from a child so that he starves than it would be to fail to provide food for a child who was starving. In the first case, the one taking the food away is actually harming, whereas in the second case, he is only failing to help.

Some people maintain that health professionals have a special duty to avoid harming that is more stringent than the duty to help. They interpret the *primum* in the slogan *primum non nocere* to mean exactly this. Not harming is a duty that is first in order of priority. To give a medical example, in deciding whether to perform a difficult, experimental operation that could cure the patient or injure him severely, they would feel a special obligation at least to avoid doing more harm to the patient. Only after the health professional has assured herself that she will not hurt the patient is she ethically justified in trying to help.

The two nurses who are convinced that they will do more good than harm in hiding their illnesses so that they can provide intensive nursing care for their patients will decide differently what they ought to do depending on whether the duty to avoid harming is more stringent than the duty to help. If their duty is to maximize the expected net benefits for their patients and they are convinced that staying on the job will do more good than harm, they are justified in staying. In fact, they have a duty to stay. If, on the other hand, they feel that avoiding harm is a duty with a special priority, they might feel obliged to avoid the risk of injuring the patients or giving them an additional medical problem even if the benefits they anticipate from their continued nursing care exceeded the amount of harm they thought they would do.

Act vs. Rule Consequentialism

A third complication in the ethics of doing what will benefit the patient arises when there are general rules in place covering nursing practices. Those rules often can be justified on the grounds that they spell out practices that will generally tend to benefit patients. As long as it appears that the rule will, in fact, produce behavior that will benefit the patient in the specific instance, no problem arises. What should happen, however, when a nurse believes that a particular patient presents an exception to the rule? If the moral mandate of the nurse is to act always so as to benefit the patient, it would appear that rules should be violated whenever violating the rule will do more good than following it. On the other hand, rules may serve important moral purposes. The next case poses the problem of when rules governing nursing care ought to be violated.

Case 15: Do Patients Always Have to Be Turned?*

Bessie Watkins was a 5′10″, 70-year-old, white-haired, retired school teacher who was admitted to a general medical–surgical floor of a small community hospital. She was diagnosed as having metastatic cancer that had spread from her left breast to her spinal column and ribs. She was a single woman and had been living in her own home with her only sister. She was admitted to the hospital because she had become too weak to walk and could barely feed herself. On the advice of her personal physician, she had decided not to have chemotherapy. Her admission orders noted that she was in the terminal stages of can-

*Case supplied by Marie E. Ridder, R.N. M.S.N. Used with permission

cer and that she was to be kept comfortable with medication (narcotic) by continuous intravenous infusion.

Mrs. Watkins had many friends on the unit. Staff and visitors delighted in her bright wit, charm, sparkling eyes, and story-telling ability. However, as her cancer spread throughout her body, she would cry and beg the staff not to move her by turning her. Because Miss Watkins was tall and thin, her bony prominences became more pronounced as she became sicker. The skin over her coccyx became red within a few days and then began to break down from the pressure of her body against the linens and mattress. The staff tried to coax her into letting them turn her every 2 hours, but Miss Watkins cried out from the pain so much that the staff wondered if they were really helping this patient with their nursing interventions.

Finally, the staff met to decide what they should do. Mrs. Twomey, the head nurse for 4 years, insisted that Miss Watkins be turned at least every 2 hours. After all, she pointed out, that was routine and minimal nursing care for all bedridden patients. If the staff did not turn her, the skin over her coccyx would become necrotic and could possibly cause sepsis. This would be a very serious problem for Miss Watkins in her already severely compromised condition. Mrs. Hanks, a nurse's aide on the floor for almost 15 years and a long-time acquaintance of Miss Watkins, said that she could not stand to see this patient cry every time she was turned. She said that furthermore she would refuse to take care of the patient until some reasonable decision for her care could be made. Miss Benson, a recent graduate, voiced her opinion that the patient should have some say regarding her care. After all, she was terminal, and not turning her would hardly make a difference in the overall outcome of her illness. Mrs. Culver, the evening charge nurse, thought that her physician ought to be the one to decide whether Miss Watkins was turned. Then the nurses could just follow his orders. The rest of the nurses strongly objected to this suggestion. Turning a patient is a nursing measure, they argued, and they should decide together whether they were comfortable *not* turning a patient even though it was "routine and minimal nursing care." How should they decide?

Commentary

Mrs. Hanks, the nurse's aide on the floor, is apparently convinced that turning Miss Watkins is doing more harm than good. She would like Mrs. Twomey to set aside the rule for this special case. If her duty as a nurse is to benefit her patient (and especially if she should protect her patient from harm), she should not insist that Mrs. Watkins be turned. Is there any reason to follow the rule when it appears to do more harm than good?

Mrs. Hanks might hear two counterarguments. First, at least in some cases, we may be more likely to do good following the rule than in using our own judgment. Many medicomoral choices are complex. They are often made under emotional circumstances and without the benefit of full information. In some cases, if people are free to use their judgments to overturn existing rules, they will make mistakes. They may even make enough mistakes that the patients would be better off if the rule were always followed.

Consider the rule that informed consent should always be obtained before surgery.

If surgeons were permitted to waive the rule whenever they thought patients would be better off without the consent process, they might waive it so often that more harm than good would result. That, after all, is the same principle that is used at traffic lights. We might have a policy of waiting at red lights only if traffic is coming, but proceeding on if the coast is clear. If drivers were infallible, that would be a better policy, but in a world of fallible human beings, we are probably better off if we always follow the rule.

Whether that would apply in the case of turning patients is hard to tell. Since turning patients who are suffering is a potentially unpleasant task, nurses might underestimate the harms of not turning the patient. Of course, there might be checks against such miscalculations. Some rules, however, can be defended as appropriate even in cases where it appears that following the rule does greater harm than breaking it.

One test is whether the nursing staff would be willing to substitute a new rule, one that had exceptions built into it. For instance, would they accept a rule that states that patients should be turned except when the nurse believes that the patient would be better off not being turned? If they accept this (and if such a rule can gain general acceptance), then a new rule is created. If, however, the nurses fear that the modified rule would permit too many mistakes to occur, it would seem to follow that an exception should not be made in this case either.

A second defense of rule-following is somewhat different. Miss Watkins may be what philosophers call a rule utilitarian. Such persons hold that the goal of moral conduct is to produce good, but that that criterion should be used only to choose a set of rules by which people should interact.[8,12,13] They would choose the rule that produces more good than any other rule, but then, in the individual case, simply follow the rule. That might mean that in individual actions the greatest good might not always result, but over the course of time, more good would come from following the rule than from following any other rule. Of course, if there seems to be a group of cases in which exception to the rule would always produce greater good, the exception could be incorporated into the rule. "Never go through a red light except to turn right" is an example of this. If a relatively simple, easy-to-apply exception cannot be incorporated into the rule, however, rule utilitarians would insist that the rule be followed even when it seems that breaking it might do more good. Could Mrs. Hanks propose a rule that contains such an easily applied exception?

Miss Benson seems to be suggesting another kind of exception. She might have in mind "Always turn patients every 2 hours except when they protest." Mrs. Culver, on the other hand, seems to be proposing the alternative, "Always turn the patient every 2 hours except when the physician decides against it." It is conceivable that either of these variants could be defended on the grounds that it is a rule that would do more good than any other rule. Honoring patients' wishes might increase the amount of good done (but it might not). Giving physicians decisive authority might work, but that assumes that physicians know more than nurses about the benefits and harms of turning (an unlikely assumption). In fact, Miss Benson may have another basis for her proposed exception. She might believe that even though turning will do good, patients have a right to refuse such benefits. If that is her reasoning, she is not basing her proposal on benefits and harms but on rights grounded in autonomy, a principle to be taken up in Chapter 5.

In exploring the alternative rules with and without exceptions, see if they would produce acceptable outcomes in other cases in which patients or the agents might oppose turning: after surgery (turn, cough, and deep breath in the recovery room), following childbirth, in the case of the comatose patient, and so forth.

BENEFIT TO THE INSTITUTION

Thus far the cases in this chapter all deal with problems of beneficence when the good to be done is strictly for the client. The problem has been to decide whether to limit the horizon to health benefits or to take into account total welfare of the client; whether avoiding harm (nonmaleficence) takes precedence over benefiting (beneficence); or whether individual case decisions or operating rules are the proper focus of assessments of benefit and harm. In real-life nursing practice, the focus often cannot remain exclusively on the benefits and harms to the individual client. Whereas the ethics of the health professions often demands that calculations of benefit and harm be limited exclusively to those affecting the client, many other ethical systems that focus on consequences impose no such limits. Classical utilitarianism holds that actions (or rules) are assessed on the basis of their overall benefits and harms without any limit on who receives them. One possible conflict is between the welfare of the patient and the welfare of the institution. The following case is one in which the nurse is required to determine whether the welfare of the institution can ever justify an action that is not in the interest of the patient.

Case 16: Cost Cutting for the Indigent Patient

Cora Martin was a staff nurse at a small, church-supported nursing home in a suburban community. One day, Mrs. Martin and the rest of the staff were informed that they would no longer be able to use the disposable, plastic-backed pads commonly used as "linensavers," as necessary for their patients. Each patient would receive six pads a day as part of the routine linen supplied by the nursing home. The additional pads used would be charged to the patient. The staff were to count the pads in the linen room each nursing shift and keep an accurate record of the number of pads that were used for each patient.

The reason for the new policy was related to rising costs associated with long-term care of the patients and the need for all personnel to be aware of these costs. The nursing home had had serious budget deficits for the past 2 years. It was felt that eliminating unnecessary use of services and products would be the best way to bring finances into line without any real risks to patients.

Mrs. Martin wondered how the staff could adequately care for some of the indigent patients in the home without the free use of the disposable pads. The pads were indispensable in the care of patients who suffered from frequent urinary or bowel incontinence, or drooling onto the pillow. The use of the pads protected the linen and prevented frequent changes of linen. Whenever linen needed to be changed on a bed, it involved staff time and effort to move and position the patient in the bed. Frequent and fortuitous placement of the pads usually prevented linen changes and enabled the staff to keep patients clean and dry with minimal effort. For those patients who could afford the extra charges for the pads, the new policy was not a problem. For the indigent patients, however, the new policy was a considerable burden. How could Mrs. Martin and the rest of the staff be expected to fulfill the policies of the institution without violating their commitment to the "welfare" of the indigent patient?

Case 17: The Patient Admitted on Friday Afternoon

June Summers, a part-time nurse who always works on weekends, has just finished a pleasant telephone conversation with Dr. Holmes, a private physician with admitting privileges at Community Hospital. He had called to inform Ms. Summers of a new admission and to let her know how glad he was that she would be working all weekend. He always complimented her on the excellent nursing care that she gave his patients. Dr. Holmes brought candy and other goodies to the nurses whenever he made rounds on the weekends. It was not surprising that Ms. Summers went out of her way for Dr. Holmes' patients during a time when most other units in the hospital ran short staffed with a low patient census. When she talked with nurses from the other units on break, she could never figure out why her unit remained full on the weekends and other units always seemed low.

One day, one of the nurses suggested that Dr. Holmes admitted patients on Friday afternoons in order to help the generally low census of the hospital and to collect fees from his well-insured patients. Now that Ms. Summers thought about it, Dr. Holmes' patients *were* always well covered by health insurance and never did require much medical intervention or nursing care over the weekends. Is it possible that she was being manipulated by the institution and by Dr. Holmes to benefit the institution at cost to the patient? Surely, this could not be right!

Commentary

Both Cora Martin and June Summers were asked by others to engage in actions that are motivated primarily out of concern for the welfare of the institution, not the welfare of the patient. In either case, it is possible that the behaviors would actually promote the patient's welfare. Possibly June Summers' patients are benefiting from the weekend hospitalization. If so, her problem is not a real one. It is, however, unlikely that they really are better off on balance. It is even less likely that Mrs. Martin's patients are benefiting from the new policy of limiting access to pads. The only way that they would benefit would be if the money saved were used for something that would benefit these patients even more.

The more likely explanation is that the institution will benefit from these behaviors, but that the patients will not. If, however, the nurse's duty is to serve the health, welfare, and safety of the patient, these practices can hardly be on the nurses' agendas. Still, many health care institutions are in serious financial jeopardy today. If cost-saving measures and measures to increase revenues are not implemented, some hospitals will fail. One approach would be to modify the duty of the nurse–clinician. The ANA *Code for Nurses,* for example, says that "Individuals are interdependent members of the community. Taking into account both individual rights and the interdependence of persons in decision making, the nurse recognizes those situations in which individual rights to autonomy in health care may temporarily be overridden to preserve the life of the human community."[3(pp 2–3)] The code gives the use of triage when a disaster has occurred as an example.

The financial crises these hospitals are facing, however, are hardly akin to a war or some other disaster justifying triage. Changing the duty of the nurse so that he or she becomes a cost-containment agent for the hospital has radical implications. Nurses could be asked to eliminate marginal services (such as the use of disposable pads) or to assist in providing extra insurance reimbursement (through weekend admissions). In doing so, they would become the institution's agents rather than the patient's. Some have made a good case for this on the basis that clinicians may be the ones who know exactly where cuts can be made or extra services billed while doing minimal harm to patients.

On the other hand, asking the nurse to take on the institution's perspective results in a significant change in the traditional role of the nurse. It means asking the nurse to abandon the patient, at least marginally, and to engage in a style of care that cannot be justified in the name of patient welfare.

One possibility is that both nurses and administrators acknowledge the two separate moral roles involved. The administrator will necessarily have to promote the more socially oriented perspective of the institution, while the nurse could be asked to remain in the role of patient advocate. This would mean serving the interests of patients or at least doing what is possible to ensure that their rights are protected, even in cases when doing so does not promote the welfare of the institution.

If the nurse is to remain an advocate for the patient, then Cora Martin would argue for the pads she needs to benefit her patients. She might, however, recognize that she ought not to win all of those fights. If she can show that it is in the institution's interest (as well as in the patient's) to use more pads, she might hope that the problem can be resolved. If, however, the administrators are correct in believing that they can serve institutional interests by reducing the use of the pads, the administrator and the nurse may end up in different moral roles. The administrator might have to promote the welfare of the institution while the nurse could remain an advocate for the patient. If that is the case, they ought to disagree. The nurse ought, sometimes, to lose the argument.

June Summers' case is somewhat different. It involves not only a potential conflict between the interests of the patient and those of the institution, but also the possibility of cheating an insurance company. As such, the ethical choice Mrs. Summers must make is one that may involve questions of honesty in addition to the conflict between the patient and the institution. June Summers may feel that the weekend admissions are morally dishonest or even illegal. If she believes that she has a duty to avoid being part of such dishonesty or that she has a duty to be faithful to the laws of her state or nation, she may feel an obligation to speak out against the practice of weekend admissions, not only because they are not in her patients' interest, but also because they involve dishonesty, cheating, or breaking faith. These latter questions will be addresssed in the cases in Chapters 6 and 7. In any case, the nurses involved in these cases have confronted the potential conflict between the welfare of their institutions and the welfare of their patients. They will have to choose whether they will modify their roles so that they take into account the institution's agenda or whether they wish to remain advocates for their patients, recognizing that sometimes they will not be able to get everything they desire or need.

BENEFIT TO SOCIETY

Similar problems arise when the conflict is between the patient's welfare and the welfare of society as a whole. Often a procedure's net benefits to a patient are clear, yet when the decision is viewed from the societal perspective, the benefits are not as great as those that would come from using the resources in some other way. The tension often arises when cost containment is the issue. It also arises in research settings where what is best for the society may not be what is best for the individual patient.

Case 18: When Providing Benefit Might Be Costly

Samuel Tatum is a 6-year-old boy with acute leukemia who has had several relapses while on chemotherapy. The possibility of his undergoing a bone marrow transplant to improve his condition has been suggested. This procedure is the only treatment that offers him a reasonable hope of survival at this point. Although Samuel receives Medicaid assistance, the bone marrow transplant is a costly procedure, involving months of treatment for which his family must travel to a distant medical center. It is not an experimental treatment, but it is not expected to offer a chance of total cure for Samuel's disease. The estimated cost of treatment would use more than two thirds of the annual Medicaid budget allotted for Samuel's entire state.

Samuel's family asks his primary nurse, Mrs. Compton, what she thinks they should do. What should she tell them? Should the nurse make a judgment on how much "doing good" should cost and at what expense to others?

Commentary
One might approach this case first by asking whether more good can be done by spending the funds on Samuel, even though they represent two thirds of the state's budget. If it should turn out that spending the state's resources this way does more good than any other approach, there would be a convergence of the nurse's clinical commitment to be an advocate for the patient and the broader perspective of trying to maximize the good done overall with the society's resources.

If that is the case, there may remain a conflict over whether it is fair for one citizen, even a desperately ill citizen, to command such a disproportionate share. If resources are distributed on the basis of need, he may have a claim, but if everyone is entitled to a more nearly equal share, he is surely getting more than his allowance. This problem— that of what is a fair allocation—is the subject matter for the cases in Chapter 4. The problem to be addressed here—the potential conflict between benefiting the patient and maximizing the benefit for the society—disappears if it turns out that benefiting this patient also produces greater benefit in total than could be produced by other uses of society's resources.

The case becomes more difficult if Mrs. Compton concludes that giving Samuel the bone marrow transplant does not result in the greatest possible good the use of the resources can produce. Two thirds of the state's budget is a great deal for one patient to receive. It seems quite likely that the good that could be done with those funds, if spent for larger numbers of patients, would be greater than the good done for Samuel, even if Samuel were to have great potential for benefiting from treatment.

It is interesting to ask whether the fact that Mrs. Compton is Samuel's primary nurse is crucial to what her moral role ought to be in this case. Would Mrs. Compton's response be the same if she were asked about expenditures for Samuel when she was administrator of the state's Medicaid program? Clearly, someone in the system must take the system's point of view. Someone must be asking what is the morally appropriate way to spend state funds. Some people would say that the appropriate way is to spend them in the way that will produce the greatest overall benefit. Others may take more directly into account what is the fair or equitable way to spend the resources, considering the various needs of potential recipients. In either case, if Mrs. Compton were the administrator taking the system's point of view, she would give no special priority to Samuel's claim.

However, Mrs. Compton is not the Medicaid administrator; she is Samuel's primary nurse. We saw in the commentary on the previous cases that, when faced with problems of scarce resources, the primary nurse might still take the broader perspective. She might ask herself the same kinds of questions the administrator would ask: What is the use of the resources that would produce the greatest benefit overall? Or, what is the fairest way of allocating the resources? On the other hand, clinicians may be viewed as having a primary responsibility to be advocates for their patients. They might take on a special "role-specific" duty, that of pressing their client's case in the strongest possible manner. If they do this, clinicians should recognize that they will sometimes lose the battle—they ought to in cases where their client's claim is not a strong one. Nevertheless, they could take on the role of loyal advocacy for their clients.

This raises the question of what Samuel's family thinks they are doing when they ask Mrs. Compton for advice. Are they asking for her thinking as an advocate for Samuel. If so, Mrs. Compton is in a position not unlike the parents. Presumably, the parents should not be forced to deal with broader social issues such as whether Samuel should surrender his claim because someone else could benefit more from the resources. The parents should stand with their child, fighting for his interests and leaving it to someone else to set some limits.

If Mrs. Compton is, like the parents, an advocate for Samuel, then the question she is asked is relatively trivial. Mrs. Compton and the parents might be asking whether Samuel would be better off with the treatment than without it. That is a reasonable question for an advocate to address. It is the kind of question that requires balancing subjective considerations that feed into the concept of Samuel's overall welfare, taking into account the burdens of the transplant as well as the likelihood of its success.

Mrs. Compton might have a unique perspective to assist the parents in answering this question.

It is much more problematic whether Mrs. Compton ought to be asked by the parents whether they should sacrifice Samuel's welfare for the good of society. Neither the parents nor Mrs. Compton (if she is an advocate for the patient) is in a good position to deal with that issue. They are fundamentally in a different position from the administrator whose task it is to deal with such social issues.

BENEFIT TO IDENTIFIED NONCLIENTS

It might be argued that clinicians have a special duty to clients that takes precedence over consideration of the welfare of society as a whole, because specific patients (such as Samuel in case 18) are given moral priority over unidentified statistical persons who might benefit from alternative uses of resources. In fact, even bureaucrats and administrators may feel this pull toward "identifiable lives." They might, for example, have given Samuel a greater proportion of the state's Medicaid funds than considerations of overall benefit would justify simply because Samuel was a very concrete patient. The fact that he was a critically ill youngster who could generate public sympathy might give him even greater consideration.

The problem would be different if, in addition to Samuel, the administrator had to consider another identifiable person who needs state Medicaid funds. If that were the administrator's dilemma, the dimension of whether the life was identified would cease to be a consideration. The administrator would have to balance the claims of the two identifiable persons in some fashion. Does a clinician have to do a similar balancing act? Does the nurse in the clinical role have the responsibility of comparing her own client's needs with those of another patient who is not her client? That is the issue that arises in the next two cases.

Case 19: When Benefit to the Client Is Constrained by Benefits to Others

Ginny Wilson, a community health nurse in a large urban area, had recently located Mrs. Burns, a tuberculosis patient whom the health clinic had been following for many years. Mrs. Burns had moved several times during the past few years and had not had her yearly chest x-ray and sputum cultures for quite some time. Finally Miss Wilson located Mrs. Burns and has encouraged her to attend the chest clinic at the local health clinic. Mrs. Burns has agreed to an appointment, despite her seeming reluctance to discuss her past health problems and her current health status.

As Miss Wilson left the row house apartment building where Mrs. Burns lived, she noticed two small boys playing in the hallway near the front door. The older child, about 3 to 4 years of age, was eating a raw potato. The younger child, about 2 to 4 years of age and wearing a very filthy and wet diaper, was crying and begging a bite of the potato from his brother. He held up a bandaged and swollen hand to wipe the tears from his eyes. Miss Wilson stopped to talk to the boys for a minute and encouraged the small boy to show her his hand. Underneath the crude bandage was an infected, angry-looking sore about the size of a quarter. The child was obviously in pain and his skin was very warm. Miss Wilson asked the older boy if his mother was at home. The boy said that she was at work but that his sister would be home from school soon. Through the open door of the apartment, Ginny could see a litter-filled room with a pot-bellied stove in the very middle. There was no heat in the apartment despite an outside temperature below 40 degrees. She asked the boy what else he had had to eat that day. He said, "Potatoes," and pointed to a large, 100-pound bag of potatoes in the corner of the room. No other food seemed to be available.

Miss Wilson returned to the apartment of her patient, Mrs. Burns. She asked Mrs. Burns if she knew anything about the family on the first floor. Mrs. Burns firmly stated that she knew nothing about the family—the affairs of her neighbors were none of her business. She quickly ended the conversation and shut the door.

Several hours later, Miss Wilson returned to the children's apartment to find the older sister (16 years old) home from school. She chatted with the girl and asked her to tell her mother that the nurse had visited and that the smaller boy's hand needed medical attention. She showed the girl how to soak his hand in warm water and apply a clean bandage. The next day, Miss Wilson returned to the apartment when the mother had come home from work. Miss Wilson explained her concern about the small boy's hand and the effect on the children of the lack of food and heat in the house. The mother claimed that she was doing the best that she could and would see that both needs were taken care of. Miss Wilson gave her the health clinic's telephone number and invited her to come in for the well-baby clinic and other services that would help her situation.

Two days later, Miss Wilson returned to Mrs. Burns' apartment to give her an appointment at the chest clinic. Mrs. Burns had refused to open the door or talk to the nurse because she interfered in the business of the family downstairs.

Apparently, the children's mother had blamed Mrs. Burns for the community health nurse's intervention in her affairs. Mrs. Burns stated that if Miss Wilson did not leave the other family alone, she would move again and then, "You'll never find me again." Miss Wilson wondered whether her responsibility as a nurse was simply to Mrs. Burns or whether she should attempt to serve the mother and small children as well.

Case 20: Institutionalizing a Retarded Child: Benefit or Harm?

James is a 9-year-old, moderately mentally and physically disabled child. He has lived at home with his mother, Mrs. Hardy, since birth and has been well cared for. During the past year, however, his mother has developed rheumatoid arthritis and is finding it difficult to care for James by herself. James has made steady progress in achieving some motor and cognitive skills, yet his disabilities prevent him from taking advantage of group teaching and other services available in his community.

Mrs. Aikens, a nurse with the rehabilitation center that follows James' case, is attempting to help Mrs. Hardy make decisions for his long-term care. Although Mrs. Aikens recognizes the comfort and high level of care that James receives at home, she also recognizes that his mother may not be able to provide this care as her own disease progresses. Mrs. Hardy clearly relies on the information that Mrs. Aiken supplies and trusts her judgment because she has been James' nurse for several years. Mrs. Aikens finds it very difficult to advise Mrs. Hardy, since any action that benefits Mrs. Hardy may result in harm to James and vice versa. Should Mrs. Aikens take it as her responsibility to strive to do what will produce the most good for both Mrs. Hardy and James, or is her job simply limited to promoting James' welfare?

Commentary

In both of these cases, the nurse might ask exactly who her client is and what difference it makes. In the case involving mentally retarded James and his mother, Mrs. Aikens seems to think of James as her client. She then faces the problem of reconciling the interests of the client with someone who is not her client—James' mother. In the case involving Miss Wilson, the community health nurse, Mrs. Burns is the original client. Have, at any point, the two boys and their mother also become Miss Wilson's clients?

Assuming that there is only one client in each case, does the nurse have a primary responsibility to that client? In the previous sections, we saw that many were arguing that when the nurse is in the clinical role he or she should limit attention to the client's welfare. That would mean, in this situation, that the two boys and their mother, as well as Mrs. Hardy, assuming they are not clients of the nurses involved, have no claim on the nurses' attention.

In both of these cases, the nurses involved are in positions in which they could expand their notion of who their clients are. Since Miss Wilson is a community health nurse and the two boys are part of the community, Miss Wilson might reason that they are also her clients. Does the fact that the boys' mother appears to want nothing to do with Miss Wilson exclude them from client status? If so, does that exclude them from Miss Wilson's agenda?

Mrs. Aikens, if she is working in a family care model of nursing, might decide that both James and his mother are her clients. If so, the traditional Hippocratic maxim that the health care professional should work for the good of the client (in the singular) is irrelevant. The question becomes one of what to do when the interests of two clients conflict.

What would happen if the nurse encountered clinical situations where the interest of another party clearly conflicted with the client's interests and there was no plausible way that the nurse could conceptualize the other party as an additional client? For example, what would happen if Miss Wilson was a hospital-based nurse caring for Mrs. Burns, and Mrs. Burns, while actively contagious with an infectious disease, wanted to go home. Miss Wilson might have never met the boys, but have only heard of them through Mrs. Burns. If the two boys were in close interaction with Mrs. Burns and Mrs.

Burns had a strong psychological need to return to her home, their interests would likely conflict with those of Mrs. Burns. It is very difficult to suppose that Miss Wilson could think of these two boys, whom she has never seen, as her clients. Certainly, neither they nor their mother has ever engaged Miss Wilson. No nursing care has ever been rendered. If the primary nurse has a special responsibility for the welfare of her client and it is in her client's interest to go home, does Miss Wilson then have a duty to block from her mind the welfare of the nonclients who will be at risk? She would if her obligation is the welfare of her client. Is it either permitted or required for the nurse to consider the welfare of nonclients in situations like these?

BENEFIT TO THE PROFESSION

Another potential conflict the nurse faces when considering the morality of actions in terms of benefits and harms is the conflict between service to the client and service to the profession. Whereas the nurse may have no particular loyalty to the society at large or even to specific nonclients, she surely does have an obligation to her profession. Normally, the profession has as its goal the service of clients and the improvement of nursing care that clients receive. In special circumstances, however, the profession's aim of improving client care and improving its own position to serve clients may come into conflict with specific clients whom a nurse is serving. The following case illustrates this problem.

Case 21: The Duty to Participate in Collective Action*

As Mrs. Marge Tomlinson, the evening charge nurse on A-wing, completed her charting, she wondered who would be taking her place during the remainder of the week. She and most of Memorial Hospital's nurses would be on strike starting 8:00 AM the next morning. The decision to strike had been reached several days ago by nurses in this private, urban hospital after many hours of meetings, conferences with hospital administration, and heated discussion among fellow nurses.

Mrs. Tomlinson strongly supported her colleagues' efforts to increase salaries, fringe benefits, and general working conditions for all nurses employed by Memorial Hospital. She had personally experienced many frustrating evenings in recent months because of loss of nursing staff dissatisfied with long hours and poor salaries. She had also experienced decreased support services for the consistently high number of elderly patients assigned to her 35-bed unit. Yet now that the strike was imminent, Mrs. Tomlinson wondered whether further reducing the available nursing services to her patients by striking was in their immediate best interests.

During the past 2 days, some patients had been sent home early in prep-

*From Fry ST: Ethical issues: Politics, power and change. In Talbott S, Mason D (eds): Political Action: A Handbook for Nurses, pp 133–140. Reading, MA, Addison-Wesley, 1985

aration for the strike. Several others whose care was too involved for families to manage had been placed in nursing homes, much to the distress of the patients, as well as their families. Other patients, however, like Mr. Ralph Osborn, a 63-year-old recent amputee with diabetes mellitus and congestive heart failure, could not be moved. Mr. Osborn and other patients without families or other resources were very dependent on the nursing staff of the hospital to meet their daily physiological and physical needs. A patient on Mrs. Tomlinson's unit for 5 weeks, Mr. Osborn was just beginning to assume control of his physical care in preparation for his eventual discharge to a nearby rehabilitation center. There were no means by which Mrs. Tomlinson could guarantee the availability of the kind and level of care he needed during the next few days or even weeks. Like the other nurses, she could only hope that the collective efforts of the nursing staff would quickly bring about improved working conditions for the benefit of future patients.

As some of her nurse colleagues often quoted, the ANA *Code for Nurses* stated that "the nurse participates in the profession's efforts to establish and maintain conditions of employment conducive to high quality nursing care." Yet Mrs. Tomlinson questioned whether these efforts should be carried out when nursing services were already operating at minimal levels of care and safety for the identified patient, and whether the profession itself, through its ethical code, should direct the actions of individual nurses. The expectations of patients like Mr. Osborn and the obligation to provide the best possible care under any conditions caused her to think that the ANA *Code for Nurses* created conflict by encouraging nurses to "collective action ... to determine the terms and conditions of employment conducive to high quality nursing care ...." Mrs. Tomlinson wondered what to do when the code called for service to the profession to maintain its high standards and also insisted that the health, welfare, and safety of patients should be the nurse's first consideration.

Commentary

The possibility that the nurse's obligation to the profession might conflict with the obligation to the present client is a perplexing one. To some extent, the profession itself says that the primary ethical duty is to serve the client. Yet, at least historically, the profession has made demands on the individual practitioner that go beyond serving the present client.

For physicians, the Hippocratic Oath placed many demands on members of the Hippocratic group. Hippocratic physicians were expected to show respect for their teachers, even to the point of giving them money if the need arose. They were to teach their teachers' offspring without fee. They were to keep the secret knowledge of the cult, revealing it only to fellow initiates. Clearly, none of these things could always work for the benefit of specific patients.

The Florence Nightingale Pledge, patterned after the Oath of Hippocrates, drops all of these, but it does retain the pledge to "maintain and elevate the standard of my profession." In an era when many health professionals are not even members of professional groups, does it make sense to place benefit to the profession on the nurse's agenda? If so, does it still make sense when working to benefit the profession will compromise the care given to patients like Mr. Osborn?

The strike is perhaps an ambiguous case. It involves working for the benefit of the profession and in this particular example deals with very concrete issues of self-interest to nurses, such as long hours and poor salaries. In an indirect sense, however, the strike being considered by Mrs. Tomlinson can be defended as being undertaken to improve conditions for patients of the future. Although the cynic might raise an eyebrow, even efforts to improve salaries and working conditions might be defended as eventually improving patient care. After all, if nurses cannot be recruited, then patients will suffer. To the extent that the strike is really for better patient care, Mrs. Tomlinson's problem reduces to one of comparing the welfare of present, identifiable patients with the welfare of future, unidentified patients, an issue addressed in earlier cases.

The case also raises another issue, however—that of whether the welfare of the profession itself has a claim on nurses and whether any such claim can ever compete with patient care.

BENEFIT TO ONESELF AND ONE'S FAMILY

There is one final possible conflict between benefit to patients and benefit to others that ought to be considered: benefit to the nurse and the nurse's family. All of the professional codes speak as if the very essence of being a professional is commitment to the client. We have explored several possible competing claims, including the institution, the society, identified non-clients, and the profession. At some point, however, all nurses sacrifice their clients for themselves and their loved ones. They go home at night, they spend parts of their waking hours doing something other than care for patients. They play other roles: parent, spouse, citizen, friend. Each of these, in one way or another, is a competing claim on the nurse's time and energy. The final case in this chapter examines the limits of the justifiable claims of the patient.

Case 22: Is There a Limit to Benefiting the Patient?

Sheila Morgan is a critical-care nurse in the surgical intensive care unit (SICU). She has received additional education to prepare her for the performance of her job and has always found her job exciting and challenging. Recently, however, Mrs. Morgan has been asked to work double shifts or put in a few hours of overtime because of a consistently high patient census, very ill patients, and the resignation of one of the other nurses. No other skilled nurse has been found to fill this position, and Mrs. Morgan and the other nurses have had to fill in the gaps whenever necessary.

Ordinarily, Mrs. Morgan would not mind the extra work. She enjoys her work and welcomes the extra money at the end of the pay period. Yet Mrs. Morgan has obligations to her family, especially to her 9-year-old son, Sean. Sean plays soccer after school and looks forward to having his mother watch his games. During the past 2 weeks, Mrs. Morgan has missed most of the games because she has been working overtime. Although her skills are necessary for beneficial patient care in the SICU, Mrs. Morgan is wondering how much benefit her employer should expect from her when family benefits are also at issue. How much benefit should she be expected to give in the role of nurse?

Commentary

When the ANA *Code for Nurses* states that the client's health, welfare, and safety shall be the nurse's first consideration, does it really mean that it is immoral for the nurse to spend any time taking care of her son whenever there are patients whose health, welfare, and safety could be served with the nurse present on the hospital floor? Sheila Morgan is exploring the limits of the nurse's commitment to the client.

We have seen that some people believe that the nurse should be given a special "role-specific" duty to serve patients and not worry about broader societal issues such as resource allocation, at least when in the role of the clinical nurse. Regardless of whether one accepts that argument, an argument that removes many societal benefits from the nurse's agenda, the nurse still must face the competing claims on her time and energy when she is in some other role, such as that of mother. Surely, there is some limit to how much patients can expect of the nurse.

One possible limit is the limit of exhaustion. At some point the nurse becomes so exhausted that, in the name of patient care, she ought to go home and rest. That answer comes from within the commitment of serving the patient and therefore is an easy answer.

Is there ever a time, however, when the nurse's other obligations justifiably compete with those to the patient? The question is really one concerning the nature of those other obligations. Some of them, the obligations associated with the roles of parent, spouse, and family member, surely are as fundamental as some of those related to the nursing role. Other roles, such as those of citizen, church member, and even friend, can hardly be placed categorically below that of health professional.

It is striking that nurses and other professionals almost never discuss the nature of these conflicts inherent in the lives of persons who take on more than one fundamental commitment. Part of the answer may lie in the collective responsibility of the professional group to patients. A nurse who has been on duty for 12 hours can reasonably pass the nursing responsibility on to someone else. The nurse who must stay home with a sick child may be able to call on colleagues to help provide coverage. It seems unrealistic, however, to assume that colleagues can always provide the needed coverage. Some nurses, such as Sheila Morgan, may have to sacrifice benefit to their patients for the welfare of other persons to whom they are deeply committed.

Finally, Sheila Morgan's case forces us to examine the nature of the obligation the nurse owes to herself. The idea of a duty to oneself is controversial. Some people see the duty as really to one's God or one's community, but the nurse must reflect on the limits of her obligation to the patient when it is simply her own welfare that is competing. What should Sheila Morgan have done if she had had tickets for the symphony or if she were enrolled in an adult education class to read poetry? Can she leave her SICU patients to go to the concert only if she is convinced that she is so "burned out" that her patients will be better off if she leaves or does she have some claim for her own welfare that can compete with that of the patient?

References

1. Edelstein L: The Hippocratic Oath: Text, translation and interpretation. In Temkin O, Temkin CL (eds): Ancient Medicine: Selected Papers of Ludwig Edelstein, pp 3–64. Baltimore, The Johns Hopkins Press, 1967
2. Tate BL: The Nurse's Dilemma: Ethical Considerations in Nursing Practice, p 72. Geneva, International Council of Nurses, 1977
3. American Nurses' Association: Code for Nurses with Interpretive Statements. Kansas City, American Nurses' Association, 1985
4. Ross WD: The Right and the Good, p 22. Oxford, Oxford University Press, 1939
5. Beauchamp TL, Childress JF (eds): Principles of Biomedical Ethics, 2nd ed, pp 106–108. New York, Oxford University Press, 1983
6. Feldman F: Introductory Ethics, p 47. Englewood Cliffs, NJ, Prentice-Hall, 1978
7. Bentham J: An introduction to the principles of morals and legislation. In Melden AI (ed): Ethical Theories: A Book of Readings, pp 367–390. Englewood Cliffs, NJ, Prentice-Hall, 1967
8. Rawls J: Two concepts of rules. The Philosophical Review 44:3–32, 1955
9. Brandt RB: Toward a credible form of utilitarianism. In Bayles MD (ed): Contemporary Utilitarianism, pp 143–186. Garden City, NY, Doubleday & Co, 1968
10. Jonsen AR: Do no harm: Axiom of medical ethics. In Spicker SF, Engelhardt HT Jr (eds): Philosophical Medical Ethics: Its Nature and Significance, pp 27–41. Boston, D Reidel, 1977
11. Veatch RM: A Theory of Medical Ethics, pp 159–164. New York, Basic Books, 1981
12. Lyons D: Forms and Limits of Utilitarianism. Oxford, Oxford University Press, 1965
13. Ramsey P: Deeds and Rules in Christian Ethics. New York, Charles Scribner's Sons, 1967

Chapter 4

Justice: The Allocation of Health Resources

Once the possibility of taking the welfare of other parties into account has been introduced, so that an ethic is in some sense social, the next question is likely to be how the benefits and burdens ought to be distributed. Some of the most interesting problems arising in health care ethics recently have involved questions of justice or equity in allocating health resources. In Chapter 3 we looked at cases that pose problems for the nurse in deciding between benefiting the individual client and benefiting others—either society as a whole or certain other identified persons. Much of the debate in health care ethics, however, goes beyond this problem of the conflict between the individual client and others to deal with the question of how scarce resources—such as the nurse's time and energy, as well as nursing budgets—should be spread among those who could benefit from them.

In the cases in this chapter we shall see that it is not always obvious that the nurse should automatically choose the course that will do the most total or combined good. An intriguing debate rages in philosophy over the proper meaning of the ethical principle of justice. That debate has direct implications for how this chapter's case problems will be resolved. Several kinds of problems of justice might arise.

In the first group of cases the nurse is forced to choose how to allocate his or her time among those that the nurse already considers to be clients. Here the question is this: Once the nurse has made a commitment to serve the interests and protect the rights of more than one client, what should happen when those interests or rights conflict? In the second group of cases, the problem of allocating scarce resources is slightly different. These cases pose conflicts between the nurse's obligation to a client when it conflicts with the needs or interests of nonclients. Here we shall have to ask whether there is such a thing as a right to health care for some or all who are not now receiving care. Finally, a group of cases involving more social health policy questions shows that the nurse may sometimes have to deal with ethical problems at the policy level as well as at the clinical level of individual clients. In all three groups of cases the critical ethical problem is whether merely producing as much good as possible (or avoiding as much harm as possible) is the only morally relevant factor in deciding about allocation of the nurse's resources.

In the philosophical debate over the ethics of justice, three more or less standard positions have emerged for deciding how resources should be allocated. The debate is made more complicated by the fact that sometimes the word *justice* is used to describe the ethically correct allocation even when the allocation is based on one of the ethical principles such as beneficence or autonomy. In other writings, justice refers to an independent principle of allocation (usually having to do with equality, need, or merit). According to those who use the term in this latter way, deciding what is the ethically right allocation may involve balancing the principle of justice against some or all of the other principles.

The most easily understood position simply answers the allocation question by reverting to the principles of beneficence and nonmaleficence—of trying to produce the most good on balance. This is the answer that is given by the classic utilitarians such as Jeremy Bentham[1] and John Stuart Mill.[2] Their strategy when trying to decide between two or more courses of action was to count up the amount of good each course would provide for each person and subtract the amount of harm it would do. The sum of all of these factors tells us the net amount of benefit for each course of action. The decision-maker is morally obligated to choose the course that produces the most good.

We have already seen in the cases in earlier chapters that some people believe there are ethical principles that count against simply choosing the course that maximizes the good. If, for example, a nurse had promised to help one of her patients, but then realizes that she might do more good, on balance, by helping another one, some would argue that the promise counts as a reason for the nurse to proceed in the direction of helping the first patient. That would result in a head-on conflict between maximizing benefit and keeping promises. Many people would not give promise-keeping an absolute priority; it is simply a moral factor countering the consideration of benefits and harms. On the other hand, if the extra net benefit that would come from temporarily breaking the commitment to the first patient is small, it may be that the promise should be kept. We shall see that the principle of truth-telling or respecting autonomy also pulls against the principles of benefiting and avoiding harm.

Whereas one group of ethical theorists insists that questions of resource allocation should be solved by simply calculating benefits and harms, a second group, sometimes called the libertarians, believes that the principle of autonomy—or liberty, as they sometimes refer to it—provides an important counterweight to consequences. They believe that resources should be allocated according to the free choices of those who rightfully own or control them. The most important philosophical contributor to this debate, Harvard philosopher Robert Nozick,[3] argues that people are entitled to what they justly possess, by acquiring it from resources not previously possessed or by trade, gift, or inheritance. If health care is provided to those who are in need, it is not because they have a right to it. It is because they have made an acceptable bargain with a provider willing to provide the care or because the provider is willing to give the care out of a sense of charity. Either way, the free choices of those involved dominate the decision-making.

The utilitarians and libertarians have in common the fact that they solve resource-allocation problems by appealing to other ethical principles: beneficence and nonmaleficence in the case of the utilitarians and autonomy or liberty (to be discussed in Chapter 5) in the case of the libertarians.

A third important group of thinkers rejects both of those answers. They believe that resources should be allocated according to another principle—the principle of justice. It is sometimes said that people have a right to health care, that health care should be allocated on the basis of need, or that equality should be the goal of resource allocation decisions. These are all rather crude reflections of the belief that neither maximizing benefits nor granting total liberty is an adequate way to allocate resources. The most important recent holder of this position has been John Rawls. In an elaborate theoretical construction in a volume entitled *A Theory of Justice*,[4] Rawls concludes that for the basic principles establishing the practices of a society, resources should be allocated according to two basic principles. First, liberty is so fundamental that each person should have an equal right to the most extensive total system of equal basic liberties compatible with a similar system of liberty for all. Then, when it comes to allocating other basic social and economic goods, justice requires that there should be equality unless two conditions are met. First, inequalities must be to the benefit of the least well off, and, second, there must be equal opportunity for all to gain the advantages of treating people unequally.

Transferring those basic principles of justice to a specific health care decision for a nurse standing at the bedside can be very difficult.[5-7] If, however, the idea can be used to establish some basic practices for nursing, the implications will be radical. The principle of justice would require allocations that are not necessarily those that produce the most good or respect autonomy the most. Deciding whether to turn away from one patient to help another or to help someone who is not a patient may be contingent not only on what will produce the most good and what agreements have been made between the parties, but also which of the parties is least well off (that is, in greatest need).

Some defenders of the view that justice is an independent principle go even further. They argue that justice is a principle that requires producing equality when possible. Sometimes called egalitarians, they agree with Rawls and his supporters that equality is a fundamental ethical requirement of practices in the health care sphere. They differ, however, in their interpretation of what should happen when everyone (or at least the least well off) will be better off if there are inequalities. This dilemma is illustrated by the hypothetical case of an airplane accident in which many of the injured need help and whoever is helped first will be helped most; however, one of them is a physician or nurse who, if helped first, could help others who would not otherwise be helped. The Rawlsian principle of justice, if extended to the specifics of a practice related to this allocation decision, would seem to say that justice permits (or even requires) treating the health care professional first—because even the least well off will be better off if the health care professional is given this unequal advantage.

The more radical egalitarians might arrive at the same decision but would interpret it very differently. They would say that justice requires that everyone be given an equal chance to be treated first, that no one has more of a claim of justice to the special benefit of first treatment than another. They might still, however, conclude that priority should go to the health care professional, but not in the name of justice. Since justice is only one among several ethical principles, when those principles conflict, some trade-offs may have to be made, or it may be necessary to set some priority rules. If treating the health professional first maximizes the benefit (satisfies the principle of beneficence) while giving all the accident victims an equal chance satisfies the principle of justice, then perhaps justice can be overridden by beneficence. If so, the health care professional gets priority in spite of justice rather than in the name of it.

That is one way the egalitarians might handle the problem. Another is to acknowledge that the right to equal treatment in the name of justice is a right that can be waived. Probably a prudent accident victim who knew that giving someone else a special chance for priority care would increase his probability of being better off in the long run would waive his right to have an equal chance for first treatment. Using this logic, even if beneficence can never take precedence over justice when they conflict (a position held by some strongly committed to the deontological or formalist principles), still, justice can be overcome through the consent of the least well off.

Thus there are three major positions on how the nurse's time, energy, and other resources should be allocated: One position stresses maximizing of net benefits grounded in the principle of beneficence; a second position stresses the freedom of providers and clients to bargain for whatever they can get grounded in the principle of autonomy; and the third position stresses equality of outcomes grounded in an independent principle of justice. Among those opting for the independent principle of justice, some (the Rawlsians) would sacrifice equality in the name of justice whenever it benefits the least well off to do so. Others (the more radical egalitarians) might sacrifice equality, but never in the name of justice. These three major positions provide alternative frameworks for dealing with the case problems of this chapter.

JUSTICE AMONG THE NURSE'S CLIENTS

One situation in which the clinician cannot avoid dealing with matters of resource allocation is the one in which more than one of the nurse's clients are competing for attention. In almost every clinical nursing role (full-time private duty nursing is the exception), the nurse may have more than one patient needing attention at the same time. For the nurse to cite the traditional ethic that the health professional's duty is to the patient does not help. In the classic ethical codes, *patient* is in the singular, yet *patients* is plural. Choosing among patients is the issue for the first group of cases in this chapter. In some cases, choice is necessary because two patients are making conflicting demands that cannot both be met, or at least cannot both be met well. Two patients coding at the same time is only a dramatic example. In other cases, time can be allocated among the nurse's patients, but there still remains a question of what a fair allocation is. In either case, the nurse must appeal, at least implicitly, to some notion of allocation.

Case 23: Allocating Nursing Time According to Benefit

After reviewing the needs of all patients on a medical–surgical nursing care unit, night nurse Clora Bingham decides that she has to set priorities for her time among four needy patients. One, Mrs. Robertson, is an 83-year-old woman with a CVA, who is semicomatose and will inevitably die, but who needs suctioning every 15 to 20 minutes. The second, Mr. Jablowski, 47 years old, was admitted for observation and has already had several bloody stools. The third, 52-year-old Mr. Hanson, is a recently diagnosed diabetic with very unstable blood sugar levels, who is receiving insulin intravenously and requires frequent vital sign checks. The fourth, 35-year-old Mr. Manfra, is a patient who learned today that he has inoperable cancer with metastasis to the spine. He has been suicidal in the past. Ms. Bingham realizes that these patients have different needs. Moreover, the amount she can do to help is different in each case. Should her decision be based entirely on how much she can benefit each patient? On how much need each patient has? Should she spread her time equally among all the patients? How should she decide how to allocate her time?

Commentary

Ms. Bingham knows that the traditional commitment of the nurse is to benefit her patient. She would very much like to do that. The trouble is that she has four patients, each of whom could benefit to some degree from her attention, and she simply cannot meet all of their needs fully. One strategy would be to spread her time evenly among each of her patients. Their needs for nursing care are very different, however. If she were to distribute her time equally, certainly the amount of good she would do would be very unequal.

One approach would be for her to ask where she could do the most good. This approach necessarily leads to difficult subjective judgments. Is it a great benefit, for example, to prevent a suicide in a previously suicidal patient with inoperable metastasized cancer? Just how much good does she do suctioning an inevitably dying, semicomatose woman. Still, some comparisons can be made. Mr. Jablowski, admitted for observation, will probably benefit less from close supervision than Mr. Hanson, the unstable diabetic.

Making comparison of benefits requires some subtle, controversial judgments. For example, younger patients whose lives are saved will live longer statistically than older patients. If "years-of-life added" is the criterion of benefit, younger patients will get much more benefit from a life-saving intervention than older patients. Moreover, if future contribution to the labor force or even more general contribution to society is the criterion, then younger patients will benefit more. By that standard, possibly Mr. Jablowski will benefit more from Ms. Bingham's attention than Mrs. Robertson, even though Mrs. Robertson's condition is much more critical at the time.

If Ms. Bingham approaches her problem by trying to find out who will benefit most from her nursing care, she faces all of the questions addressed in the previous chapter's cases. She might, however, ask a somewhat different question: Who has the greatest need, regardless of how much he or she will benefit? Sometimes those who have the greatest need will also benefit the most from a nurse's care; however, in other situations, patients with great need can be helped but not as much as those with lesser needs. This is where the problem of justice arises.

Mrs. Robertson's situation is probably the most desperate of the four patients. She is facing imminent death. Failure to suction her could easily result in a mucous plug blockage of her bronchi and respiratory failure. Yet even with careful attention to suctioning, it is not clear how much benefit Ms. Bingham would be offering. Surely, she should do what she can. Humaneness seems to require that. Some additional facts might be relevant in determining exactly how much benefit Ms. Bingham can offer Mrs. Robertson with particularly rigorous nursing scrutiny. Is Mrs. Robertson suffering from her situation? Is the suctioning primarily to make her comfortable or to prolong her life? If it is to prolong life, did Mrs. Robertson (or her family, if she was not able to express her wishes earlier in the course of her illness) want aggressive life support? It is possible that, although Mrs. Robertson's condition is very grave and therefore her needs are great, Ms. Bingham has relatively little to offer that will really benefit her. If so, on benefit grounds, Mrs. Robertson might not get as much of Ms. Bingham's attention.

Age is another complicating factor. Whereas age may help determine how much benefit will result, it can also be relevant to need. Eighty-seven-year-old Mrs. Robertson, 52-year-old Mr. Hanson, and 35-year-old Mr. Manfra all seem to have great needs, yet they are of substantially different ages. If Ms. Bingham is to base her time allocation on need, should age be relevant in defining need as it might be in defining possible benefits? On the one hand, all three patients can be said to have significant immediate nursing care needs. On the other hand, need might be viewed in an "over-a-lifetime" perspective. The older the patient, the more of a life plan that has been completed. If we are considering what is needed to complete a life plan, then the younger the patient, the greater the need.

One thing seems clear from these four patients, meeting need and maximizing benefit are different moral tasks. If Ms. Bingham tries to do one, she may not be able to do the other.

Case 24: Choosing Between Two Infants with Multiple Handicaps

Baby J was a 16-hour-old neonate who had been transferred from a local medical facility to the NICU of a tertiary care center. She was the firstborn child of a state legislator and his wife, and the product of in vitro fertilization (the couple had attempted to conceive three previous times unsuccessfully at $5000 an effort). At the time of transport, Baby J was having mild to moderate respiratory distress and had been anuric since birth. On examination, it was noted that the infant had an enlarged thymus, low-set ears, questionable lung size on x-ray, and a history of no amniotic fluid present on delivery. Completed testing indicated that she had no kidneys, ureters, or bladder, and that her small lung size was indicative of pulmonary hypoplasia. The pediatric staff offered the diagnosis of Potter's syndrome, a condition known to be fatal within a few weeks.

Consultation with infant renal transplant centers indicated that, because of pulmonary complications, there had never been a successful renal transplant done in an infant with Potter's syndrome. All but one center declined to offer treatment, stating that renal transplant in such an infant would be purely experimental. The primary physician, Dr. A. Smith, after consulting with other health team members, discussed the prognosis with Baby J's parents. They wanted a few hours to think about whether they wanted their infant transported to the one center that offered to treat her on an experimental basis.

While the parents were making their decision, the unit was notified that it would be receiving another admission. There were no more beds in the unit unless, of course, Baby J was transported. But Baby J's parents were waiting for another neonatologist to visit their infant and give a second opinion about Baby J's prognosis. They did not plan to make any decisions for their daughter's care for several hours. When members of the health team pressured Baby J's physician to speed up their decision-making process or to order Baby J's transport, he refused. According to him, Baby J's parents were "paying customers" and should be able to purchase the type of care they needed or, for that matter, wanted. There was also the fear of legal recourse if Baby J's condition should deteriorate if she was transferred against her parent's wishes. If the unit must receive another admission, another infant would have to be moved—but not Baby J.

Within an hour, it was decided that the unit would transfer Baby T, an infant with Down's syndrome and a hypoplastic left heart, to the pediatric step-down unit. Baby T was awaiting surgery, her only opportunity to survive. Baby T's mother, 18 years old and unmarried, lived 50 miles away in a rural community. Because she did not have a telephone, she could not be notified immediately of the decision to transfer her child. The mother had been discharged from the hospital 5 days earlier and had not called about her baby since leaving. There was a note on Baby T's chart that the mother would be placing the infant for adoption if she lived.

The decision to transfer Baby T demoralized the nursing staff, especially Becky Turner, Baby T's nurse. She knew that Baby T needed close cardiac monitoring and that the step-down unit would be hard pressed to provide close supervision of the infant. Even though Baby T had a very poor prognosis, even with surgery, Miss Turner felt that the transfer would place this infant at greater risk than she was presently experiencing. Miss Turner and the other nurses could not agree to the decision to transfer Baby T. Somehow it seemed that some infants, because of circumstances beyond their control, were not as "deserving" of care and services as other infants. Surely, this was not right.

Commentary

This case raises problems similar to those of the previous one. Both Baby J and Baby T have desperate need. From the standpoint of need alone, they seem equally critical. If need were the only criterion, it is hard to imagine how the person responsible for the NICU would choose. Even the person committed to using need rather than benefit as the criterion might, under such circumstances, be inclined to look at potential benefit as a possible "tie-breaker." The person who believes that the proper basis for allocating nursing care should be potential benefit would, of course, be even more comfortable with a benefits assessment.

In this case, Baby T seems to stand a much more obvious chance of benefiting. With intensive care until surgery, Baby T stands a chance of surviving. Without it, Baby T will die. On the other hand, the chances of Baby J benefiting from the NICU are remote. In fact, when the burdens of the experimental, heretofore unprecedented transplant surgery are taken into account, Baby J might simply be worse off with the temporary NICU care than without it.

If the benefits assessment is extended beyond the medical benefits, the judgment might become more complicated. Someone might argue that saving Baby T, with Down's syndrome, would count for less benefit than saving a presumably more normal Baby J with Potter's syndrome. Such an assessment of benefits, however, requires a premise that a baby with Down's syndrome is somehow less valuable than a more normal one. Without that judgment, this conclusion would not be possible.

Dr. Smith adds another dimension to the decision. He appears to bring two assumptions to the cases. First, he accepts the idea that Baby J's parents as "paying customers" should have the right to buy whatever care they need or desire. He seems to be committed to the notion that NICU care, including nursing care, can be sold as a commodity to anyone who has the ability to pay. He has a free market view of allocation in which persons should be able to buy whatever providers are willing to sell. This view is linked to the view on allocating resources that was described in the introduction to this chapter as libertarian. Autonomous individual buyers and sellers should be free to make whatever bargains they can. If other persons, not blessed with equal resources, cannot make such a deal for themselves or their children, it is unfortunate, but not unfair or unjust.

Even if that view of allocation of resources were accepted, Dr. Smith brings to the case another assumption that needs to be examined. He seems to assume that he, as the attending physician for one patient, should be the one to make a deal with Baby J's parents on behalf of the hospital. Even with a libertarian position on allocating health resources, it is not clear that an individual physician is in a position to bargain away the hospital's NICU beds. By that logic, Becky Turner, Baby T's nurse, might also have the authority to deal with Baby T's parents.

A good case can be made that neither Dr. Smith nor Ms. Turner should have any absolute control over the NICU beds. Rather, that would appear to be an institutional decision under the control of the trustees of the hospital or its sponsoring agency.

If neither need nor potential benefit justifies "bumping" Miss Turner's patient, and ability to pay is not acceptable as a basis for allocating the bed, Miss Turner may find herself in the position of being witness to what appears to be an immoral allocation decision. If she is to be thought of as an agent for her patient's rights and welfare, that leads her to reflect on how she might intervene to attempt to serve her patient's interests, in this case, keeping Baby T in the NICU bed. Seeking discussion and review of the decision with Dr. Smith, other physicians, nursing colleagues, nursing supervisors, and administrators of the hospital have all been proposed. Many institutions have hospital ethics committees available to nursing staff to help review such ethically controversial decisions. Finally, Miss Turner may have to consider outside review: reporting the case to child abuse authorities under federal regulations governing such reporting or to other police authorities. What would be the effect of these alternative strategies?

Whereas in the last case it appeared difficult to establish which infant had the greater need, often it is much more clear. In the following case, the pattern of needs may appear clearer.

Case 25: The Last Bed in the CCU on a Weekend

It had been a very busy week in the coronary care unit at University Hospital (a major tertiary referral medical center). Karen Pence, RN and administrative co-ordinator of the CCU, was very glad it was Friday afternoon. One of her final tasks of the day was to review the staffing for the coming weekend. Karen's review showed two things: first, seven of the available eight beds in the CCU were full and these patients had great need for intensive nursing care; second, it would be possible to provide safe and quality care for these seven patients for the next three shifts. However, this was accomplished only after a great deal of time had been spent reworking and switching her staff's time schedules. This was an unpleasant task but one that was often required to provide adequate coverage for a full CCU on weekends.

At this point, Dr. North approached Ms. Pence and related the following situation. Dr. North's patient, Mr. Dombrowski, a 52-year-old white male with documented three vessel coronary artery disease, was in need of coronary artery bypass (CABG) surgery. Mr. Dombrowski's surgery, scheduled 2 days ago, had been canceled because of inadequate blood supply in the blood bank. Mr. Dombrowski had naturally been upset over the cancellation. Dr. North was satisfied that the medical risks of waiting a few days were not great, but this assurance did little to relieve Mr. Dombrowski's anxiety over the surgery. He was anxious to "get this surgery over with." A few minutes ago, Dr. North was notified by the blood bank that the blood was finally available for Mr. Dombrowski's surgery. Dr. North asked Ms. Pence if the CCU could provide the necessary coverage for Mr. Dombrowski's care over the weekend if he were to begin the surgery later that afternoon. In other words, could Mr. Dombrowski occupy the last bed in the CCU over the weekend?

Ms. Pence was aware that this is the only unit in the hospital equipped to provide appropriate nursing and medical care for Mr. Dombrowski postoperatively. Since the step-down unit for the CCU is also full, there is little likelihood that any of the present patients in the CCU can be transferred, even if they could be ready for transfer in 8 to 10 hours. Mr. Dombrowski will require one-to-one nursing care for approximately 16 hours postoperatively. His admittance to the CCU will fill the last available bed early on a Friday evening. Should Ms. Pence tell Dr. North that her unit can adjust to provide adequate care for Mr. Dombrowski (and adequate coverage for the needs of the other patients in the unit)?

Commentary

It may be helpful to ask how Ms. Pence might analyze her moral problem taking each of the three positions about allocating resources outlined in the introduction to the chapter. If her goal is to produce as much benefit as possible, it seems clear that her existing seven patients could benefit greatly from the care of her nursing staff, but that adding Mr. Dombrowski at this time does not increase the amount of good the nurses will do by very much. If Mr. Dombrowski were critically ill and would not likely survive the weekend without the surgery, then the calculation would be different, but it seems that little would be accomplished by rushing Mr. Dombrowski to surgery. He would have his mind put at ease but would receive very little, if any, medical benefits from having surgery on Friday rather than Monday. On the other hand, the other patients could suffer harm from having their nursing care diverted to Mr. Dombrowski.

The analysis from the standpoint of need seems to lead to a similar conclusion. If Ms. Pence's goal were to use her nurses to benefit the sickest or least well off patients, it seems likely that her existing patients would have a higher priority than Mr. Dombrowski. Therefore, from the more egalitarian standpoint of distributing on the basis of need, Ms. Pence would apparently reach the same conclusion that she would have reached were she simply trying to maximize benefits.

That would not be the case if the existing CCU patients were so debilitated that the nursing care was unlikely to help them whereas the same nurses could be used to benefit much healthier patients. If the healthier patients would benefit more than the sicker ones, a person trying to do as much good as possible would divert the nurses from the very sick to the better-off patients, whereas the egalitarian would still feel obliged to help the sick even though it would not produce as much benefit. In Ms. Pence's case, however, she is in the happy position that helping the sicker patients also does the most good.

Ms. Pence might also consider the third basis for distribution outlined in the introduction to this chapter: letting autonomous people make whatever agreements they can, using their financial and other resources to influence the choices as they see fit. We have no data in this case about the ability to pay of either Mr. Dombrowski or any of the other patients in the CCU. If we did, a real libertarian supporting free market mechanisms for allocating health care resources would let the CCU units go to the one who could pay for them. There might even be different rates for one-on-one nursing and nursing that was shared by other patients. It appears that neither Ms. Pence nor Dr. North took this approach as a serious option. Some patients may, in effect, have the opportunity to buy special, high-quality care, however, by using their resources to buy into a particularly luxurious private hospital with low patient-to-staff ratios.

In this particular case, the nurse was highly respected and had worked with the staff for over 4 years. Knowing the needs and capabilities of her staff, she informed the physician that she wanted to talk to the patient scheduled for CABG. She did (with the physician's permission) and told the patient about her staff, the needs of the other patients in the unit, and the kind of care that he would need after surgery. The patient decided to wait until the following Monday to have his surgery.

JUSTICE BETWEEN CLIENTS AND OTHERS

In all of the cases in the first section, the nurse faced the problem of allocating care among clients. The notion of doing what will benefit the client (in the singular) was unhelpful, in fact, irrelevant, because doing what would benefit one client meant failing to do what would benefit another client. Sometimes, however, the nurse must choose between his or her own clients and the interests of third parties who are not the nurse's clients. Whereas, in the first group of cases, the nurse had to determine some basis for choosing among clients—whether it was on the basis of meeting needs, maximizing benefits, respecting autonomy, or some combination of these—in the cases in this section, the nurse could, in principle always act to maximize the client's welfare and rights. The question is whether the nurse always ought to do that even when it means failing to meet greater needs of others who are not his or her patient and even if it means failing to do as much good as possible. This can arise when those who are not the nurse's clients are, in fact, patients or potential patients within the nurse's institution, or it can arise when the other parties are not patients at all.

Case 26: The Elderly Patient Who Was Transferred

Mrs. Sally Grissom, the day supervisor of a skilled nursing facility, has just learned that several of the home's patients will be transferred to other homes. Mrs. Grissom hates to tell one of the patients that this will occur. The patient, 74-year-old Mrs. Lewiston, has lived at Ferndale Care for 3 years. Mrs. Lewiston has no relatives, is quite alert, and considers Ferndale her home for the rest of her life. Although confined to a wheelchair, Mrs. Lewiston no longer requires skilled nursing care and has been singled out for transfer as a means to control costs of patient care in higher priced skilled nursing homes across the state. Mrs. Lewiston is a recipient of public assistance. The administrators are insisting that care not be funded at a level beyond what is necessary.

After learning of the planned transfer, Mrs. Lewiston calls a public-assistance attorney and asks him to represent her and other patients in a legal suit to block the move. She argues that the state has no right to move her and other patients without notice and without a hearing about the benefits of present level of care and potential harms and benefits at another hospital with a lower level of care.

Mrs. Grissom is undecided whether she should support the patients' legal suit. Aside from the detrimental effect such an action might have on her job, she is truly uncertain whether an elderly resident of a nursing home can "select" his or her home and level of care when the state pays for all costs of the care. Certainly, each patient is entitled to some level of care, but who decides what level of care is appropriate for each patient and how much input does the patient have?

Case 27: The Patient Who Could Not Get Admitted to the Hospital*

Mrs. Jean Wyman is the emergency room nurse for a small private hospital in the suburbs of a large metropolitan area. She has worked at this particular hospital for 7 years. Because of recent cuts in federal monies to her institution, the emergency room has been asked to screen admissions very carefully. For example, patients who do not have health insurance are to be referred to other nearby hospitals for emergency care whenever possible; maternity patients are

*Adapted from Cushing M: Expanding the meaning of accountability. Am J Nurs 83:1202–1203, 1983

not to be admitted if they are not the patient of any of the staff physicians, except in extreme emergency.

One Friday night, a pregnant woman at term came to the emergency room. The woman thought that she might be in labor, but since this was her first pregnancy, she was not sure. The patient was unmarried and accompanied by her mother. She was not the patient of any of the staff physicians and had not received regular prenatal care during her pregnancy. The woman had been referred from the emergency room of another private hospital several miles away. She could not pay, and the other hospital wanted to admit only paying patients; she did not qualify for Medicaid. After checking the woman's vital signs, Mrs. Wyman telephoned the acting chief of obstetrics. Since Mrs. Wyman noted no abnormalities and the patient did not appear to be in active labor, the acting chief of obstetrics told Mrs. Wyman to tell the family to transport the pregnant woman to the county medical center where she could be admitted without any trouble.

Mrs. Wyman wheeled the pregnant woman to the emergency room entrance and helped her into her mother's car. A few minutes later, the mother returned and asked for an ambulance. She thought her daughter was becoming ill. Mrs. Wyman went outside to the car and examined the pregnant woman. She noted that, aside from being in advanced pregnancy, the woman had vomited, she was lethargic, her skin was moist, and her respirations were rapid. There were still no signs of labor. The mother asked the nurse to call a specialist because she was concerned about her daughter. Mrs. Wyman returned to the emergency room and again called the acting chief of obstetrics. He firmly told Mrs. Wyman to refer the patient to the county medical center. Even when she expressed concern about the patient's condition, he told her to send the patient to the other hospital. Although she did not agree with the acting chief of obstetrics' decision, she felt that she could do nothing but again recommend traveling to the county medical center—a 15-minute drive. She told the mother that she would call the emergency room of the county medical center and inform them of their impending arrival.

The next day, Mrs. Wyman learned that the young woman was in critical condition at the county medical center, because of a ruptured uterus. Her fetus had died. There was a strong possibility that the family of the pregnant woman would sue Mrs. Wyman, the acting chief of obstetrics, and the hospital for their failure to provide emergency care to the woman. Mrs. Wyman was furious. A careful and respected practitioner, she felt that her otherwise prudent and expert nursing judgment was being constrained by the economic position taken by the hospital concerning emergency admissions. Whereas it was certainly acceptable for a hospital to be concerned about the cost-effectiveness of its services, could any institution make regulations that potentially constrained the moral (and legal) judgments of its nursing staff?

Commentary

Both of these cases pose problems of the ethics of resource allocation. In both cases it seems clear that the interests of the patients are in conflict with the interests of others.

Seventy-four-year-old Mrs. Lewiston would prefer to stay in the Ferndale Care center where she had lived for 3 years. However, the economic interests of others, in this case the tax payers providing the public assistance that is supporting Mrs. Lewiston's care, are quite different.

In the case of the young woman turned away from the private hospital apparently because she did not have insurance coverage, it is less clear exactly whose interests were in conflict with those of the patient. Presumably, if she had no insurance and was not on Medicaid, the private hospital would absorb the costs if she were admitted. Since it is a for-profit institution, the owners of the hospital would either have to subsidize this patient's care or pass the extra costs on to other paying patients. In either case, someone else has an interest in making sure that only true emergency patients are cared for without charge. The result is that nonpaying patients who are not deemed to be emergencies are referred to a public institution.

As in the previous cases, someone or some group will have to make a judgment about how scarce resources should be allocated. The libertarian, who is willing to let free market forces determine how resources are allocated, might not support formal public assistance programs such as those funding Mrs. Lewiston's care. In the case of the private, for-profit hospital, the institution would be under no obligation to provide care. At most, it would be an act of charity. If that charity is funded by stockholders or by other patients who have not agreed to be charitable, a health professional offering such charity might actually be seen as being unfair.

The decision-maker approaching the problem from the standpoint of trying to do as much good as possible with limited resources would have an easy time justifying transferring Mrs. Lewiston. The skilled nursing care is not providing adequate benefit. To be thorough, those calculating the benefits and harms would have to take into account Mrs. Lewiston's emotional distress from the move, but even so, it is not implausible to conclude that the funds could be used better elsewhere.

The benefits and harms of the policy of turning away the young pregnant woman are harder to determine. She may well have been put in jeopardy by the referral, and someone must pay the costs of her care in any case. Surely, however, some moral limits must exist on the obligation of a private hospital to provide charity care.

The egalitarian would ask not who is willing to pay or how benefits can be maximized, but rather who is in the greatest need. Both Mrs. Lewiston and the young pregnant woman seem to be persons having significant claims of need. Mrs. Lewiston's need, however, is presumably not as great as those of patients requiring skilled nursing care. In the case of the pregnant woman, a physician made a judgment that she could be transferred safely. In doing so, he made a judgment call about the level of her need.

The real question for the nurses in these cases may not necessarily be the question of what counts as a just or fair allocation of resources. Mrs. Grissom and Mrs. Wyman could not help being aware of the resource allocation question. It can be debated, however, whether it is their job to solve the ethical and policy questions raised by such allocation issues. They have special obligations to their patients. When their patients' interests conflict with others in the system, someone must deal with the allocational problem, but nurses should ask whether that is their responsibility. Some would argue that their first duty is to their patients. This would mean that they become advocates for their patients. Presumably someone else—the public assistance administrators in Mrs.

Lewiston's case and the owners of the hospital in the case of the pregnant woman—will advocate on behalf of the interests of the other parties. If this notion of special "role-specific" duties is adopted in which the clinician is an advocate for the patient, it makes sense that sometimes they ought to lose their cases. Sometimes the advocates for the interests of other parties will be closer to being right. Under this model, nurses should not feel angry or distressed if what they advocate does not happen (for example, if Mrs. Lewiston is moved even though Mrs. Grissom, her nurse, had argued that the move was not in Mrs. Lewiston's interest).

If this special advocacy role is not assigned to clinicians, then Mrs. Grissom and Mrs. Wyman would presumably be responsible for considering the broader question of what are the fair limits on the use of the skilled nursing home or the private hospital emergency room. If they are to deal with these social ethical questions, then in some cases, not necessarily these, but at least in some others, they will have to be the ones who decide that their clients' interests must be sacrificed for the more weighty moral claims of other parties. In cases where there is a conflict of interest between a clinician's patients and other parties, one of the critical questions is whether clinicians should attempt to decide what the fair limits of care are for their patients or whether they should simply advocate for their patients and let someone else make these allocation decisions.

JUSTICE IN PUBLIC POLICY

In the cases presented thus far in this chapter the nurse is clearly paired with at least one identified client. In the first group, the problem was that more than one client had needs that conflicted. In the second group, the client's interest conflicted with those of other persons—stockholders or the public at large. In the latter cases we raised the question of whether the nurse should be in the role of deciding how resources should be allocated. The alternative was to take on the role of advocate for the client, leaving the allocation decisions to others. The cases in this section deal with nurses in other than clinical care giving roles where the nurse, by the very nature of the role being played, must make allocational choices.

Case 28: The Problem of Justice in Policy Decisions

Marcia Forsyth is the director of nursing of a community health nursing agency in a large Midwestern county. Periodically, she meets with her two associate directors to discuss the budget for agency programs for the next fiscal year. Together, they determine how the agency will allocate its nursing resources during the coming year and discuss the agency programs that will be initiated, terminated, or changed in order to meet health needs of their community.

During the most recent meeting, one associate director, Jann Beech, requested that the agency give her the resources to initiate a primary care clinic for adults that would be staffed by nurse–practitioners. Her data in support of this program included an increase in the adult population in the community over the past 5 years and a decrease in the number of family physicians serving the county during the same time period. She argued that adult care clinics had resulted in dramatic improvements in community health statistics where such programs had been tried.

The other associate director, Susan Chinn, also made a request at this meeting. She requested that the agency provide counseling services for pregnant teenagers. Citing increased numbers of teenage pregnancies in the county during the last 3 years, she argued persuasively that counseling of the pregnant teenager will help prevent future pregnancies in this age-group and that both the mothers and their children are potentially among the most needy residents of their community.

Mrs. Forsyth reminds her associate directors that there is a ceiling on the amount of agency funds available for new programs. Only one new program can be initiated this year and then only if the agency is willing to support the program for a minimum of 3 years. Therefore, the associate directors should carefully consider the type of policies that may be formed by the focus on specific programs and populations within the county and the amount of financial support each program request may require in order to be operative. They must also consider the amount of nursing time and expertise that will be required by the residents of the county. Mrs. Forsyth is at a loss to choose between them without further study and data. What should be the determining factors in deciding to fund one program and not the other?

Case 29: Screening School Girls for Urinary Tract Infections*

Sheila Goberman was a community health nurse. After receiving an advanced degree in child health care, she began working for the Warren County Department of Health and is now employed as the Director of School Health Maintenance. She and others specializing in public health for school-age populations have been concerned about the high incidence of urinary tract infections in school-age girls in her county. Approximately 15% of girls with asymptomatic bacteriuria (ASB) are reported to have renal scarring when first detected. It is believed that early detection might prevent progressing renal damage. Ms. Goberman is in the process of developing a program that will screen school-age girls in the county.

She was aware of two strategies for screening school-age populations. The first method involved sending an explanatory letter to parents a week before screening. A health department nurse was then to be sent to the school. She would distribute kits containing a dipslide and a letter of instructions, which each child would take home. At home, the parent would assist in collecting a midstream urine specimen on the slide. The slides were then to be returned to the school the following day and analyzed in the Health Department laboratory. The second strategy involved sending a Health Department mobile unit to the

---

*Adapted from Rich G, Glass NJ, Selkon JB: Cost-effectiveness of two methods of screening for asymptomatic bacteriuria. Br J Preven Soc Med 30:54–59, 1976

school, where the specimens were collected under the supervision of a Health Department nurse.

Ms. Goberman was aware that in previous studies the first, home-administered test was considerably cheaper. One study in Britain reported that the cost per child screened for the first approach was 0.26 pounds while the second method, using the mobile unit and Health Department personnel was 0.77 pounds per child screened.

Whereas the home-administered method was thus about one-third as expensive, and thus very cost-effective, Ms. Goberman was also aware that the home testing was not equally successful for all socioeconomic groups. Specifically, failure rates were three times as great in the home-administered test for children in the lower socioeconomic groups as in the upper classes. This has been attributed to both a greater incidence of failure to return a slide and greater incidence of spoiled slides among lower class families.

Ms. Goberman realized she had an ethical choice to make. As a health officer for the county, was it her mission to find as many cases of ASB as possible per dollar invested (in which case she would use the home-administered test) or was it to see that girls of all socioeconomic classes had an equal opportunity to have their ASB detected (in which case she would have to use the more expensive test or some mix of the two methods)? If resources were unlimited, Ms. Goberman would simply opt for the second method, but she knew that she would not have enough funds from the Department to do the screening as often as would be desirable in any case.

Commentary

These cases both pose problems of nurses who are in administrative positions rather than one-to-one patient relations. In both cases the nurse is in a position to make ethical policy determinations when the key question is what constitutes a fair use of limited resources.

Marcia Forsyth is in the unenviable position of having to choose between two programs where both would be valuable, but only one can be funded. She might notice that Jann Beech and Susan Chinn, the two associate directors, have made somewhat different appeals for their proposals. Ms. Beech based her appeal on data showing that aggregate community health statistics improved dramatically when nurse–practitioners provided a primary care clinic for adults. Ms. Chinn, on the other hand, based her appeal on the fact that adolescent pregnant women and their children were among the most needy residents of the community. Both are arguments commonly heard in debates about health resource allocation, but they are morally different appeals. In the first case, it is the amount of improvement in aggregate health statistics that is the basis of the argument. In the second case, it is not the total community health improvement that is being cited, but the health of one particular segment of the community—the most needy.

Possibly each nurse–administrator could have reframed her argument in the terms that the other used. Ms. Beech might have argued that the clients of the primary care clinic would be among the most needy of the community and Ms. Chinn might have argued that her adolescent pregnancy program might produce dramatic improvements in aggregate public health statistics such as rates of mortality and morbidity. The problem here is which kind of appeal is ethically most appropriate. Is the goal to produce the most benefit in aggregate or to help the most needy? A similar issue arises in the bacteriuria screening program.

Ms. Goberman has no direct one-on-one client relationships. Although her staff will eventually visit the schools, she will never see any of the clients herself. The cases in the previous section posed problems of conflict between the nurse's client and society, but in this case Ms. Goberman's client, in a way, is society. She needs to know whether her ethical obligation is to find the most cases in her population with the limited resources she has for the screening program or, alternatively, whether she should screen less efficiently, but in doing so give socially and economically deprived school girls a better chance to have their cases of ASB detected.

Since her funds for the project are limited, she will have to compromise in some way. She will probably opt for an arrangement in which the testing is done at much less frequent intervals than would be desirable. If she opts for the second method in order to give the socially and economically deprived school girls an equal chance of having their cases found, she will be able to screen even less frequently and will thus find fewer cases overall.

The three major alternative approaches to the ethics of resource allocation presented in the introduction to this chapter give three very different answers to Ms. Goberman's dilemma. The more libertarian approach, insofar as it supports free market policies, would simply make information about screening available so that any parents who wanted to and could afford it would have their daughters screened. Possibly, such a person would even use the Health Department to offer the screening, but on a fee-for-service basis.

The approach that considers a fair distribution to be one that gets the most benefits in total for the investment would clearly favor the home-administered test. It is the essence of the approach that the distribution of benefits and burdens, in principle, do not count ethically. Since it is the community's health in aggregate that is the goal of the Health Department, the funds available should be used to lower the incidence of ASB regardless of its distribution.

The more egalitarian approach, on the other hand, is very concerned about matters of distribution. Who receives the benefits is ethically important. Each girl in the community ought to have an equal chance to have her urinary tract infections diagnosed. That would mean spending extra money, if necessary, to detect cases among the lower class school girls.

Possibly a compromise strategy could be developed. In-school screening could be used for lower class students while the home-administered test could be used for upper class girls. If, however, this were done on a school-by-school basis with schools in upper class neighborhoods using the home-administered method, some lower class students in primarily upper class neighborhoods would still lose out. If the differentiation were done on a student-to-student basis, awkward, potentially stigmatizing discriminations would have to be made. Ms. Goberman has encountered a situation where doing what is efficient in community health terms will be quite different from doing what will give people equal opportunity to have their health problems addressed.

JUSTICE AND OTHER ETHICAL PRINCIPLES

The cases thus far in this chapter deal exclusively with distribution of scarce nursing resources on the basis of the needs of the patient (egalitarian justice), the amount of benefit to be done (beneficence), and the freedom of persons to make agreements (autonomy). The final case suggests that occasionally there are other moral principles that may influence the morally right decision. In the following case, a nurse has made a promise to one of her patients. She must decide how her duty to keep a promise is to be reconciled with her duty to be fair, to do good, and to respect autonomy. In this case, it may turn out that doing what is right may be different from doing what is fair, benefit-maximizing, or autonomy-respecting.

Case 30: When It Is Hard to Keep Promises*

Peter was a 15 year old with acute myelocytic leukemia. As his condition deteriorated, Peter began to realize that he was dying. He was in pain, angry, afraid, and largely dependent on others to meet his physical needs. However, the nurses on his unit promised that he would not be allowed to suffer and that he would not be alone as he became sicker.

During a 6-month period, Peter was in and out of the hospital four times. Although Peter was often difficult to get along with, the nursing staff had begun to care about Peter, and he had learned to trust them. The fact that Peter had lived in foster homes most of his life explained some of his difficult behavior. Of greater concern was the fact that his natural parents had slowly withdrawn themselves from him during his illness. Over time, the staff of the nursing care unit realized that they were, in many ways, Peter's "family"—the nursing staff would be the ones who would care for him and be with him when he died.

As Peter's condition worsened, his needs for physical and emotional care increased. The staff decided that he should be assigned a primary care nurse, Sheri Martin, RN, who would coordinate and plan the increasing amount of care that he would need. Within a few days, Peter could no longer walk because of the pain from the effects of his illness. He was often feverish and suffered from nausea, vomiting, and diarrhea. He experienced constant fear—of pain, of the effects of morphine, and of the possibility that he might not wake up once he fell asleep. Nighttime was especially difficult for Peter and his nurses. He was in near-constant pain but often refused his morphine. Instead, he asked that his nurse stay in the room, talk to him, read to him—anything to distract him from his pain.

*Adapted from Leff E: Keeping a promise. Am J Nurs 82:1136–1138, 1982

One evening, he asked Miss Martin to stay with him even though she had already worked all day. She switched her hours with another nurse and stayed on the unit to take care of Peter. There was a real possibility that Peter was near death. Unfortunately, another staff nurse called in sick. There was not enough staff to take care of all the patients, especially if Miss Martin spent most of her time with Peter. Miss Martin could not decide what to do. She had promised Peter that she or one of the other nurses would stay with him, especially when he died. Yet it did not seem fair to the other patients, some of whom needed careful preparation for surgery the following day, to forgo their needs in favor of Peter's needs. Yet if no one stayed with Peter, he would feel abandoned at the time when he needed someone the most. If this happened, the nurses would surely feel guilt, frustration, and anger at being unable to respond to Peter's important needs. Should promises to Peter be met when nursing resources were strained to the limit and other patients' needs were equally important?

Commentary

The moral problem in this case seems to arise from the fact that nurse Sheri Martin is convinced that there are other patients who could benefit greatly from her nursing care, and yet she has made a promise to Peter to stay with him in his time of need.

We have already seen in the other cases in this chapter that not everyone is convinced that the morally correct thing to do is always to use resources in ways that do the most good in total. Some people would say that justice requires identifying the people with the greatest need and using resources that way even if some other use would do more good. If Peter has very great need, and it appears that he does, then perhaps Sheri Martin, if she is governed by the principle of justice in addition to or in place of beneficence, will conclude that she should go where the need is the greatest, quite possibly to Peter. That would mean that justice would require the same thing that keeping the promise would require. Her moral dilemma would disappear.

Some people hold, however, that it is more morally correct to do the most good than to help the people with the greatest need. If Sheri Martin is one of those people, she still has a problem with Peter. If he has the greatest need, but she can do more good helping others, than she would normally have a moral duty to abandon Peter.

If she holds this view, the fact that she had promised him that she would stay with him could become morally important. In effect, there are three moral dimensions to the case: doing good, serving the most needy, and keeping promises. The resolution could depend on how one ranks these various principles. If doing good counts as definitive, the matter will be settled in favor of abandoning Peter and breaking a promise. That position would be the same as saying that normally needs should be met and promises should be kept, but only because usually that does the most good. In cases where it does not, one should do the most good anyway.

Others might give priority to the other principles. Someone like Immanuel Kant would hold that the duty to keep promises is unconditional. That might have settled the matter for Kant. Others might hold that the duty to serve the most needy is unconditional. One final position is worth considering. Serving the needy and keeping promises are related duties in the sense that they are not simply duties related to the amount of consequences produced. Philosophers sometimes call such duties "deontological" or "formalist," meaning simply that it is the form or nature of the action rather than its consequences that is morally important. One might hold that these duties take precedence over simply producing good consequences. Holders of that view would recognize that both serving the needy and keeping promises would bind Ms. Martin to staying with Peter, whereas only the lower priority principle of doing good authorizes her to leave him. It is to these other principles that we now turn.

References

1. Bentham J: An introduction to the principles of morals and legislation. In Melden AI (ed): Ethical Theories: A Book of Readings, pp 367–390. Englewood Cliffs, NJ, Prentice-Hall, 1967
2. Mill JS: Utilitarianism. Priest O (ed). New York, Bobbs-Merrill, 1957 [1863]
3. Nozick R: Anarchy, State, and Utopia. New York, Basic Books, 1974
4. Rawls J: A Theory of Justice. Cambridge, Harvard University Press, 1971
5. Green RM: Health care and justice in contract theory perspective. In Veatch RM, Branson R (eds): Ethics and Health Policy. Cambridge, Ballinger, 1976
6. Daniels N: Just Health Care. Cambridge, England, Cambridge University Press, 1985
7. Engelhardt HT: The Foundations of Bioethics. New York, Oxford University Press, 1986

Chapter 5

Autonomy

We have now seen that acting so as to produce the greatest possible net benefit is not necessarily acting in such a way that the good produced is justly or equitably distributed. Many who reflect on ethical theory believe that even though a particular distribution may not do the greatest possible good in aggregate, it may nevertheless satisfy the principle of justice. Anyone who holds that view is committed to the position that just or equitable distribution is one right-making characteristic of actions independent of the amount of good produced. Most contemporary ethical thinkers are convinced that there is much more to ethics than simply producing good consequences. This turns out to hold not only for social questions such as the way goods are distributed, but also for ethics focused more at the level of the individual. For example, what should the nurse do when he or she is convinced that a patient who has signed himself out of the hospital is leaving too early for his own good? If the nurse could persuade, pressure, coerce, or trick the patient into staying, should he or she do so? Suppose the nurse, by lying or deceiving the patient, could induce him to change his mind and thus make the patient better off. Would it be an acceptable behavior simply because it would make the patient better off?

Often the goal of doing good for the patient and avoiding harms—the principles of beneficence and nonmaleficence—conflicts with other ethical principles such as the principles of respect for autonomy, truth-telling, promise-keeping, or avoiding killing. The group of cases presented in this chapter all raise problems related to one of the most important of these additional principles, the principle of autonomy. The principle of autonomy affirms that individuals are to be permitted personal liberty to determine their own actions according to plans they themselves have chosen. Part of what is entailed in the idea of respect for persons, according to those who accept the principle of autonomy, is an acceptance of the individual's own choices regardless of whether such choices are in their interests.[1–3,4(pp235–273)]

Of course, not all persons are capable of autonomous choice. Some, such as small children or the severely retarded, have never had the capacity for substantially autonomous choices. The first case in this chapter examines the conflict between autonomy and patient welfare for a patient with diminished capacity for autonomy—an aging person who can no longer live alone.

Other persons, while they may not be lacking in the capacity for autonomous choice, are nevertheless in environments that make autonomous decision-making very difficult. The next group of cases deals with clients in such environments—persons in nursing homes and in the military.

The final three cases explore the grounds on which a nurse might decide to override the client's autonomy because it would be in the patient's interest to do so.

DIMINISHED CAPACITY TO CLAIM AUTONOMY

In several of the cases presented in earlier chapters, the conflict between the autonomy of the patient and the welfare of the patient has been presented. It is now widely accepted that autonomy, like justice, is an independent principle that helps determine whether actions are right or wrong. It stands beside the principles of beneficence and nonmaleficence. Anyone who holds this position would be quite prepared to say that an intervention will benefit the patient but may still be wrong because it violates the patient's autonomy.

One of the problems that arise in analyzing autonomy is that persons appear to be autonomous in varying degrees. No one is perfectly autonomous. No one is perfectly capable of choosing a plan for himself or herself free from internal and external constraints. However, some persons are capable of being substantially autonomous in their decisions. Others are clearly not capable of such inner-direction. If persons who are capable of substantial inner-direction ought to be able to act on their own plans, it is important to explore the limits of the capacity for autonomous choice.[4(pp 274–297)] The first case presented in this chapter poses such a problem.

Case 31: When Aging Parents Can No Longer Live Independently*

Joyce Fisher, a home health agency nurse, has just received a telephone call from the daughter of a patient, 82-year-old Mr. Sims, whom she had visited some months previously. The daughter was very distraught, telling Ms. Fisher that her father had fallen at home but refused to be seen by a physician. Mrs. Sims, her mother, had called the daughter at her place of business and pleaded with her to come to the home and stay with them. The daughter was exasperated by the frequency of these calls from her parents in recent weeks and was appealing to Ms. Fisher for help in making some long-term decisions for the care (and safety!) of her parents.

Ms. Fisher well remembers the conversations that she had with Mr. and Mrs. Sims and their daughter several months ago following Mr. Sims' last hos-

*Adapted from Scott RS: When it isn't life or death. Am J Nurs 85:19–20, 1985

pitalization. The Sims live alone in a small home and are frequently visited by their married daughter, who buys their groceries and takes them to their various health appointments. Mr. Sims has always been the decision-maker of the family, but allows this amount of assistance from the daughter "for Mama's sake." Another daughter lives in a nearby city but has chronic health problems that prohibit her active involvement in her parents' affairs. A son lives on the West Coast and travels constantly in his line of business. He supports his parents by sending money for their expenses to his sister. (Mr. Sims has refused direct financial aid from any of the children.) All three children are concerned about the future welfare of their parents, but have been unsuccessful in persuading them to change their mode of living.

The present problem is caused by the fact that Mr. and Mrs. Sims are losing their ability to live independently and make their own decisions. Mr. Sims' unexplained falls are also increasing and are a continued source of worry for Mrs. Sims and a genuine concern for their married daughter. They all look to Joyce Fisher as the person who can help them make and support a decision that will preserve some autonomy for the aging parents and respect their choices and life-style. Yet Ms. Fisher doubts that what is best for all concerned (parents as well as children) can avoid infringing on the choices and self-respect of the Sims. Is there no happy medium for aging parents when they can no long live independently? What is the role of the home health nurse in assisting individuals reach decisions with which they can live?

Commentary

Mr. and Mrs. Sims both are people whose capacities for autonomous decision-making are beginning to be compromised. The critical decision, both for Ms. Fisher and for the Sims' daughters, is whether they will treat the Sims as autonomous agents. If they do and if they are convinced that it is in the Sims' interest to change their living arrangements, they may try to persuade them of the wisdom of a change. They will present reasons why a change would be appropriate; they may try to argue with them.

If Ms. Fisher and the daughters have doubts about the Sims' capacities to be substantially autonomous decision-makers, they may try to test them. They may try to determine if the Sims comprehend the risks, the alternatives, and the advantages and disadvantages of each.

If one or both seem incapable of making reasonably autonomous choices, Ms. Fisher and the daughters will face a critical point. They might simply take over the decision-making, but, even though they might get away with it, that kind of unilateral "declaration of incompetency" is problematic both ethically and legally.[5,6] Legally, the daughters have no authority to take over decision-making for their parents, even if they are well motivated. Certainly, a health care professional has no such authority. If there is to be a declaration of incompetency, the only agency with the legal authority to make the declaration is a court of proper jurisdiction. Where does that leave the daughters and Ms. Fisher ethically?

They might first approach the problem by looking at the consequences of going beyond persuasion and offering of reasons for the alternative they favor. The daughters may argue that they have seen the dangers increasing and know their parents well enough to realize that they are at risk. Ms. Fisher might argue that she has seen elderly people similarly situated so that she knows the risks they are taking.

The consequentialist argument for respecting the liberty of the parents to make their own decisions rests on at least two considerations.[7] First, probably neither the daughters nor the nurse is in a particularly good position to know the disadvantages of a more protected living arrangement. The parents are probably in a better position than anyone else to know the psychic trauma of a major life-style change. Second, the mere fact that they would be losing control would appear to be an important disadvantage of a more protected arrangement. Mr. Sims appears particularly distressed by that possibility. Thus, even on consequentialist grounds alone, there are good reasons for the Sims to retain their freedom of choice.

Added to this is the fact that a general practice of permitting adult children or health professionals to take over decision-making for elderly persons would run the risk that some people authorized under such a policy would not be as caring as Ms. Fisher and the Sims' daughter seem to be. A general policy would have to determine what the authority of the second daughter and the son would be. In some cases, and the Sims' case may be one, not all people of equal degree of kinship are equally committed to the elderly person's welfare. In some cases, there might be not only a single nurse, but several health professionals, each with a unique idea about what would best serve the welfare of the person who was being made their ward. A general policy that permitted relatives or health professionals to take over decision-making without the benefit of judicial review could lead to serious problems.

Finally, even if these hurdles could be overcome in arguing that some mixture of family and health care professionals could do what is best for such persons who have never been declared incompetent, those committed to an ethical principle of autonomy would still argue that it would be wrong to take over the decision-making. According to the principle of autonomy an action is wrong insofar as persons with substantial capacities for autonomous decision-making are not permitted to exercise that autonomy.

What should happen, however, in cases where persons are clearly totally lacking in autonomy—where they are infants, profoundly retarded, chronically senile, or comatose persons, for example? Where autonomy is lacking, it cannot be a violation of autonomy to take over decision-making. There still may be very good arguments that the interests of the nonautonomous one can best be served by using rigorous due process, but no one can seriously disagree with the goal designating a decision-maker whose assignment is to promote the welfare of the nonautonomous person. Several questions are worthy of debate: At what point along the continuum of capacities for autonomous decision-making ought decision-making authority be taken from the one whose autonomy is compromised? Is there some identifiable point where autonomy is so obviously lacking that transfer of decision-making authority can legitimately take place without due process of court review? If so, who is the one who ought to be given that authority? Are there any circumstances under which it would be acceptable for a nurse or physician to take over that role? By law, parents already have that authority for their minor children. Several states have now also given that responsibility to the next of kin even in cases where the nonautonomous one is not a child.* What is the justification for such a policy and what are the potential dangers? Are there adequate safeguards (such as court reviews) to protect against those dangers?

EXTERNAL CONSTRAINTS
ON AUTONOMY

The elderly couple in the previous case had their capacity for autonomy questioned because of doubts about their inherent abilities to act on their own agendas. What limits there were arose from organic and psychological factors that were basically internal. They were not seriously constrained by external factors. That is not to say that persons with compromised capacities for autonomy cannot have what capacity there is enhanced by external considerations. Patient explanation of alternatives, efforts to overcome limitations in vision and hearing, and support with financial and physical resources all may increase their capacity to act autonomously.

Other persons have no such internal constraints, but are still unable to act as autonomous agents because of external constraints. The next two cases illustrate the problem.

Case 32: The Patient Who Wanted to Eat Alone

Sylvia Gambino, Nursing Supervisor of Bayside Elderly Care, gave a quick look at the dining room where the majority of Bayside's 30 residents were eating lunch. She noticed that Miss Phoebe Merryweather was gazing out the window and had not touched her lunch. A quiet, dignified woman of 78 years, Miss Merryweather has been living at Bayside for 2 1/2 months. In recent weeks, however, Mrs. Gambino and the rest of the staff have begun to notice that Miss Merryweather is becoming withdrawn, does not eat much of her food, and is noticeably thinner.

Mrs. Gambino is troubled by Miss Merryweather's behavior and concerned about her nutritional status. Although this patient has some left-sided weakness due to a mild stroke some 12 years earlier, she has seemed alert and in good health for her age until recent weeks. Miss Merryweather had apparently lived an active life as an interior decorator in a Southern city until her retirement. About 2 years ago she came to Brooklyn to live with her one remaining relative, an unmarried sister. When the sister died quite suddenly, members of her sister's church persuaded Miss Merryweather to live at Bayside Elderly Care. Well known for its small resident population, excellent facilities, and the fact that most of the residents need minimal nursing supervision, Bayside seemed to be the ideal place for Miss Merryweather to live. The residents of Bayside are almost

*These states include Arkansas, Louisiana, New Mexico, Texas, and Virginia for certain decisions.

entirely drawn from the large Italian–American community surrounding Bayside, seem to know one anothers' families, and receive excellent community support.

Miss Merryweather, however, has not joined in the activities and comradery of Bayside. She seems to prefer reading, crocheting, watching a few select television programs, and eating alone in her room. In fact, she strongly objects to eating her meals in the main dining room with the other residents. On several occasions, she has even wrapped her food from her tray in a napkin and surreptitiously carried it to her room. When this practice was discovered, the staff scolded Miss Merryweather for bringing food to her room. She was told to "count her blessings" in that she could walk to the dining room and eat her meals with other people and did not *have* to eat all alone in her room like some elderly residents.

It seems that Mrs. Gambino and her staff firmly believe that the health of elderly persons is directly related to opportunities for community involvement, contact with other people, and shared daily activities such as eating meals. Bayside operates its daily activities on a Partnership Model, which fosters partnerships between residents, residents and staff, and residents and community members. Having been reared and educated in Bayside's community, Mrs. Gambino considers the Partnership Model in resident elderly care to be a close approximation to the kind of life-style Bayside's residents had enjoyed in earlier days. Thus, the Partnership Model is heartily supported by the residents, the staff, and community groups. Yet Miss Merryweather does not seem interested in this overall plan and the goal of resident involvement.

Deciding to talk directly with Miss Merryweather about her eating behavior, Mrs. Gambino learns that this elderly woman detests eating meals with the other residents. As Miss Merryweather states, "I lose my appetite when I see others drop their food all over their trays and clothes. Some have suffered strokes like me and cannot help but be messy eaters. Others have trouble guiding forks and spoons to their mouths. I cannot stand to watch others eat like this. So I prefer to eat alone. Is that too much to ask?"

Mrs. Gambino is stunned by the vehemence behind Miss Merryweather's words. Certainly, this elderly patient could be more tolerant toward others and learn something from them, despite the deficiencies in their feeding skills related to physical handicaps. After all, one of the goals of the Partnership Model is to increase social opportunities for elderly residents. In Bayside's community, mealtimes are considered the major social activities of the day. Since Miss Merryweather has no friends or relatives in Brooklyn, her social involvement is entirely dependent on activities at Bayside. Moreover, the Bayside administration has had serious maintenance and sanitation problems when residents have kept food in their rooms. They have had to adopt a policy of permitting food in rooms only for patients who were too ill to come to the dining room and then food is permitted only under the strict supervision of the staff. Should Mrs. Gambino continue to enforce Bayside's requirement of eating meals in the dining room for all residents who are able to walk, including Miss Merryweather, or should she give up some of her beliefs about resident elderly care in this patient's case?

Case 33: The Recruit Hospitalized for Weight Control

Phyllis Somerville is a civilian nurse who works in a U.S. Naval Hospital. A 19-year-old patient, Pvt. Barnes, has just been admitted to the medical ward for enlisted personnel with the diagnosis of obesity. He is moderately overweight, weighing 205 pounds at 5' 10" in height. In admitting the patient, Mrs. Somerville learns that Pvt. Barnes has a long-standing weight problem, predating adolescence. He managed to survive basic training after losing 60 pounds in a 4-month period. Now that he has been assigned to his first duty station, he has relaxed the near-starvation diet imposed on him during basic training. Unfortunately, he has gained 20 pounds and has been unable to keep up with the rest of his platoon during morning marches and forced runs. His platoon leader, 2nd Lt. Harris, desperately wants his platoon to excel in platoon competition and basic military skills. Because of his previous weight problem, he has ordered Pvt. Barnes to lose weight, a feat that Pvt. Barnes has not been able to accomplish in the last few weeks.

At today's early morning formation, Pvt. Barnes wondered how much longer he could endure 2nd Lt. Harris' belittling comments and the 100 push-ups he inevitably was ordered to do each time he blinked an eye. To his surprise, his name was called to check in for sick-call. He soon learned that 2nd Lt. Harris wanted him to be hospitalized for the purpose of weight reduction. Pvt. Barnes was adamantly opposed to the plan because he would begin his specialized training—the entire reason for his enlisting in the military—within a few days. It soon became apparent that Pvt. Barnes really did not have any choice in the matter. Since he had not lost the required weight in recent weeks, 2nd Lt. Harris had the power to admit him to the hospital for "weight reduction." Pvt. Barnes would lose the opportunity for the specialized training, an opportunity that might not occur again during his 3-year enlistment. In discussing the rigor of the diet ordered by the admitting physician, Mrs. Somerville could not help but feel sorry for the fact that Pvt. Barnes had absolutely no control over his present situation and future success in the military, particularly with a very basic life mechanism such as eating. Even more disturbing, she would be the agent to enforce the regulation imposed on Pvt. Barnes and deny his choices on a day-to-day basis.

Commentary

Both Pvt. Barnes and Miss Merryweather lack the capacity to choose life-styles based on their own internalized norms. They lack autonomy. However, unlike Mr. and Mrs. Sims, in the first case in this chapter, they have no inherent physical and mental limitations that constrain their autonomy. They are constrained by being in institutional environments where their choices are limited. Like many residents in what are sometimes called "total" institutions (that is, institutions that involve one's total life, such as prisons, boarding schools, and religious communities) they are confronted with institutional policies that shift many aspects of decision-making away from the individual toward supervisory figures vested with authority to make decisions.

The first question faced by nurses Gambino and Somerville is whether there is any justification for them to practice their profession in an environment where such external constraints on autonomy are part of the fabric of everyday existence. In both cases, especially in Mrs. Gambino's case, one might argue that part of the duty of the nurse is to be an advocate for the patient. In more traditional times, that probably would have meant that the nurse was to be an advocate for the medical well-being of patients—for their care and safety. More recently, however, the nurse, in taking on the role of advocate for clients, has focused on their rights, as well as their well-being. If one of their rights is to act as autonomous decision-makers within their inherent capacities, the nurse may sometimes find herself advocating for decision-making freedom for patients rather than merely for their care and safety.

Mrs. Gambino might have some leeway to do just that in the case of Miss Merryweather. Perhaps institutional policies have been too rigid. Perhaps commitment to the Partnership Model may have been overdone. Perhaps exceptions should be made in institutional policy pertaining to residents having food in their rooms. If the nurse is an advocate for the autonomy of the client, as well as her medical welfare, these are all legitimate questions for Mrs. Gambino.

Mrs. Somerville must face similar questions. For at least some of her patients, institutional policies may be unnecessarily constraining. If these policies are unreasonably depriving participants in the institutions of their freedom to make basic life-style decisions, perhaps the only answer, if the nurse is unsuccessful in advocating for changes in those policies, is for the nurse to leave, seeking a more acceptable institution in which to practice her profession.

However, at least some policies in some institutions make sense. The institutions are serving legitimate purposes, and the policies are plausibly necessary to accomplishing those purposes. Whereas Bayside Elderly Care may not really need to be quite as rigid in imposing its Partnership Model, some limitations on food in rooms may be reasonable in some environments. Certainly, some limits on personal choice are reasonable for those in the military, especially when the requirements are necessary to accomplish important institutional objectives. Placing some limits on weight may be such a limit.

One way to analyze the relationship between autonomy and such external institutional constraints on freedom of choice is to ask whether the participants in such total institutions have freely waived their personal decision-making freedom. If Miss Merryweather and Pvt. Barnes can meaningfully be said to have waived their freedoms in the relevant decision-making areas as part of the price for being in the institution, it makes no sense for them to complain or for the nurses to worry about their complaints. The real question, of course, is whether the clients in either case really consented in any way to the policies under which they are now suffering.

The notion of persons autonomously relinquishing their autonomy has puzzled philosophers at least since the time that Ulysses agreed to have himself bound to the mast of his ship to keep him from resisting the temptations of the sirens. The notion that one can autonomously surrender one's autonomy is generally believed to have some moral limits.[8] It is often held to be morally unacceptable, for example, to voluntarily sell oneself into slavery or other forms of permanent servitude. However, Miss Merryweather's decision to enter Bayside is hardly a surrendering of autonomy of that order of magnitude. Even Pvt. Barnes would appear to be within what most people would consider the reasonable limits of surrendering one's autonomy. Thus, if Miss Merryweather or Pvt. Barnes have knowingly consented to limits and those limits serve some reasonable purpose, it is questionable whether the nurses involved have any reason to pursue the matter further.

There is one additional issue raised by these two cases. The two limits placed on these persons are both at the fringes of what could be called medical decisions. It is because they are vaguely related to health care that nurses find themselves in the decision-making position in the first place. Yet, the choice of where one eats, even if it means challenging the Partnership Model, is not normally considered a "medical" choice. Likewise, obesity is a problem having health implications, but the rigid diet proposed for Pvt. Barnes is not exactly a core medical intervention either.

This can become important when one realizes that the right of refusal of medical intervention, which we shall explore more fully in Chapter 13, is often considered to be preserved even in settings of total institutions where other constraints are the norm.[9] Medical interventions are normally offered for the good of the patient. To the extent that the interventions are only for the patient's good, they are plausibly seen as subject to the autonomous decision-making of the client. Thus even in prisons and military institutions, persons are often seen as having freedom of choice regarding medical intervention, even if they are severely constrained in many of their other choices.

What appears to be interesting about the policies that are constraining Miss Merryweather and Pvt. Barnes is that it is not clear that either is being enforced for the client's welfare. The extra costs and other risks of having food in residents' rooms are surely institutional concerns, not driven out of concern for Miss Merryweather's welfare. Even more so, the concern driving 2nd Lt. Harris is an Army concern, not one exclusively about the health and well-being of the private.

In both cases, nurses find themselves in awkward positions. If the only concerns were the rights, health, and welfare of their clients, and if the nurses were committed to maintaining the clients' autonomy, no problem would exist in respecting the client's wishes. However, in both cases, the nurses may be caught in situations where agendas not focused on the clients' health are driving policies that constrain the nurses as well as the clients. Nurses in such situations must recognize that they are being asked to use their nursing skills for nontraditional purposes. If they cannot resolve the tension by having policies changed in ways that do not jeopardize important institutional objectives, the nurses will have to determine whether they are willing to be used in such programs having objectives well outside the tradition of nursing.

OVERRIDING AUTONOMY

If autonomy is accepted as an independent principle of ethics in addition to the principles of beneficence and nonmaleficence, it is inevitable that eventually it will come into conflict with these principles. There will be circumstances faced by the nurse in which he or she is convinced that what is best for the patient and what the patient is choosing are not the same. In such circumstances the critical question is how autonomy and beneficence (as well as nonmaleficence, if it is a separate principle) relate to one another. Any ethic for nursing must address the question of how these two ethical considerations become intertwined in cases of conflict between them.

One strategy is to give one of them priority over the other. Philosophers sometimes refer to this as lexical ordering (as in a dictionary all "A's" come before any "B's"). A full lexical ordering would place the principle of doing good always superior to or subordinate to autonomy. An alternative strategy is to hold that both are legitimate moral concerns and that neither can be totally subordinated to the other. Holders of such views might insist that the two concerns be balanced, depending on the circumstances of the case. The problem of relating beneficence to autonomy is sometimes avoided because it often turns out that granting persons the freedom to act on their own plans, in fact, also does the most good. That, at least, is what liberal philosophers such as John Stuart Mill have maintained. The interesting cases, however, are those where it is plausible to believe that granting the client a free hand to act on his or her own agenda will result in doing more harm than good. The following cases illustrate this problem.

Case 34: The Patient Who Refuses His Pills

Jesse Hodges is a 21-year-old young man who resides in a halfway house for psychiatric patients. The home has nine residents in a family-type arrangement (men, women, and young adults) and is under the direction of Abe Brown, a social worker, and Mimi Donaldson, a registered nurse. All residents attend school or have jobs and have a high potential to be fully productive members of the community. Jesse is very pleased to be a member of the home and is receiving technical training at a local job training center.

Ordinarily, Jesse presents few problems for Mr. Brown and Ms. Donaldson. He is well-mannered, manages his training and financial allowance with minimal assistance, and might soon be able to live in a less protected environment. During the past few weeks, however, Jesse has had several agitated outbursts at the other residents. One night, he picked a fight with Mr. Brown that resulted in Mr. Brown's physically restraining Jesse and taking him to his room to "cool off." When questioned, Jesse admitted that he was not taking his medication, a mild tranquilizer, that had been prescribed for him since living at the home. The medication was prescribed to help combat the anxiety that Jesse experienced when he first started living at the home and traveling to the training center. Because taking the medication had been a condition of his continued placement in the home, Ms. Donaldson was surprised to learn that Jesse has not been following through with this otherwise routine procedure in his life. Jesse apparently did not like the idea that he *had* to take the medication and did not want his newfound friends at the training center to think that he was "on something" or had a "mental problem."

Ms. Donaldson tried to explain why the medication was necessary for Jesse, but could not induce him to agree that he would take it in the future. When Jesse continues to have agitated spells at home as well as at school, Ms. Donaldson considers limiting Jesse's movie privileges until he demonstrates his willingness to cooperate with his prescribed regimen. It is obvious to her that Jesse needs the medication until he is well adjusted to living in the home. Jesse, however, feels he should decide whether he takes his medication. Does the nurse have the right to limit Jesse's privileges in this manner?

Case 35: The Elderly Patient Who Fears Constipation*

Mr. Johnstone, a mentally alert and physically fit 82-year-old man, was admitted with the diagnosis of acute upper respiratory disease. During the course of his recovery, Mr. Johnstone experienced an uncomfortable episode of constipation. The problem was corrected, however, and the patient soon returned to his normal state of good health.

When it was time to prepare Mr. Johnstone for discharge, Janis Forsyth, his primary nurse, noticed that Mr. Johnstone was having frequent diarrheal bowel movements. When questioned, Mr. Johnstone just chuckled and said that it was no problem. "Better this than being constipated," he stated. Ms. Forsyth and his physician were not convinced that he was entirely well and decided to keep Mr. Johnstone hospitalized for a few more days. Mr. Johnstone loudly objected to this and asserted that he was "just fine."

The physician suspected that Mr. Johnstone might be causing the diarrhea by taking laxatives. Mr. Johnstone denied the charge. Ms. Forsyth, however, thought that the physician's suspicion might be correct. In fact, she had noticed that Mr. Johnstone had a small bag that he kept in his suitcase in the closet. The previous day, he had quickly closed his suitcase and put it in the closet when she walked into the room. When she asked if he needed anything, he was quite defensive and quickly turned on the television.

After relating this episode to the physician, Ms. Forsyth was asked to "do a little detective work" and search for laxatives when Mr. Johnstone was out of his room. Should she search Mr. Johnstone's personal belongings? If she finds any laxatives, can she take them from Mr. Johnstone or prohibit him from taking them? After all, doesn't the patient have some choice over his bowel functions? Or does the fact of hospitalization take away this type of choice?

Case 36: Inflicting Agony to Save a Life

Sally Morganthau was an experienced nurse in the care and treatment of patients suffering from body burns. She was newly assigned as the primary nurse for James Tobias, a 32-year-old man who had been on the burn unit of Parsons County Hospital for 4 weeks. He had suffered 60% body burns (40% first and second degree; 20% third degree) after being trapped in a house fire.

It was clear to the staff that Mr. Tobias would survive his injuries, but his treatment process would be a long and painful one. He would be hospitalized

*Adapted from Morreim H, Donovan A, Huey R, Brimigion J, Fine E: The patient's right to privacy. Nurs Life 2(May/June):35–38, 1982. Used with permission

for months and would face a number of operations. He would probably lose his sight and have limited mobility due to extensive muscle damage in the lower extremities. Of greater concern to the staff was Mr. Tobias' mental distress from his tankings and dressing changes. He often screamed in agony as the staff worked on his dressings. He demanded that they stop, but the team, used to the screams of its patients, continued their efforts, day after day. This particular burn team had an excellent record of pulling patients through for whom survival would have been unprecedented only a few years ago.

One day after his daily tanking and dressing changes had been completed and he had returned to his room, Mr. Tobias asked for Ms. Morganthau. He insisted that no further treatment be performed. He made it clear that he understood that this would mean his possibilities of surviving his injuries would decrease and that if he did survive, his contractures would be worse and his problems even more severe. Yet he insisted that the agony was too much for him and he did not want any further treatment.

Ms. Morganthau spoke with her nursing colleagues and discovered that Mr. Tobias had been demanding that they stop the treatments for over a week. A psychiatric consultant had confirmed that Mr. Tobias was mentally lucid and understood the significance of his decision. Dr. Albertson, the chief of the unit was well aware of Mr. Tobias' feelings. He had seen patients like Mr. Tobias before. Some who had considered refusing further treatment thanked Dr. Albertson and the staff years later for going on with the treatments. Dr. Albertson knew that Mr. Tobias' life was on the line. He was not going to lose a patient he knew he could save. What should Ms. Morganthau do?

Commentary

All three of these cases pose problems of nurses who are considering overriding the autonomy of their clients. The first question to be faced by each of them is whether they are dealing with substantially autonomous clients. If they are not, then whatever the ethical problem is, it is not one involving the conflict of autonomy with other ethical principles such as beneficence.

It is clear that all three patients have made choices that many rational people would not make. Omitting the tranquilizer seems unreasonable, especially if it contributes to the disruptions in living that Jesse Hodges is facing. Mr. Johnstone's behavior, though it involves a relatively trivial problem, does not seem to make much sense. James Tobias' treatment refusal, on the other hand, is literally a matter of life and death. Most reasonable people probably would not make the choices that these patients are making.

Moreover, all three of them are facing conditions that call their mental capacities into question. Jesse Hodges is a psychiatric patient. Mr. Johnstone is elderly, perhaps facing the confusion and disorientation that troubles some of his age-group. James Tobias has recently experienced a major, life-disrupting trauma. It would not be surprising if depression, anxiety, and loss of hope clouded his ability to reason about his treatment. The severe pain may make it impossible for him to compare short-term suffering with the long-term benefits of the tankings.

It is possible that each of these patients suffers from debilities that make them not substantially autonomous decision makers. That is possible, but there is nothing in any of the case reports that supports that conjecture. Jesse Hodges has not been committed to a mental institution. He has not been adjudicated incompetent. In fact, he is living in a halfway house with reasonable hope of gaining even more independence. Mr. Johnstone has not been diagnosed as facing any problems of senility or other mental debilitation that might accompany age. James Tobias has been found mentally competent by a psychiatrist. Furthermore, no effort has been made on behalf of any of these patients to have court interventions to remove their presumption of competence.

It might be argued that the substantive decisions that each has made is good evidence that they are not acting autonomously. The choices are seriously disruptive of their life plans and, in Mr. Tobias' case, likely to result in his death. The fact that persons make unusual choices, choices that most reasonable people similarly situated would not make, however, is not grounds for presuming that they cannot act autonomously. They may, in fact, be incapable of autonomous choice, but there is nothing in any of the case reports to support that conclusion. If Mr. Brown and Ms. Donaldson limit Jesse Hodges' privileges in order to pressure him into taking his medication, they are acting so as to infringe upon his autonomy; they are acting paternalistically. If Miss Forsyth cooperates in a plan to determine whether Mr. Johnstone is taking laxatives and then helps keep him in the hospital beyond the time Mr. Johnstone is ready to go home, she is infringing upon his autonomy and acting paternalistically. If Ms. Morganthau cooperates with Dr. Albertson over the wishes of Mr. Tobias, then Mr. Tobias's autonomy is being infringed upon, and she is acting paternalistically.

That does not necessarily mean that any of these nurses would be doing the morally wrong thing. That would be the proper conclusion if, and only if, it is always wrong to infringe upon a person's autonomy. If autonomy is the more stringent principle, if it "trumps" beneficence, there seems to be little justification for the actions the nurses are contemplating. If, on the other hand, promoting the client's welfare is the dominant moral principle, or even if beneficence and autonomy need to be counterbalanced against each other, presumably on some occasions infringing upon autonomy is acceptable. What conditions must be met for autonomy to be overridden?[10,11]

The most obvious is that there must be good reason for the nurse to be convinced that the patient will really be better off with the paternalistic action. That is possible, but in each of our cases there is some reason to doubt that the patient will be better off. Jesse Hodges will at least lose some of his privileges. He may feel stigmatized if forced to take his medication. Although the medication would appear to help him, it is not absolutely clear that he will benefit from his caretakers' planned intervention. Likewise, Mr. Johnstone might benefit from being separated from the means to perform inappropriate self-medication. On the other hand, he may discover the clandestine search and feel infringed upon. He may simply sign himself out of the hospital and continue taking the medication he thinks he needs. Mr. Tobias seems to have the most to gain from Dr. Albertson's and nurse Morganthau's paternalistic forced treatment. He will in all likelihood live because of it, whereas without it he might die; but he will live in great agony. We shall see in the cases in Chapter 14 that many people hold that it is morally acceptable to refuse treatments that are gravely burdensome, even if the result of such refusal is death. Mr. Tobias will be better off with the forced tankings, provided living is always better than dying, but that is a controversial evaluative judgment. In all cases, the judgments that the patients will be better off with the nurses' interventions need careful assessment.

Even if the patients will be better off with the intervention, it is not immediately clear that the intervention is justified. If the patient is only slightly better off, while his or her autonomy is infringed upon, then those who balance the competing principles might not consider the additional benefit sufficient to tip the scales. Given the controversial and subjective nature of the judgments involved and the fact that a patient's freedom is being infringed upon, many would argue that even if the paternalism is justified, the justification cannot be solely on the basis of the private assessments of a private citizen, even if that citizen happens to be a physician or a nurse. The concern is not primarily over the good intentions of the decision-makers; it is more over the high risk of error in making very complicated, very subjective judgments. Perhaps those who have given their lives to health care and preserving life are not in a good position to judge whether the health benefits justify infringing upon the patient's autonomy. Many would insist that there be some due process, some formal review, before overriding the patient's autonomy.

That review might come from a group like a hospital ethics committee, but such committees normally have no more authority to override autonomy than do individual physicians or nurses. They may have biases as a group, especially those biases that are associated with the health care professions, such as the commitment to the preservation of life. Should a more public review be necessary, such as a court review, before autonomy of patients is overridden?

The final question the nurses in these cases must face is whether even with the best possible conditions it is justifiable to override autonomy. Suppose that in each case, a careful assessment of patient benefit and harm was made and that assessment could be confirmed by some due process (such as judicial review). Assuming that there is no further evidence that the patients involved are incompetent, would a decisive judgment made with formal due process that the patients would be better off if their autonomy were infringed upon justify overriding the patients' wishes? On what grounds?

References

1. Beauchamp TL, Childress JF (eds): Principles of Biomedical Ethics, 2nd ed, pp 59–105. New York, Oxford University Press, 1983
2. Childress JF: Paternalism in Health Care. New York, Oxford University Press, 1982
3. Dworkin G: Moral autonomy. In Engelhardt HT, Callahan D: Morals, Science, and Sociality, pp 156–171. Hastings-on-Hudson, NY, The Hastings Center, 1978
4. Faden R, Beauchamp TL (in collaboration wtih King NNP): A History and Theory of Informed Consent. New York, Oxford University Press, 1986
5. Allen RC, Ferster EA, Weihofen H: Mental Impairment and Legal Incompetency. Englewood Cliffs, NJ, Prentice-Hall, 1968
6. Roth L, Meisel A, Lidz C: Tests of competency to consent to treatment. Am J Psychiatry 134:(3):279–285, 1977

7. Mill JS: On Liberty. New York, The Liberal Arts Press, 1956
8. Winston ME, Winston SM, Appelbaum PS, Rhoden NK: Can a subject consent to a "Ulysses Contract?" Hastings Center Rep 12(4):26–28, 1982
9. Gobert JJ: Psychosurgery, conditioning, and the prisoner's right to refuse "rehabilitation." Virginia Law Review 61:155–196, 1975
10. Gert B, Culver CM: The justification of paternalism. Ethics 89:199–210, 1979
11. Dworkin G: Paternalism. In Wasserstrom R (ed): Morality and the Law, pp 107–126. Belmont, CA, Wadsworth, 1972

Chapter 6

Veracity

Telling the truth in personal communication is another characteristic of actions that many people believe is morally required for reasons other than producing good consequences. Just as the principle of autonomy requires that there be respect for the self-determination of substantially autonomous individuals independent of the fact that such respect will often have good consequences, so the principle of truth-telling requires that the nurse assess whether communication is honest. If truth-telling is a right-making characteristic of actions independent of consequences, then we may have to face cases where being honest will be inconvenient to the nurse, distressing to other health professionals, and even harmful to patients. The cases in this chapter raise problems of honesty in communication.

citation

The problem raised by the first case is that of what the nurse should do when she has information that she is not yet sure is accurate. Assuming that the nurse would feel she has a moral obligation to disclose a piece of information, in this case about the effectiveness of an unusual treatment modality, what should she say during that period when she is still in doubt? Are there some guidelines about when we should feel confident enough about the information that we should act on the duty to disclose?

The next two cases tackle directly the problem of situations where telling the truth may lead to consequences that are bad for the client. Sometimes it is argued that withholding of information is morally different from lying.[1] We say, "I didn't lie—I just didn't tell the whole truth." In these cases, we shall see whether omitting the truth can be morally different from outright lies.

Two special complications arise in the debate over the ethics of telling the truth in health care situations. One is the case in which the competent adult patient makes a specific request of the health care professional to not be told a piece of information that most patients would want to know about or might find material to their decision to participate in a course of treatment. The patient may plead that he does not have the time for the detailed discussion of the complicated research protocol that is being proposed.

He may say that he trusts the research team and is willing to proceed without the details. Or another patient may, when having a breast mass diagnosed, say she would rather not know the details of what is found. She may simply authorize the medical team members to treat in the way they think is reasonable. Should the patient be permitted to waive his or her right to know? If so, does this not violate the duty to deal truthfully with the patient?

The other complication is when family members—often the family of an elderly patient who is perhaps still competent but not fully in charge of his or her day-to-day critical living decisions—ask the nurse or other health professional not to disclose to their ill family member the true gravity of the disease. Does the family have the right to waive the requirements of the principle of truth telling? If so, what does the nurse say to the patient who then asks about his or her condition?

Finally, in this chapter we shall look at the truth-telling problem from the client's perspective. How should the nurse respond to the patient who wants to know his blood pressure reading? Does the patient have the right to the truthful and immediate communication of this kind of information? In many jurisdictions, hospital charts are, by law, available for patients to read.[2,3] Is there a right to health record information, and what should a nurse do who observes the patient reading his chart?

THE CONDITION OF DOUBT

Before tackling the difficult substantive issues of the ethics of truth-telling, a preliminary issue must be addressed. Even if one were to acknowledge a duty to be truthful with well-established and confirmed information, in health care there is a constant evolution of suspicions, trial diagnoses, hunches, and speculations. Information about diagnoses and prognoses gradually evolves, and different members of the health care team have different knowledge during that evolution. There is often a period when physician, nurse, and others are in doubt about what the truth is. This period of uncertainty might be called "the condition of doubt." The following cases show problems the nurse may face when she is confronted with new, preliminary, and uncertain information.

Case 37: The Nurse Epidemiologist and Newborn Morbidity Statistics*

Christine Smith was the Director of Nursing in a county health department that served a population of 350,000 people. In the course of her work, she reviewed statistical data on maternal and infant mortality and morbidity within the county. One day she was struck by the findings that in one large hospital, where 554 women deliverd 559 infants during a 3-month period, 211 multiparous women had episiotomies with fourth-degree extension tears of the perineum. In addition, 10% of the infants born to primiparous women had Apgar scores of zero at 1 minute and at 5 minutes, and 10 of the infants had a score of zero at 10 minutes. All of these infants had been born to women who had had a no-risk-factor

*Based on Smith CS: Outrageous or outraged: A nurse advocate story. Nurs Outlook 28(Oct):624–625, 1980

pregnancy, no significant problems in pregnancy, and an uneventful labor that fell within the norm for the primigravida on the Friedman labor scale. During the postpartum period, there was a 10.3% infection rate for the total group of 559 mothers. Since the infection rate in postpartum women for the United States at that period of time was 3.8%, Mrs. Smith viewed the rate as significant or at least as a rate that warranted further investigation.

In investigating the data and additional literature, Mrs. Smith learned that episiotomies with extended maternal injuries can be caused by a number of variables that would have to be studied to determine ways to reduce the incidence. However, in reviewing high-risk factors for infants, she found that vacuum extraction was identified as a significant factor in newborn morbidity. This method of delivery had been used in delivering all the newborns with zero Apgar scores at the hospital in question.

In presenting her findings to nurses and physicians in the health department and in the community, Mrs. Smith found no support for further study of the problem. Everybody agreed that the data indicated problems in the delivery care at the hospital in question. No one, however, wanted to speak up or take action. Based on her preliminary data and the need for further study, Mrs. Smith was uncertain how far she could (and should) go in reporting the risk factors of delivering a baby in that one hospital.

Case 38: The Nurse Discovering a Possible Arrhythmia

Mortimer Haley had recently joined the North Country HMO through his employment. At 39, he felt healthy, but the HMO asked him to come in for a routine intake physical examination. After the routine history and physical examination were completed by physician Daniel Wordling, Mr. Haley was asked to move to a room down the hall where nurse Jennifer Spandler would take an EKG.

When the leads were attached, Ms. Spandler began the tracings without incident. Mr. Haley's heart rate was slightly elevated, but there was nothing to be alarmed about. Suddenly there was a jump of the needles and a clear abnormality in the pattern. Watching the tracing, Ms. Spandler was startled. She instinctively checked the leads as she had done hundreds of times before. A few seconds later there were two more lurches of the needles in succession, tracing a pattern similar to the previous one. Ms. Spandler was sure that she recognized first a PVC and then a run of two ventricular arrhythmias. She also realized that her slight arousal at the unexpected finding had alerted Mr. Haley. He asked her, "Is anything wrong?" She was fairly sure that there was. How should she respond?

Commentary

These cases pose problems of nurses who have reason to suspect that something is wrong. Were they completely certain, they might very well know what to do. They would apparently not be afraid to speak up if they were certain of their facts and their judgments, but in all three cases, the nurses were in on the process of discovery. Ms.

Spandler was the first to discover what she thought might be PVCs and ventricular tach-ycardia. Mrs. Smith began to be convinced that she had discovered a pattern of increased mortality in newborns involved in instrument-assisted deliveries.

In Ms. Spandler's case, when she was asked by Mr. Haley if there was anything wrong, the easiest and most unobtrusive response would have been, "No, nothing at all." It would also have been untruthful. Ms. Spandler was suspicious that something unusual was taking place and that it was not a result of equipment error. On the other hand, were she to come right out and say to the patient, "You have PVCs and a dangerous ventricular tachycardia," she would be saying more than she was capable of saying. The reality of the situation is that she was in doubt. She was not expected to interpret EKGs, and a hard-and-fast diagnosis on the basis of one PVC and one two-beat run is not possible anyway. Yet she knew that this was something that she normally did not see.

The cases reveal a variety of ways in which nurses can be in doubt. Mrs. Smith was in doubt primarily because in epidemiologic research of this kind, preliminary patterns may emerge that are simply statistical flukes. They may disappear as more data are collected. As a skilled researcher, Mrs. Smith presumably has the capacity to understand and interpret the data such as they are. The problem here is that preliminary data are inherently ambiguous. Were she to go public too early, she would cause needless alarm, damage the reputation of the hospital and its staff, and look foolish in the process. If, on the other hand, she were to hold out and avoid speaking up even when the pattern became clearer, she would be exposing more and more newborn babies to substantial risk.

It is interesting to note that there is some truthful statement that could be said throughout the entire process of data-gathering from the very first discovery of an infant death to the point at which the data are confirmed and reconfirmed by additional investigation. One argument often heard when data are ambiguous is that, since the health professional cannot know for sure, it is wrong to say anything. It is surely wrong to say more than one knows. It would be wrong for Mrs. Smith to report to the newspapers that instrument-assisted delivery has injured babies at a certain hospital when she has not established that fact. She could, however, speak truthfully by describing the appearance of the pattern, together with the degree of uncertainty that exists. If she has done her statistical analysis, she could honestly say, for example, that, after examining this number of patients, an infection rate that is almost three times as high as expected was unlikely to occur by chance. She could honestly say something like this. Whether it is morally correct for her to do so is another matter, but she cannot rely on the fact that the data are not "certain" to justify her saying nothing. Uncertain data justify avoiding a claim of certainty, but only some other kind of moral argument would justify withholding the statement of the facts, such as they are.

Mrs. Smith might argue that the duty to be truthful is subordinated to an assessment of the benefits and harms that are likely to come from speaking up and remaining silent. We shall see in the next sections that it is ethically problematic to subordinate the duty of veracity to calculation of consequences. She might claim that, while she would have a duty to be honest, that does not include a duty to speak up if she is not asked. She might say, "I didn't lie. I simply withheld the truth." Whether this justification of non-disclosure is adequate will depend on whether one believes that withholding the truth is somehow different ethically from actually telling a falsehood. If that is the basis of Mrs.

Smith's willingness to remain silent, then she is in a predicament should anyone, for example , a reporter, happen to ask her if she has found any unusual patterns in her newborn morbidity study.

Most people would acknowledge that at some point, Mrs. Smith has no duty to speak, that, in fact, she probably has a duty to remain silent. For example, if she had found one death at the hospital in question, but none at the others after examining 10 records at each institution, she clearly ought not to go to the press. The suspicion of high risk at this hospital is simply not warranted. The question posed by Mrs. Smith is at what point a piece of information becomes reliable enough that something should be said.

Ms. Spandler is in a slightly different position. The data she has are preliminary, but they will never be subject to a definitive statistical analysis that will convey the level of confidence in the findings. Rather, they will be subject to a much more vague "clinical judgment." Part of Ms. Spandler's problem is that she has much too small a sample on which to base a finding, but equally important is the fact that Ms. Spandler is not the person charged with the interpretation of the data. At the same time, she knows enough about EKGs to know that what she sees is not normal and that the abnormality is probably the patient's rather than that of the equipment. It is simply not truthful to say to Mr. Haley that nothing is wrong. When asked by him if anything is the matter, if Ms. Spandler is to be honest, she will have to avoid saying that everything is fine. She might say any of the following. Which is the most honest answer? Which answer is the most appropriate morally?

1. "There is a pattern in your heart rhythm that needs to be called to Dr. Wordling's attention."
2. "I think I see a ventricular arrhythmia. I am going to have Dr. Wordling check this."
3. "I am not sure what is happening here. I'll have Dr. Wordling come in."
4. "I know ventricular tachycardia when I see it, and you have it."

On what moral grounds, if any, could Ms. Spandler convey that nothing was wrong? What would be the result if she simply refused to answer Mr. Haley's question?

DUTIES AND CONSEQUENCES IN TRUTH-TELLING

Lying and Patient Welfare

Whereas in some cases the ethical problem of truth-telling is trying to decide what the truth is and when it should be disclosed, in many other cases, the truth is only too apparent. The patient is dying, has a serious genetic disease, is diagnosed as being mentally ill, or is facing a possible future of pain and suffering. The traditional pattern of ethics in the health professions has been one of doing what will benefit patients and protect them from harm. That is what the Hippocratic Oath and the tradition of the Florence Nightingale pledge tell us. Yet sometimes clinical professionals have believed that the way they can benefit patients or protect them from harm is to withhold the truth or to tell an outright lie.

More recently, this pattern has been challenged on two grounds. First, there has been increasing doubt that withholding information from patients really benefits them.[4-6] Second, even if, hypothetically, it would benefit them, some maintain that people have a "right to the truth."[7] The following cases explore these controversies.

Case 39: Lying to Protect the Patient*

Cleo Wimmers, a 70-year-old diabetic, developed cyanosis of a toe (left extremity) following a recent below-knee amputation (BKA) of the right extremity. Because of his depression and sense of hopelessness prior to the BKA, the nursing staff lied to the patient when they received a wound culture report of *Pseudomonas* (it was unclear whether the culture report referred to the BKA wound or the toe). They placed an "infection control" sign over his bed and told him that he had a urinary tract infection. They reasoned that since he had been through a great deal of stress, they did not want to contribute to his fears of losing his other leg. It soon became apparent that the infection was definitely in his cyanotic toe. The nursing staff wondered if and when they should tell him the truth. They decided not to tell him anything. Eventually his left foot became gangrenous and required amputation.

Several months later, the nurses decided to present the incident to the Ethics Committee. The patient was invited to tell how he had felt once he learned that the nurses had lied to him. The patient described how his nurses and doctors had reacted when he asked them direct questions about his health. He claimed that they "hid behind their medical authority," and the patient experienced fear and false impressions about what was really going on. He stated, "If I had been told, 'Yes, there is some infection, but we are going to treat it,' it would have been easier for me." Instead, he was afraid that he had a terrible infection that was going to get progressively worse. He understood that the nurses were keeping the truth from him out of the desire to help, but their actions were *not* helpful. They had just made him feel alone.

Case 40: When the Physician Asks Not to Tell

Nurse Patricia Alexander admits patient Donald Vespucci to his room following surgery. His diagnosis is metastatic cancer. The family members have apparently talked with the physician, Dr. Ernest Hester, and know the diagnosis. However, the physician has written an order that the patient should not be told his diagnosis. During the first 2 days following surgery, the patient frequently asks the staff about the results of the surgery, results of laboratory reports, and so on. The physician visits the patient twice but has still not told the patient his diagnosis.

---

*Adapted from Harris E, Schirger-Krebs MJ, Dericks V, Donovan C: Nothing but the truth? Am J Nurs 83:121–122, 1983

The wife and children are finding it difficult to avoid the questions that their family member asks. They keep asking the nurse when the patient will be told his diagnosis (they want the physician to tell him), and the nurse feels caught between the patient's requests, the family's requests, and the physician's order. The nurse firmly believes that the patient has a right to know his condition but does not believe that it is her responsibility to tell him. Should the nurse be put in a situation that requires her to lie when others on the health care team do not follow through with their responsibilities?

Case 41: Deceiving the New Mother Who Asks About her Baby*

Baby T is a healthy, 2-day-old female infant who suddenly stops breathing. Immediate suctioning by the nurse results in spontaneous respirations within 2 minutes. Two hours later the baby is breathing normally and is taken out of the nursery to the mother for a scheduled feeding. The nurse decides not to tell the mother that her baby had stopped breathing. At the end of the feeding time, the mother asks the nurse if there is something wrong with her baby—the baby has slept throughout the feeding time. The nurse reassures the mother by saying, "It is OK for the baby to sleep; sometimes babies just do that."

Commentary

All three of these cases involve what is sometimes called benevolent deceptions. All three patients are told lies, but the motivation of the one doing the lying is benevolent. In all cases, the health professional wanted to protect the patient from the trauma of the bad news. The central ethical question is whether either good motive or the accurate judgment that the patient would be better off not knowing justifies the deception.

It is important in analyzing these cases to distinguish between good motive and right action. Benevolence is acting out of a will to do good. If we were asked to assess the intentions of each of the three health care teams, we would surely find them well motivated. On the other hand, beneficence is a principle of action, not a motive. It holds that one characteristic of actions that tends to make them right is that they will do good.

In the case of Cleo Wimmers, the 70-year-old diabetic suffering from a cyanotic toe, the nurses were sensitive to the trauma that Mr. Wimmers had experienced, and they clearly were motivated out of a concern that he be spared the agony of anticipating another amputation. They were clearly benevolent. It is not as clear that they were beneficent, that they were acting so that they really benefited him. He claimed during the ethics committee meeting that he experienced fear and "false impressions about what was really going on." He says that if he had been told it would have been easier for him. He imagined that something even worse was happening. All of these concerns of the patient suggest that even if a nurse is benevolently motivated, she can still end up harming the patient by withholding the truth.

The same empirical questions arise in the cases of Donald Vespucci (the cancer patient) and Baby T (the infant with respiratory problems). Calculating the full range of

*Case supplied by Ann Cavazos Chen, R.N., B.S.N. Used with permission

possible consequences from disclosing or withholding information is terribly complicated. It is increasingly recognized that even well-motivated health professionals are
likely to err in making such calculations. Since any of these disclosures would be emotionally difficult for physicians or nurses, the health professional has a vested interest in
having the calculation of consequences come out against disclosure. Perhaps that explains why controversial decisions often come out against disclosure.

There are other compounding factors in calculating whether disclosure does more
harm than good. Often health professionals are inclined to apply the so-called golden
rule. They ask, "If I were in the patient's position , would I want to be told this bad
news." The golden rule, applied in this way, can be very dangerous, however. At best, it
discloses what the health care professional would want to happen. The health professional, however, may have very different values from those of the patient. They may
have different psychological makeups. For instance, it is reported that physicians may
have an unusually high fear of death. That might have led Dr. Hester to write the order
against disclosure. He might have truthfully been able to say, "If I were in the patient's
position, I would not want to be told."

One problem with the golden rule is that, if one really adopts the patient's position,
one must be certain to adopt the value system, the psychological profile, and the social
characteristics of the patient. That, of course, is difficult, perhaps impossible, to do. On
the other hand, asking what a person with the physician's or nurse's values would want
done about a disclosure is clearly not the right question.

Aside from the difficulties in resolving these issues by calculating what will do the
most good for the patient, many people would argue that that is not really the relevant
question in the first place. Some would hold that the patients in these cases have a right
to the truth regardless of whether the truth makes them better or worse off. If truth-telling is a characteristic of actions that makes them right, then perhaps it is wrong to lie,
even if it were granted that in a particular instance it would do good. Many philosophers
(Immanuel Kant is probably the most famous one) hold that one's ethical duty in such
situations cannot be determined solely by the consequences. They give various accounts
of why it would be wrong to lie, even to obtain good consequences. Some say, for example, that there is an implied promise when relationships are established that communication will be honest and open. Purposeful deception, such as that experienced by
Cleo Wimmers when he was told that he had a urinary tract infection, violates the trust
that is presumed by both parties of a communication.

Health professionals are shifting in their assessment of this problem. Physicians,
for example, used to hold that deceiving the patient is acceptable, even required, provided it will benefit the patient. Increasingly, however, they are shifting in the direction
of recognizing that there is an ethical duty to tell the truth, independent of consequences. The American Medical Association's 1980 revision of its principles of ethics,
for example, boldly says, "A physician shall deal honestly with patients...."

Nurses have been more committed to providing patients with honest information.
The first principle of the American Nurses' Association (ANA) *Code for Nurses* includes in its interpretation that "Each client has the moral right...to be given the information necessary for making informed judgments, to be told the possible effects of care,
and to accept, refuse or terminate treatment." While the professional codes of either

physicians or nurses do not necessarily settle the question of what is morally right for members of the group, each profession's code raises questions that are worth addressing in conjunction with these cases.

Even if the nurse does not accept the trend in the direction of honoring the principle of truth-telling, a more pragmatic problem arises when patients such as Cleo Wimmers, Donald Vespucci, and Baby T's mother are not given significant information about their cases. Nurses and physicians have legal obligations, as well as ethical ones. Among these is a requirement that patients be treated with informed consent. Have any of these patients given an adequate consent to the treatment they are receiving? When Dr. Hester writes an order that requires withholding the cancer diagnosis from Donald Vespucci, he is not only treating the patient without an adequately informed consent, he is also requiring Patricia Alexander and her colleagues to do so as well. There probably are times when treatment of patients in violation of the law is called for and is ethically justified. Do any of these cases fall into such a category? If not, what responses are available to the nurses in these cases?

Lying and the Welfare of Others

The previous cases have dealt with the problems of lying for the welfare of the patient, a goal clearly central to the traditional ethics of the health care professions. Sometimes problems of telling the truth arise when one is motivated not out of concern for the welfare of the patient, but rather the welfare of other parties. The next three cases examine, in turn, lying to protect a fellow student, a colleague, and oneself.

Case 42: Covering Up for a Fellow Student*

Student A was the team leader on a medical unit. Student B was a part of Student A's clinical group. A newly divorced woman and mother of two children, Student B has experienced a personality conflict with the clinical instructor during the clinical rotation. Student B was advised that she was in danger of failing her clinical experience.

On the day that Student A was Team Leader, Student B was assigned to an elderly man with a history of cardiovascular disease and poor venous access. He was hospitalized for treatment of diabetes mellitus. That day he was scheduled for an oral glucose tolerance test requiring five blood samples at intervals of 30 minutes, 1 hour, 2 hours, 3 hours, and 4 hours. Since the hospital lacks transportation services for this type of testing, the nurse is responsible for taking the patient to the laboratory for the appointed blood samples. Student B failed to remember to bring the patient to the laboratory for the 1-hour and 3-hour samples. She did not inform anyone of this fact until the end of the day.

When reporting to Student A, Student B beggged her friend not to inform the clinical instructor of the forgotten blood samples and the fact that the test would have to be repeated the following day. Student A agreed not to tell the

*Case supplied by Leslie G. Potter, R.N., B.S.N. Used with permission

instructor, since the students were friends and she did not want Student B to receive any more criticism from the instructor. When the instructor asked Student A for her final report of the day, she specifically asked if the patient's test had been completed without incident. Should Student A tell the truth?

Case 43: Telling the Family of the Deceased About a Mistake?

Nurse Hodges telephoned the resident on call when a newly admitted patient (for observation following car accident, age 46, history of asthma) developed severe shortness of breath and cyanosis. By the time the sleepy and somewhat disoriented resident came to the unit, the nurse had alerted the ICC and was beginning to intubate the patient. The resident took over and decided to do a hasty tracheotomy before transporting the patient to ICU. In doing the tracheotomy, he severed a major blood vessel, and the patient lost a great deal of blood. A tracheal tube was put in place, however, and the patient was quickly transported to the ICU. At that point, the nurse realized that the portable oxygen tank did not seem to be functioning properly. The patient remained cyanotic and was brought to the ICU. The patient never regained consciousness and died 2 days later. Death was not related to injuries from the car accident.

When the husband comes to the unit to pick up the deceased's belongings, the nurse struggles with whether or not she should tell the husband the truth about the "mistakes" that were made in the care and treatment of his wife.

Case 44: Lying to Cover Up Your Past

Janet Miller has recently completed a 6-month rehabilitation program for alcoholism. Having been an experienced and competent critical care nurse at Memorial Hospital for many years, Janet applied for a new position in another part of the city. She was aware that she was under investigation by the license registration body in her state, but she also knew that while the investigation was in progress, she was still regarded as a fully licensed RN.

In speaking to potential employers, Janet is open about her reasons for leaving her previous employment and about her subsequent treatment. However, she experiences difficulty securing employment because of the reference being given by her previous employer. She begins to wonder if she should lie about her alcohol problem and her employment at Memorial Hospital.

Commentary

In these three cases, unlike the ones in the previous section, the nondisclosures being contemplated are not directly for the benefit of clients. The student who asks that her fellow student withhold information about the failure to take the patient to the laboratory, was motivated out of her own interest, possibly even to the detriment of the client whose omitted tests might go unnoticed. When Nurse Hodges contemplates withholding the truth about the resident's mistake, it is surely not for the benefit of the client. Conceivably it could be argued that it was for the benefit of the client's family. (It would spare them the agony of knowing the truth about the irreverisble disaster that had taken place), but realistically it is primarily for the benefit of the resident. Withholding the information for the family could, in fact, prohibit them from taking actions that are very much in their interest, such as suing for damages. Janet Miller's proposed plan to lie about her history of alcoholism is obviously for her own welfare, not that of patients.

If this is true, then none of these dishonesties and nondisclosures is open to the most obvious defenses of the earlier cases. It cannot realistically be argued that at least the lie was for the benefit of the patient. The question then becomes one of whether nurses have the right or even the duty to violate the principle of truth-telling when the welfare of any of these other parties is at stake.

One possible justification of dishonesty is that the one to whom the lie was told is not deserving of the truth. Kant and many other philosophers have contemplated this dilemma. An example is whether a Nazi era German hiding a Jew in his house should respond truthfully when asked about it by a Nazi. Some have argued that lying is acceptable in such a case because the Nazi has no right to the truth. There has been no bond established in which truthfulness is expected. There is no right to information to be used for evil purposes.

Whether or not one accepts this qualification of the truth-telling principle, it is hard to see that it would apply in any of our cases. Possibly the student could argue that she was unfairly in jeopardy because the clinical instructor "had it in for her." It would be hard to introduce a similar argument in the other two cases.

That would leave the defender of the deceptions in these three cases only with arguments based exclusively on consequences. We have already seen that even if it could be shown that the consequences would be better, on balance, with the deception than with the truth, many people hold that there is a duty to be truthful.

COMPLICATIONS IN TRUTH-TELLING

When the Patient Asks Not to Be Told

Case 45: Please Don't Tell Me I'm Blind

Gregory Hanson was a 22-year-old man admitted to the burn unit of a large acute care center. He had been burned by igniting chemicals at a small chemical processing plant outside the city limits. Quickly transported to the medical center, Mr. Hanson was found to have second- and third-degree burns over 25% of his body, mainly on his upper torso, face, and neck. Several of his co-workers had died in the fire, while others would have long-term disabilities from their burns. Mr. Hanson, however, was considered lucky. It did not appear that he would have any loss of limb or muscle function. He would have severe facial disfigurement and would need extensive restorative repair to his ears, nose, and lips. His left eye was removed shortly after the burn incident, and there was some doubt whether the sight in his right eye could be preserved. Despite these problems and uncertainties, it was felt that Mr. Hanson would recover from his injuries satisfactorily. Depending on whether his sight could be preserved, there was reason to believe that he could return to work and remain a contributing member of society.

Marsha Bannister had given nursing care to Mr. Hanson for several weeks. They had developed a good relationship, and Mr. Hanson shared some of his concerns about his condition and the painful treatment for his burns. While depressed over his facial disfigurement and the prospect of multiple surgical procedures to reconstruct his nose, ears, and lips, he was most concerned about the strong possibility of losing his sight and being blind for the rest of his life. The possibility of blindness was so disturbing to him, that he told his physicians and Miss Bannister that he did not really want to know the condition of his sight at the present time. He felt that he could not emotionally deal with the prospect of blindess while going through the painful burn treatments and the healing of the facial scars. "If you find out that my eyesight is lost," he said, "please don't tell me. It would be more than I can bear at the present time. Please allow me to hope that my eyesight might be preserved. I don't know what I'd do to myself if I thought that I would be blind for the rest of my life. Please don't tell me this."

As the days went by, it became more apparent to the consulting opthalmologist and to Miss Bannister that Mr. Hanson's sight could not be restored. Miss Bannister felt that her patient should know this in order to make plans for his future, but he had emphatically told her that he did not want to know this information. Should Miss Bannister tell him anyway?

Commentary

Cases such as this, in which the patient himself asks that information not be disclosed, require additional analysis. We have seen that there are two reasons for supporting truthtelling to patients. First, often, but not always, it is the case that the expected consequences will be better if the patient knows his or her condition. Patients may worry if they do not understand their situations; they may not be able to prepare adequately for their treatment and their other life needs. Second, some people argue that truth-telling is simply a moral requirement even if it does not produce the best consequences in every case.

The situation in which the patient himself requests nondisclosure of some information that normally would be disclosed requires reassessment of both reasons supporting disclosure. Those who argue for disclosure on the grounds that it will normally produce better consequences need to take into account that the patient has some reason for not wanting the sensitive information. If the patient is saying that he does not want it, there is good reason to suspect that the consequences of the disclosure will not be good.

Of course, those who insist that telling the truth is a right-making characteristic that is still morally relevant regardless of the consequences will not be swayed by such reasoning. Is there a duty to be honest that derives from the principle of truth-telling in such cases?

The duty to be truthful, if it exists independent of the consequences, is based on the expectations of the relationship that is established between two people. One philosopher argues that lying is a breaking of the implied commitment that persons normally make when they communicate with one another. If that is so, then the duty to tell the truth would exist only when honesty is the expectation. In certain unusual situations, people actually do not expect honest and reasonably complete disclosure. No one would accuse a magician of violating the norms of truth-telling when he deceives his audience. Likewise, many would argue that health professionals are not violating any expectation of fidelity if they fail to be honest because a patient has asked that they not be. This reasoning would suggest that in cases where the patient has requested nondisclosure, there is no duty of truth-telling insofar as the patient and nurse have agreed that certain information be withheld.

Sometimes the problem is analyzed in terms of autonomy. Assuming that the patient is substantially autonomous, the patient should be free to waive any right to information that may exist. Certain rights derived from moral principles can be waived. The right to information might be one of them that autonomous persons can waive.

That seems to let the nurse "off the hook," but there are other moral issues at stake in this case. Even if a principle of autonomy permits one to waive the right to information about his condition under certain circumstances, it does not follow that it is right for the patient to do so. Autonomy gives people the freedom to act, even if their actions are not always the most conscientious and appropriate. The patient may still have to face the question of whether it is morally appropriate to waive crucial information about his condition. Just as a principle of autonomy may require that persons be allowed to engage in foolishly dangerous or otherwise immoral actions, so, too, persons may be free to refuse information, but it does not make it right for them to do so. If persons have a duty to be responsible for their own health and well-being and the information in question is necessary for responsible decision-making, asking not to be given the information might be irresponsible. Should the nurse in this case attempt to encourage the patient to accept the information and take responsibility for its use?

When the Family Asks Not to Tell

Case 46: Fetal Death in the Labor Room: Should the Nurse Tell the Patient?*

Nurse Sally Majeski has admitted a new patient: Mrs. Feedham, a 36-year-old (G-2, P-1) of 28 weeks' gestation. The admitting diagnosis is eclampsia, acute glomerulonephritis, and intrauterine growth retardation. Mrs. Feedham is placed in a quiet room and given a parenteral administration of magnesium sulfate. The admission assessment reveals that Mrs. Feedham has hypertension, proteinuria, epigastric pain, a severe headache, and blurred vision. Abdominal palpation reveals that the abdomen is soft but irritable, a uterus small for dates, and a faint, rapid fetal heartbeat. The patient is easily startled and appears tense, restless, and unable to concentrate.

Ms. Majewski learns that the patient and her husband have been planning for this baby for a long time. They have a 6-year-old daughter who eagerly looks

*Case supplied by Christine Way, R.N., M.S. Used with permission

forward to having a brother or sister. Ms. Majewski learns, from reading the physician's notes, that the physician hopes that conservative treatment will stabilize Mrs. Feedham's renal condition. If the renal condition does not stabilize, then he will propose a treatment that is, unfortunately, potentially detrimental to the survival of the fetus. Mrs. Feedham expresses concern about her baby, but does not seem to realize that the treatment of her renal condition may require medication that will be harmful to the fetus.

On the following day, Ms. Majewski is again assigned to care for Mrs. Feedham. Her condition has not improved since admission. The physician has discussed Mrs. Feedham's condition with her husband, and he has consented to the administration of the renal medication with the understanding that such treatment will greatly diminish the fetus' chances of survival. The husband has agreed not to discuss the matter with his wife because of her condition—additional stress would only increase the danger of her condition.

Ms. Majewski remains in the labor room with Mrs. Feedham during most of the day, checking on the treatment per intravenous infusion, and checking on her vital signs and those of the fetus. Mrs. Feedham, although heavily sedated, repeatedly asks, "How is the baby doing?" Ms. Majeski can see the fetus' erratic heartbeats on the fetal monitor, but does not tell the patient. Instead, she urges her to rest and not to worry. Finally, the heart rate tracings on the monitor became a flat line. Soon after this, Mrs. Feedham arouses from her semistuperous state and specifically asks , "What is the baby's heartbeat?" Ms. Majewski replies, "Sh-h-h, just try to rest." When she informs the head nurse that she does not think she can remain in the room any longer and deceive the patient, the head nurse replies, "I know that this situation is difficult, but we must do what is best for the mother regardless of the guilt that we might feel." Ms. Majewski does not find this to be an adequate explanation of the moral distress she is experiencing.

Case 47: Protecting Dad from the Bad News*

Ralph Bradley, a recently widowed man in his mid-60s , was discharged from the hospital following exploratory surgery that disclosed cancer of the colon with metastasis involving the lymph nodes. His physician referred him to a community health agency for nursing care follow-up. In reading the referral, the nurse learned that Mr. Bradley had been living with a married daughter and her family since his wife's death. An unmarried daughter apparently lived nearby, visiting him regularly and helping with his daily care. The referral did not explain what, if anything, the patient had been told by his physician concerning his condition.

During the first home visit it became apparent that Mr. Bradley did not know that the tumor removed from his body had been diagnosed as cancer and

---

*Adapted from Yarling RR: Ethical analysis of a nursing problem: The scope of nursing practice in disclosing the truth to terminal patients. Part I. Supervisor Nurse 9:40–50, 1978

that it had metastasized to nearby organs. He did not realize the seriousness of his condition. However, Mr. Bradley did express concern about his health. He complained of vague pain in the abdomen, asked for information about the results of tests performed before discharge from the hospital, and wanted to know how soon he would be able to return to his work as a cabinet maker. When the nurse avoided a direct answer to these questions, Mr. Bradley asked directly, "Is everything all right?" The married daughter, who was present when her father was asking these questions, assured him that, of course, everything was all right and he would be up and around the house in no time at all.

Walking the nurse to her car when the visit was over, the married daughter confided that it was the family's wish that their father not be told how serious his condition was. She said that their mother's recent death had been very difficult for him to accept. They did not want him to be further burdened with the knowledge of his condition. The nurse listened, acknowledging the difficulties posed by the wife's recent death and the father's serious condition. She told the daughter, however, that it would be very difficult, if not impossible, for anyone from her agency to continue to provide nursing care to Mr. Bradley without his knowledge of his condition.

When she returned to her office, the nurse discussed Mr. Bradley's situation with her supervisor. The nurse did not want to continue visiting the patient knowing that he was being deceived by his physician and family. The supervisor suggested that she consult with the attending physician as soon as possible, explaining that Mr. Bradley was asking questions about his condition. Luckily, the nurse was able to reach the physician before it was time to make the next home visit. She asked the physician what the patient had been told about his condition. The physician said that Mr. Bradley had not been told that he had cancer at the family's request. He said that he agreed with the family that Mr. Bradley probably could not withstand the anxiety of knowing he had a terminal illness so soon after his wife's death. The physician also expressed concern about Mr. Bradley's daughters who, as he put it, "need a little time to accept the mother's death as well as accept the impending death of the old man." The physician went on to state that he would consider any act of disclosure on the nurse's part, at this time, to be inappropriate to her role as a visiting nurse and inconsistent with the well-being of his patient and the patient's family.

Commentary

The cases of Mrs. Feedham and Mr. Bradley are like the case of Mr. Hanson preceding it in that someone has waived the right of information that may exist. In these cases, however, it is not the patient, but a family member who has waived the right. Thus the question becomes one of whether the family has the authority to waive any claims to diagnosis, prognosis, and other information that the patient may possess.

As with the previous cases, in analyzing the ethical issues we might first assess the consequences of disclosure and nondisclosure. Whereas in Mr. Hanson's case, the patient's own request revealed evidence of the bad consequences that might result from the disclosure, that is not so in the cases of Mrs. Feedham and Mr. Bradley. These two cases are much like the earlier ones in which the health professionals were trying to guess at the consequences of telling or not telling the patient. We saw in the earlier cases, where health professionals were trying to make such a judgment, that there is a great deal of room for error in the assessment of consequences. The same problem exists when family members are the ones deciding that the patient would be better off not knowing. The only difference to consider is whether the family members might be better able to assess the impacts of the bad news on their loved ones than would health professionals.

Next we should assess the possible impact of a principle of truth-telling. In the case of Mr. Hanson, we saw that some would argue that the principle gives the patient a right to information, but that that right may justifiably be waived if the patient has good reason not to want the information. Do family members have the authority to waive rights claims of the patient? In some cases they might. For example, if the patient were totally incompetent, many would argue that the family has not only the right but the duty to serve the incompetent one's interests. It might be argued that totally incompetent persons have no right to information at all. If they do, could family members waive it on their behalf on the grounds that it was in their interests not to have it?

In the cases of Mrs. Feedham and Mr. Bradley there is no evidence presented that they are in any way incompetent. They are seriously ill, but apparently not rendered incapable of making autonomous choices about their care. If the information is needed to help make those choices, then the role of the family in waiving the patient's rights is suspect. Both autonomy and truth-telling appear to militate against permitting family members a role in granting nurses or other health professionals the right to withhold information or deceive patients.

Mrs. Feedham's case is complicated by the fact that the life and welfare of a 28-week fetus is also at stake. Would the interests of the fetus justify treating Mrs. Feedham differently from other competent adults? Several factors need to be taken into account in making this judgment. First, Mrs. Feedham apparently has the legal right to abort her fetus, assuming that were necessary to protect her own health. Second, even if the medical staff could obtain a court order to treat Mrs. Feedham in some special manner against her consent in order to protect the fetus, the resulting order would not be one of authorizing the risky treatment. It would more likely be one blocking it. In fact, Mrs. Feedham might actually have preferred to take the risk of more conservative therapy in an effort to save the fetus. Without knowing the choices being made about her care, that is a choice she cannot make. Withholding the information about the risk to the fetus of the more aggressive treatment deprives Mrs. Feedham not only of her right to consent to the treatment, but also of her right to determine what shall be done to protect her fetus.

In Mr. Bradley's case, these complications do not arise. The physician who made the original decision not to tell Mr. Bradley about his diagnosis and prognosis apparently felt he was justified out of consideration of Mr. Bradley's welfare or that the daughters had the authority to waive Mr. Bradley's right to know. The community health agency nurse was therefore left in a position similar to that of nurse Majewski of trying to work within a moral framework established by agreement between the physician and the family. Assuming that they find the nondisclosure objectionable, on what basis can these nurses continue to treat?

If they do continue, they should realize that they are treating patients without their consent. They might well find that not only unethical, but illegal. They may, therefore, want to appeal not only to their supervisors, but also to the legal authorities within their institutions. They may feel obliged to point out that such behavior is not consistent with the ANA *Code for Nurses* or other codes they consider authoritative. Ultimately, they may simply have to refuse to treat.

There is one final moral dimension to these cases of familial requests for nondisclosure. Traditionally, medicine and the other health professions have been bound by a principle of confidentiality, a principle we shall examine in the following chapter. There are various interpretations of that principle. Most bind the health professional, with certain limitations, to avoid revealing information about the patient to others. Mrs. Feedham's and Mr. Bradley's physicians have both broken confidentiality by disclosing the patients' conditions to their families without patient permission. It is conceivable that these were justifiable breaches of confidence, but they were breaches nevertheless. If that is the case, the nurses who cooperate in care are not only treating patients without their consent and potentially violating the norms of truth-telling, they are also collaborating in a breech of the duty of confidentiality.

THE RIGHT TO HEALTH RECORDS

In the cases presented thus far in this chapter, we have examined the consequences of disclosure and nondisclosure and the possible inherent duty to be truthful. We have seen that sometimes it is difficult to determine exactly when the nurse has enough information to disclose (she may be in a condition of doubt), but that once she has enough information, the moral dilemma is approached by assessing both consequences and the implications of the principle of truth-telling. Furthermore, patients may at times waive their right to information, in part because the duty to disclose is based on the expectations of the relationship and in part because patients should be free to act autonomously. It is much harder to establish a similar right of waiver on the part of the family of the patient. If, in some sense, patients are entitled to information about their conditions so that, among other things, they may make intelligent choices about their care, this raises important and controversial issues about the handling of medical and nursing records. The following case raises the issue of who is the moral "owner" of the information in a nursing chart.

Case 48: The Patient Caught Reading the Nursing Notes

Mr. Ellwood Berry had been hospitalized six times in the previous 2 years for treatment of cancer of the prostate that had metastasized to the pelvis. He was often in great pain and had serious red blood cell loss. He had experienced fainting spells that had led to the current hospitalization. When he was hospitalized this time, his blood pressure was 90/50. He was stabilized by a transfusion of 2 units of packed cells.

In the course of his illness, Mr. Berry had become quite knowledgeable about his condition. He knew that his blood pressure and red cell counts were important clinical indicators of his condition. When nurse Charlene MacPherson made her routine rounds, she took Mr. Berry's blood pressure, recording the reading on Mr. Berry's chart. Mr. Berry craned his neck, attempting to see the readings, but he was unsuccessful. He then asked Ms. MacPherson what they were. She became somewhat flustered, saying "They were fine." She quickly left the room.

When Ms. MacPherson came back into the room several minutes later, she found Mr. Berry reading his chart, which had been left on his bedside stand. She scolded Mr. Berry, telling him that it was against the law for patients to see their charts, which, she admitted to herself, she doubted was true. Mr. Berry apologized but explained that he was just trying to find out his blood pressure. In his mind, he thought, "Who is she to tell me I can't even know my own blood pressure? It's my blood pressure. I'm the one paying the bill for her to take it. Why can't I even know what it is?" To whom does the nursing chart information belong?

Commentary

This case follows naturally from the earlier ones dealing with the patient's right to information. The evidence is quite good in this case that Mr. Berry desired the information, that he had some basic understanding of its meaning, and that he was distressed in not receiving it. On grounds of consequences, his case seems to be a good one. On the other hand, other patients might not understand as clearly the meaning of information on the chart. They might become needlessly upset, especially if the nurse cannot explain some of the findings. From the point of view of the benefits and harms, whereas Mr. Berry might have a case, the case for a general rule allowing patients to see their charts is more controversial.

What steps might be taken to overcome the potential harms of patients obtaining information from their charts? Some in the movement for more active patient participation have suggested that it ought to become routine practice for patients to have their charts, together with an explanation of the meaning of what is in them. In fact, in many jurisdictions state law requires giving patients access to charts when they want it. Advocates of reform want to go even further. They maintain that patients would be better off if all patients, not just the curious ones, had their health records explained to them. Some have gone so far as to give the patient a copy of the record routinely so that the patient can carry it with him or her in case the patient moves or changes practitioners.

Regardless of the consequences of withholding the information for the patient, Mr. Berry might be suggesting that he ought to have a right to the information, that these are his blood pressure readings and white cell counts, that he is paying to have the information produced.

The model under which Mr. Berry is operating is radically different from the traditional one. It is one that suggests that the client has engaged the health care team for services while the client remains in charge—a radical contrast to the older, more paternalistic model. There is clearly a breakdown in understanding between Ms. MacPherson and Mr. Berry. Ms. MacPherson must now face several critical questions. First, is there any good reason why Mr. Berry should not be able to get his health care under his model? Second, if there is, should he be able to get it in Ms. MacPherson's hospital? Assuming the hospital has no principled objections to that model, is there any reason why Ms. MacPherson should not be willing to cooperate? If she insists on the more traditional understanding of communication between nurse and patient, should she be able to operate under that model, or should she have to withdraw from caring for patients such as Mr. Berry? What should she do if she is willing to cooperate, but Mr. Berry's physician is not?

References

1. Beauchamp TL, Childress JF (eds): Principles of Biomedical Ethics, 2nd ed, pp 223-224. New York, Oxford University Press, 1983
2. Hayes J: The patient's right of access to his hospital and medical records. Med Trial Techn Q Winter:295–305, 1978
3. Tucker G: Patient access to medical records. Legal Aspects Med Pract 6(Oct):45–50, 1978
4. Bok S: Lying: Moral Choice in Public and Private Life. New York, Pantheon Books, 1978
5. Novack DH, Plumer R, Smith RL, Ochitil H, Morrow GR, Bennett JM: Changes in physicians' attitudes toward telling the cancer patient. JAMA 241:897–900, 1979
6. Veatch RM, Tai E: Talking about death: Patterns of lay and professional change. Ann Am Acad Polit Soc Sci 447:29–45, 1980
7. Kant I: On the supposed right to tell lies from benevolent motives, Abbott TK (trans). Reprinted in Kant I: Critique of Practical Reason and Other Works on the Theory of Ethics, pp 361–365. London, Longmans, 1909 [1797]

Chapter 7

Fidelity

Both autonomy and truth-telling are principles that involve respect for other persons. Sometimes they are treated as aspects of the same moral requirement. Fidelity is another aspect of respecting persons. When commitments are made to others, other things being equal, most people recognize that there is a moral obligation to keep those commitments. Commitment can take many forms. One obvious example is making a promise. Insofar as the promise is made, there is an ethical obligation to keep it, according to people who include a principle of fidelity in their ethics.

This does not necessarily mean that the duty of fidelity is rigid and exceptionless. In some cases, such as when remaining faithful to one's commitments will mean that serious harm is done to another, the requirements of one ethical principle may conflict with those of another. If keeping a promise will mean that serious harm is done, then the principle of beneficence would pull in the direction of breaking the promise, while the principle of fidelity would pull in the direction of keeping it. Here, these partial or *prima facie* duties pull in opposite directions. Whether the commitment is kept or broken will depend on how one relates the demands of the two principles. If, for example, one used only calculations of benefit and harm as the criterion for resolving such conflicts of principle, then promises would never be kept when breaking them does more good than harm. Others, however, give priority to the principle of fidelity, leading to the conclusion that the promise should be kept even if breaking it would do more good. Still others argue that neither principle can take absolute priority, giving rise to an approach in which one "balances" the competing claims and is guided by how weighty the demands of each principle are in a particular case.

The cases in this chapter all raise problems of what it means for the nurse to be faithful. The first group of cases deals with promises made to patients. Sometimes those promises are explicit; sometimes they are implied. One kind of implied promise is the promise to keep confidential information that is disclosed during the course of providing nursing services. If there has been an explicit or implied promise—through the well-established practices of the nursing profession and through the codes of ethics to which nurses have adhered—then nurses have a duty of fidelity to keep such information confidential. That is the issue in the second group of cases in this chapter.

PROMISE-KEEPING

It is widely recognized that acting morally includes the keeping of promises. At least, if there is not good reason to break a promise, it is normally held that promises should be kept. Some people would maintain that this is simply a principle derived from consideration of consequences. If people did not generally have an obligation to keep promises, then the very act of making a promise would be meaningless. Promise-keeping, then, may simply be an aspect of our duty to act on the rules that will generally produce good consequences.

Other people take promise-keeping more seriously. They believe that it is a duty that has independent moral status. It is not just that keeping promises tends to produce good results. Rather, keeping promises is just like respecting autonomy and telling the truth—it is inherently a right-making characteristic of actions.

While most people acknowledge that promises should not be broken trivially, they face a moral conflict when keeping the promise will lead to much worse consequences than would breaking it. They ask whether, in that special case, it is morally permitted (or even morally required) to break the promise. That is the issue in the two cases presented here. A case posing a similar problem is presented at the end of Chapter 4.

Case 49: When Breaking a Promise Might Do Good*

Helene Shifflett was a 79-year-old woman who had been admitted to the hospital on three different occasions during the past year for her "nerves." Now she was complaining of dizziness, weakness, multiple awakenings during the night, as well as early morning awakenings, and generalized pain. Mrs. Shifflett's internist notified the psychiatrist, Dr. Muller, and Mrs. Shifflett was admitted to the psychiatric unit of a large county medical center. Brought to the unit by her son and daughter-in-law, Mrs. Shifflett was obviously quite anxious and wanted to make sure that one of her family members was within touching distance during the initial nursing assessment. Her posture was slightly slumped, and she walked with an unstable, shuffling gait. Except for mild diabetes controlled by diet and mild hypertension controlled by medication, she seemed in good physical condition. She was, however, confused and very frightened of being admitted to the psychiatric unit.

Judith Broughton, an experienced psychiatric nurse, admitted Mrs. Shifflett to the unit and learned some important psychosocial information about her patient. It seemed that Mrs. Shifflett had experienced several losses in recent times, including the death of her husband just over a year ago. She had also been re-

*Case supplied by Nancy L. Hazard, R.N. Used with permission

jected by her middle child, who had always been her favorite. She presently cared for her oldest daughter, who was disabled. She had also raised her granddaughter, but this child had recently moved away to a distant city. She had no living siblings and expressed special concern for a younger sister who had been in a state mental hospital for many years and had died there. Apparently, this sister and Mrs. Shifflett had been very close.

An extensive medical workup was completed, and the results of all tests were essentially within normal. Mrs. Shifflett was started on low doses of Norpramin and clonazepam with some results. She began to smile when spoken to by others, took a slight interest in her appearance, and began to participate in unit activities. Despite these improvements, Dr. Muller thought that a course of electroconvulsive therapy (ECT) should be considered. He asked the social worker to discuss ECT with the family while he and the nurses would begin to discuss it with Mrs. Shifflett.

Mrs. Broughton had established a good relationship with Mrs. Shifflett and felt confident that her patient would consent to ECT. She had taken care of many patients like Mrs. Shifflett who had greatly benefited from this particular form of treatment. She believed in the overall beneficial effects of the therapy in depressed elderly patients who also had good family support and care. Mrs. Shifflett, however, strongly opposed any discussion of a potential course of ECT. After both Mrs. Broughton and Dr. Muller had discussed it with her, she became very agitated and began to show marked signs of mental decompensation. She begged Mrs. Broughton to promise her that she would not "let them do that to me." Mrs. Broughton assured her that they would not harm her and that she had nothing to fear.

In discussing the matter with Mrs. Shifflett's son, it was learned that she had signed a power of attorney shortly before admission to the hospital, giving her son the authority to handle all her affairs. Since she was still the sole provider for her disabled daughter, this had seemed a wise thing to do while she was in the hospital. The social worker had informed the son that he could authorize the ECT for his mother, based on the legal powers that he already had for her care and her affairs. Yet the son was reluctant to sign for the therapy knowing how frightened it made his mother. However, he also realized that the ECT would probably improve her mental status to the point where she could return home and live without fears. He was convinced that the procedure was safe and promised great benefit to his mother. He decided to seek the advice of Mrs. Broughton in helping him to decide whether he should agree to the treatment for his mother. He told Mrs. Broughton, "If you and Dr. Muller think that ECT will help my mother, then I will sign the papers agreeing to the therapy. What do you think is best for my mother?"

Mrs. Broughton was torn between her promise to the patient that she would not let anything harm her and her knowledge of the beneficial effects of ECT. While Mrs. Broughton did not think ECT was harmful, Mrs. Shifflett certainly perceived it as something harmful. Thus, Mrs. Broughton was very uncomfortable with the son's questions. She also realized that her comments would more than likely sway the son to sign or not sign the forms. At the same time, however, she could see Mrs. Shifflett's mental condition deteriorating each day. She was uncertain how she should respond to the son.

Commentary

Several strategies of moral reasoning are available to Mrs. Broughton. One conspicuous possibility is that she could finesse the problem of keeping the promise if she reasoned that she was not actually breaking the promise she had made. She did not promise Mrs. Shifflett that she would keep the medical staff from doing the ECT. She promised that she would not let them harm her. Assuming that Mrs. Broughton concurs with Dr. Muller and Mrs. Shifflett's son that the ECT will help rather than harm, she might try to convince herself that she would not be breaking her promise if she failed to speak up against the ECT.

This may not be accurate even at face value. Mrs. Broughton realizes that Mrs. Shifflett would perceive the ECT as a harm, and she would at least be upset. So it may not really be accurate to say that she will not be harmed. She would also need to face the question of what keeping her patient from harm really means. We saw in Chapter 3 that some people, when they speak of not harming, have in mind the net amount of benefits over harms, so that a person who receives more benefit than harm could be said not to be harmed. Others, however, distinguish between harming and helping in such a way that if there was some harm (such as the discomfort of the ECT), they would say that harm was done, even though more good was done on balance. If Mrs. Shifflett takes the latter stance, she would have to admit that harm was to be done even if the end result would be good on balance. It is going to be hard for Mrs. Broughton to argue that she is not breaking her promise to avoid harm.

More critically, she may be obliged to take into account the spirit of the promise. It appears that what Mrs. Shifflett really wanted (and what she probably thought she received) was a promise to protect her against ECT. If that was what was implied, it is deceptive and hardly respecting persons for Mrs. Broughton to rationalize her way out of a moral dilemma by arguing that, technically, she never promised to prevent the ECT, only to protect Mrs. Shifflett from harm.

The core moral problem faced by Mrs. Broughton is really whether it is justifiable to break a promise (or at least an implied promise). It might be that it is acceptable to break promises when (and only when) more good will come from breaking the promise than keeping it. If that is the case, Mrs. Broughton would be justified in calculating carefully all the good that could come from breaking her promise. She would, of course, also have to take into account all the evils that could result from breaking the promise: the possibility that Mrs. Stifflett would no longer trust the staff and that she would never return to the institution in the future, as well as the possible physical harm that could result from the ECT. True consequentialists who focus on individual acts would say that promises can be broken morally whenever the benefit outweighs the harm on balance (taking into account all the subtle harms).

On the other hand, other consequentialists use another approach, one that makes promise-breaking more difficult. These consequentialists say that consequences should be used to assess moral rules and the rule should be adopted that produces more good consequences than any other rule. These consequentialists could consider two possible rules, one that required keeping promises unless more good would come from breaking the promise and another rule that required keeping promises regardless. They might conclude that the latter rule actually would lead to more good than the former even though the former appears to permit more good. They could reach this conclusion if they held that people are likely to make errors in calculations so that the rule "keep promises unless you believe more good would come from breaking them" would actually not lead to as much good as the simpler rule "always keep promises." This would be one way that Mrs. Broughton could conclude that, on grounds of consequences, the promise should be kept even if she believed it would do more good for her patient to break it.

Still another approach is to acknowledge the duty of promise-keeping grounded in the principle of fidelity as a duty independent of consequences. Just as some people hold that there is a duty to respect autonomy or to tell the truth, so they also may hold that it is simply wrong to break promises. While other considerations may be so overwhelming that the promise can be broken in a particular instance, there is still an inclination to regard breaking a promise as wrong. Some overwhelming counter-consideration would have to be brought into play to offset this. The question then becomes one of whether Mrs. Broughton made a promise to protect her patient against ECT in the first place and, if so, whether she has any duty to keep that promise when she believes her patient would be better off if it were broken.

CONFIDENTIALITY

One of the aspects of fidelity is the keeping of confidences. This is one of the classical ethical requirements of professional health care ethics. In virtually all of the codes of ethics of the health care professions, some form of confidentiality requirement has been included. However, the content of those codes is more variable and controversial than might be expected. The key provisions are summarized in the Table 7-1. Note that the Hippocratic Oath is very ambiguous. It calls for confidentiality only in reference to those things "which ought not be spoken abroad." Another group of professionally written codes, including those of the World Medical Association and the Florence Nightingale Pledge, seem to require keeping all confidences without exception. Other codes allow for certain kinds of exceptions. The most frequently cited exception, especially in the older professional codes, is breaking confidence when it is in the interests of the patient to do so. The early American Medical Association Principles of Ethics and early codes of the British Medical Association included such an authorization to break physician confidence. Both codes have been revised, however, dropping this exception. In doing so, health professionals may have run the risk that no client-centered reasons are sufficient to permit breaking confidences. This leaves anyone guided by these codes with a dilemma when, for example, he or she might break a confidence to report clients that appears to be so severely mentally ill that they are a serious danger to themselves.

It is not clear whether the ANA *Code for Nurses* would permit violating confidence in order to protect the welfare of the patient. The Code says, "the right of privacy is an inalienable right of all persons." The use of rights language indicates that this right is one that cannot be overridden simply because of consideration of benefits and harms. This statement also indicates that "only information pertinent to a client's treatment and welfare is disclosed and only to those directly concerned with the client's care."[3(p5)] It further states that "the rights, well-being, and safety of the individual client should be the determining factors in arriving at this decision," leaving the nurse in an ambiguous position if the client's rights require confidentiality and well-being and safety require disclosure.[3(p5)] The next group of cases in this chapter looks at problems of confidentiality when the welfare of the client is at stake.

A second possible exception to the duty of confidentiality is the case in which the serious welfare of other parties is jeopardized by keeping a confidence. Is it clear, for example, that the nurse should break confidence if she knows that her client is a carrier of a serious contagious disease or a parent engaged in child abuse? The earlier version

Table 7-1. Confidentiality in Codes of Medical Ethics

I . . . will hold in confidence all personal matters committed to my knowledge in the practice of my calling

—Florence Nightingale Pledge[1]

The nurse holds in confidence personal information and uses judgment in sharing this information.

—Code for Nurses
International Council of Nurses, 1973[2]

The right to privacy is an inalienable human right. The client trusts the nurse to hold all information in confidence. This trust could be destroyed and the client's welfare jeopardized by injudicious disclosure of information provided in confidence. The duty of confidentiality, however, is not absolute when innocent parties are in direct jeopardy.

—ANA Code for Nurses (1985)[3]

Whatever, in connection with my professional practice, or not in connection with it, I see or hear, in the life of men, which ought not to be spoken abroad, I will not divulge, as reckoning that all such should be kept secret.

—Hippocratic Oath[4]

A physician may not reveal the confidences entrusted to him in the course of medical attendance, or the deficiencies he may observe in the character of his patients, unless he is required to do so by law or unless it becomes necessary in order to protect the welfare of the individual or of the society.

—AMA Principles of Medical Ethics, 1971[5]

of the Principles of Ethics of the AMA permitted breaking confidence when it would protect the welfare of society. That seemed to be a very broad exception, covering virtually any case in which one would reasonably want to break confidence. It did not even require that the risk to society of keeping the confidence be a serious one. When the AMA rewrote its code in 1980, it dropped this exception entirely, leaving the opposite problem: what to do if your client confesses to you a plan to commit a mass murder and you are pledged to base your judgment solely on the basis of the client's well-being. The ANA *Code for Nurses,* in contrast, holds that confidentiality "is not absolute when innocent third parties are in direct jeopardy."[3(p4)] The second group of cases will deal with breaking confidentiality to benefit other identifiable persons or to benefit society in general.

There is a third possible exception: breaking confidentiality when required by law. The current codes of both the British and American Medical Associations endorse

---

A physician shall respect the rights of patients, of colleagues, and of other health professionals, and shall safeguard patient confidences within the constraints of the law.

—*AMA Principles of Medical Ethics, 1980*[6]

It is a practitioner's obligation to observe the rule of professional secrecy by refraining from disclosing voluntarily without the consent of the patient (save with statutory sanction) to any third party information which he has learnt in his professional relationship with the patient. The complications of modern life sometimes create difficulties for the doctor in the application of this principle, and on certain occasions it may be necessary to acquiesce in some modification. Always, however, the overriding consideration must be adoption of a line of conduct that will benefit the patient, or protect his interests.

—*British Medical Association, 1959*[7]

If, in the opinion of the doctor, disclosure of confidential information to a third party seems to be in the best medical interest of the patient, it is the doctor's duty to make every effort to allow the information to be given to the third party, but where the patient refuses, that refusal must be respected.

—*Addition to British Medical Association Principles, 1971*[7]

A doctor owes to his patient absolute secrecy on all which has been confided to him or which he knows because of the confidence entrusted to him.

—*International Code of Medical Ethics,*[8] *World Medical Association, 1949*

I will hold in confidence all that my patient confides in me.

—*Declaration of Geneva, 1948*[9]

breaking confidentiality in these circumstances. The interpretive statements of the 1976 *ANA Code for Nurses* did so, too, but that was dropped from the 1985 interpretive statements. The third group of cases in this chapter will deal with problems of confidentiality in the face of laws that may require disclosure.

The moral basis of the duty of confidentiality is not always clear. Often keeping information confidential will benefit the patient. In those cases, it might be called for by the traditional professional ethical principles that require the nurse to benefit the patient and protect him from harm. That implies, however, that in cases where the nurse believes that a patient could be benefited by a disclosure, the nurse would be justified in disclosing. Moreover, if the welfare of the patient is the criterion for deciding when to keep or break confidences, then the interests of society are excluded. The requirements of law are also excluded.

The *ANA Code for Nurses* suggests a second possibility. It implies—in an ambiguous manner, to be sure—that confidentiality is a right, perhaps a right that is independent of judgments about benefit and harm to the client. According to the *Code for Nurses,* it is grounded in a principle of privacy—a principle requiring that people not have information disclosed about them without their consent. If confidentiality is a right, then benefits to the client would not justify the disclosure.

Grounding confidentiality in a principle of privacy may lead to a strong confidentiality requirement—perhaps too strong. It would seem not to allow for breaking confidence under any circumstances either to protect the client (initiating commitment hearings for a suicidal patient) or others (reporting child abuse).

Another possibility is that confidentiality should be grounded in the ethics of fidelity. Fidelity is another principle of many ethical systems. It, like autonomy and truthtelling, may be a right-making characteristic of ethical action, binding on a person independent of the consequences. If that is the basis, then the critical question is what should health care professionals and clients promise to one another regarding confidentiality. Surely, they would not promise to keep confidences when required by law to break them. To do so would require breaking another promise—obeying the laws of the land. They probably would not promise to each other to keep confidences when there were serious threats of bodily harm to others at stake (although they might promise to keep confidential information when only minor interests of others were involved). Whether they would promise to keep confidences when it was thought to be in the interests of the one to whom the promise was being made—the client, in the case of the nurse—is not clear. If they refused to make such a promise, clients would reasonably be reluctant to disclose important information. If they did make such a promise, then it would impose a moral obligation even when the significant welfare of the client was at stake such as in commitment proceedings.

When the Patient May Be Harmed

Being faithful to a patient normally requires that information transmitted during the course of professional contact be kept confidential. In the traditions of medical ethics, however, health professionals have also been seen as having a duty to benefit the patient and protect the patient from harm. For the nurse, the pledge is to the health, welfare, and safety of the patient. That means that the nurse has a serious ethical problem whenever he or she is convinced that the only way to protect patients from harm is to disclose a piece of information that was transmitted with the assumption of a pledge of confidentiality. The next case in this chapter illustrates the problem.

Case 50: The Pregnant Teenager with Other Health Problems*

Vickie Simpson, the pediatric nurse–practitioner in an ambulatory health clinic, called 15-year-old Melinda into her office. Melinda had been referred to the nurse–practitioner by the fracture clinic. At her 6-month check-up for a difficult ankle fracture, it was discovered that Melinda's hemoglobin was below normal. Since her fracture had healed without complications and would require no further follow-up, the fracture clinic nurse had referred Melinda and her mother to Ms. Simpson for evaluation of the low hemoglobin and nutritional counseling.

During the nutrition-counseling session, Melinda confided to Ms. Simpson that she is 6 weeks pregnant. She also told Ms. Simpson that she was scheduled to have an abortion during the following week and did not want her mother to know. At the close of the session, Ms. Simpson invited Melinda's mother into her office to explain the diet and follow-up planned for the low hemoglobin. Melinda's mother expressed concern about her daughter—she seemed so tired lately, has had nausea and has not been eating well, and so on. Were these symptoms caused by her daughter's low hemoglobin? Ms. Simpson is concerned about Melinda. She is convinced that Melinda will have a very difficult time facing her abortion on her own. She believes that Melinda's mother would be understanding and that Melinda would be much better off if her mother were told about her real problem, but she is also committed to confidentiality.

Case 51: When "Doing Good" May Harm the Patient

Joan Schuller, an OB nurse on the night shift, has received an admission from labor and delivery. The patient, Miss Timmons, a 23-year-old unmarried woman, has delivered a healthy female. While getting Miss Timmons settled for the night, she learns that Miss Timmons is planning to give up her child for adoption. Mrs. Schuller is very surprised, since mothers who do not keep their babies are usually admitted to the medical unit rather than the obstetrics unit. Miss Timmons assures the nurse that she knows what she is doing—she has read about the beneficial effects of the bonding process between mother and child immediately after birth, and she wants to give the child everything she can before she gives it up for adoption. She has specifically chosen to deliver her child at this hospital because of its reputation for rooming-in arrangements for mothers and children. There is no indication that Miss Timmons will change her mind about giving the child up for adoption—her life situation simply does not include the

---

*Adapted from Mahon KA, Everson SJ: Moral outrage—Nurses' right or responsibility—Ethics for nurses. J Contin Educ Nurs 10(May/June):4-7, 1979. Used with permission

care of a child. Yet, she wants to care for and breast-feed her infant during her stay in the hospital. She asks the nurse how soon she can see her infant and get started.

Mrs. Schuller pleads for some time while she quickly reviews Miss Timmons' chart. The possibility of adoption is not included on the chart, and Miss Timmons quickly explains that she has not told anyone because she was afraid she would not be able to see and hold her infant if her plan was known. Mrs. Schuller explains that it is very unlikely that she will be allowed to see her infant, let alone have rooming-in and breast-feed the child for several days, if she plans to give the child up for adoption. The hospital has a long-standing policy prohibiting visits between children up for adoption and their natural mothers. She also expresses concern for the psychological harm that Miss Timmons might experience from the process. Giving a child up for adoption is always a difficult process for women, regardless of their circumstances. Once bonding has occurred, giving the child up for adoption often leaves deep psychological scars on the mother that persist for many years. Mrs. Schuller advises Miss Timmons to reconsider her request.

Miss Timmons insists on carrying through with her plan to have rooming-in and breast-feed the infant. She asks the nurse to keep "her secret." Mrs. Schuller realizes that she is in a very awkward position. She recognizes that early contact and bonding between mother and child is very beneficial to both. It is especially important for children up for adoption, since they are often moved from one foster home to another while an adoptive family is found. The OB unit's rooming-in arrangements with mother and child are specifically designed to foster this process. If she keeps Miss Timmons' secret, much good can result, in terms of the health of the child and the wishes of the mother. However, considerable harm could result, in the long run, as well. Mrs. Schuller is not sure whether to keep Miss Timmons' "secret" or not.

Case 52: The ER Patient Who Was Robbed

A 62-year-old woman is brought to the ER with a myocardial infarction, having been found lying by the road in front of her house in a rural community. She is a widow who lives alone and has no previous history of cardiac anomalies. The patient "codes" and is resuscitated. When she regains consciousness, the nurse attempts to gain some information about the patient. The patient asks the nurse if she can "keep a secret." The nurse says "yes," and the patient tells her that a man entered the patient's house after breakfast, robbed her of over $200, and told her that he would kill her if she told anybody. She asks the nurse not to tell the police because she is afraid of the man and thinks he will come back and kill her. In order to calm the patient and help her to rest, the nurse promises that she will not tell anyone about the robbery.

The next day, the ER nurse finds out that the patient "coded" and was resuscitated again while in the MICU. When she is conscious, she yells out in ter-

ror when anyone approaches her bed. Should the ER nurse tell others what the patient told her?

Commentary

Ms. Simpson, the nurse who learns of a young patient's plan for an abortion, seems to be caught in a moral dilemma because her judgment about what is in her client's interest leads her to want to disclose, while her commitment to a promise of confidentiality leads her to want to keep Melinda's trust by remaining silent.

One approach to this case involves an assessment of Ms. Simpson's judgment that Melinda would be better off in the long run if her mother knew about her real problem. Perhaps Ms. Simpson is wrong. Possibly, Melinda knows her mother's reaction better than Ms. Simpson does. One problem with ethical codes that authorize breaking confidence whenever the health professional judges it to be in the patient's interest is that it depends on a very difficult, subjective assessment by the individual practitioner. This would allow individual clinicians to make idiosyncratic judgments about patient interest.

In Ms. Simpson's case, however, her judgment is not unreasonable. Although Melinda might find it uncomfortable for her mother to know, in the long run she might really be better off. That raises the question of whether correct judgments of patient welfare would justify breaking confidentiality. Suppose, for example, that Ms. Simpson took her case to her hospital ethics committee, which confirmed her judgment. Suppose she did everything possible to make sure her judgment was a good one. Would she then be justified in breaking confidence or would Melinda still have a right to confidentiality? If she would, why?

One basis for viewing confidentiality as a right is that it rests on a promise made (at least an implied promise) by health professionals that information disclosed in the course of professional communication will be held confidential. Any nurse who subscribes to the ANA *Code for Nurses* has, in fact, made such a pledge. Breaking it involves more than potential injury to the patient. It also involves breaking a promise, a promise that is important to the lay–professional relationship.

It may also be viewed as violating the autonomy of the patient. If the patient is an autonomous person capable of making choices about medical and nursing care, it is paternalistic to disclose to others information about the patient on the grounds that it would be in the patient's interest to do so.

Some have argued that Ms. Simpson should seek Melinda's permission to disclose her pregnancy to her mother. If Melinda agrees, then Ms. Simpson would no longer be bound by a promise of confidentiality. She would not be acting paternalistically. But what if Melinda refuses to grant permission for Ms. Simpson to tell her mother? Then Ms. Simpson would be back in the same moral bind. If she is committed to doing what she thinks will benefit Melinda, she may feel obliged to break confidence. If she is committed to a morality that insists that promises (such as the promise of confidentiality) should be kept even in cases where breaking them would be beneficial, then she will feel a moral obligation not to disclose.

Some might argue that Melinda, a 15 year old, is, in fact, not an autonomous person who should have the right to insist upon or to waive confidentiality. If she is a minor whose parents must consent to medical treatment, do the normal rules of confidentiality apply?

There is a complicating factor. Many states have laws permitting minors to get abortions without the permission of the parent. If Melinda is in such a state, and she can, therefore, get the abortion without her mother's approval, does that imply that she also has a right to confidentiality (or to waive confidentiality)?

Anyone who concludes that Ms. Simpson has a right or a duty to break confidence in Melinda's case because of her age should turn to the cases of Miss Timmons and the woman who had a heart attack after a robbery. Miss Timmons is an adult, and presumably she could be asked to waive any right to confidentiality she might have. But it seems clear that, if asked, she would not give Mrs. Schuller, the nurse in her case, permission to disclose the fact that she is planning to place the child for adoption. When age is no longer a factor, does Mrs. Schuller have the right to disclose even against Miss Timmons' wishes?

Mrs. Schuller is perplexed, in part, because it is possible that good can come if the secret is kept. On the other hand, harm can come as well. Miss Timmons might be injured psychologically by bonding with the infant she would eventually place for adoption. If Mrs. Schuller concludes that the patients would both be better off if the secret were kept, then there is no real confidentiality problem. There remains a moral problem of whether Mrs. Schuller should be a party to the deception, but that is another matter.

The interesting problem arises if Ms. Schuller concludes that one or both of her patients would really be better off if the disclosure were made. She might possibly conclude that Miss Timmons would be better off if she did not bond with the infant she is going to place for adoption. In that case, Ms. Schuller will have to go through the same reasoning as Melinda's nurse.

It is also possible that Mrs. Schuller could conclude that the infant would be the one that would be better off if the bonding did not take place. In that case, she might be inclined to break confidence for the benefit of the infant. That brings us to the problem of breaking confidences for the benefit of other parties, which is the subject of our next group of cases.

The woman who had a heart attack after a robbery is also an adult. She also could be asked whether, for her own good, she would agree to breaking confidence. There is a good chance she would refuse, as well. In her case, keeping the tension bottled up inside her could well be life-threatening. Perhaps this case is the best test of the three for determining whether one is willing to be paternalistic or whether one will stick to the duty of confidentiality even when there is very good reason to believe that breaking confidence would benefit the patient.

When Others May Be Harmed

In some cases, the nurse may consider breaking the promise of confidentiality not to benefit the client, but to benefit third parties. The nurse may feel that the client's family may need to know some important information about the client's medical condition. The client may, for example, be a carrier of a genetic disease. That information could be important to others in his or her family. If the client refused to disclose the genetic disorder, the nurse might consider whether she has a duty to disclose. In the first case in this section, a son might benefit from learning of his father's terminal illness.

In other cases, the beneficiaries may be much more distant from the patient. The second case in this section deals with a nurse with a drug problem and whether confidential communication between her and another nurse can be disclosed in order to protect future patients, as well as the nurse. Finally, sometimes privacy may be invaded for educational, research, and other benefits for others when there is nothing unique to the patient's condition that is crucial. That is the focus of the third case in this section.

Breaking Confidence to Benefit Another Individual

Case 53: The Dying Father and His Son

Mr. Burns is dying from cancer. His large bowel is riddled with metastatic lesions, and the staff fear that a massive hemorrhage could develop at any time. A widower, Mr. Burns is fully aware of his condition and has decided not to tell his grown children the nature of his condition. He does not want to be a burden to them and has told them that he will be coming home in a few weeks.

One evening, he confides to Martha Spencer, the regular evening shift nurse, that one of his biggest disappointments in life occurred when his youngest son dropped out of college several years ago. Although he is proud of all his other children, his disappointment in the youngest son is quite noticeable and has disrupted their relationship. He expresses hope that the son will be able to straighten out his life in the future, although he will probably not be alive to see this happen.

A week later, one of the family members confides to Ms. Spencer that they have a big surprise for Mr. Burns when he comes home. Mr. Burns' youngest son, who lives in another state and has been estranged from his father for several years, will be coming home to visit his father. The surprise is that the son has been attending college part-time for the last 2 years and will graduate in a few weeks. He plans to surprise his father with his diploma for Mr. Burns' 65th birthday.

Realizing that Mr. Burns may not live long enough to learn of the surprise and that his son might be deprived of winning his father's approval before he dies, Ms. Spencer wonders whether she should break one of her confidences. Or should she break all of them?

Breaking Confidences to Benefit Society

Case 54: The Case of the Nurse Addict

Judy Boise and Claire Temple have been colleagues for a long time—they have worked together at the same hospital for 6 years. Since she obtained a divorce, however, Claire's personality has changed. She often makes silly comments or giggles at inappropriate times. At other times, Claire is very irritable and resorts to taking medication for "her nerves." Judy suspects that her friend is becoming a drug-abuser. Her suspicion is confirmed one day when Claire asks Judy to work for her while she "sleeps off" the effects of some medication. Judy confronts her friend with her suspicions. Claire acknowledges that she has been having trouble and asks Judy not to tell other nurses about the nature of Claire's problems. Judy promises not to tell. The next day, however, Claire almost falls asleep while giving afternoon report. Does Judy have an obligation to break the promise she made to Claire in order to protect both Claire and their patients from unsatisfactory levels of nursing care? How much respect for confidentiality can one expect from a fellow nurse?

Case 55: The Supervisor's Dilemma

Mrs. Phyllis Brock is the supervisor of emergency room and critical care facilities in a large, urban teaching hospital with a famous medical school. She is informed by ER nurses that on weekends, several physicians on the faculty of the medical school are setting up closed circuit video-taping of medical students doing admissions, histories, physical examinations, and so on in the ER. The tapes are being used for teaching purposes to allow students an opportunity to evaluate their own mistakes. The physicians assure the nursing staff that no one else ever sees the films, and the films help medical students give better medical care. However, the nursing staff feel that they are being coerced into participating in the physical exposure of the clients (since the nurse brings the patients into the room and asks them to disrobe), as well as the disclosing of personal information without their consent. The ER nurses appeal to the supervisor, who intercedes with the physicians. She is told that the hospital is a teaching institution, and the films will continue to be taken. If the ER nurses are uncomfortable with the practice, they can refrain from entering the room. But the nurses still know that the practice is going on. The supervisor finds that the practice of taking "training films" on weekends has been going on for several years. The previous nurse supervisor did not find anything objectionable to the practice. The supervisor feels caught between the goals of medical education in a teaching institution and upholding her nurses' obligations to protect the privacy and confidentiality of their clients.

Commentary

In none of these three cases is confidentiality to be broken strictly for the benefit of the patient. In some sense, Claire Temple, the drug-abusing nurse, is a "patient," but even in this situation, an important reason to break confidence is that the welfare of future patients is jeopardized if her problem is not addressed.

The ANA *Code for Nurses* is apparently open to the possibility that a nurse may break confidence for the benefit of others. The code says that privacy is an "inalienable right" and that "all information" should be held in confidence, but then adds that the duty of confidentiality is not absolute when innocent parties are in direct jeopardy.[3(p4)] The nurse trying to follow the code may be confused.

The situation in which an identifiable individual, such as a family member, has a real interest in having the confidentiality broken is perhaps the most powerful case for breaking confidences. Would one stand by with information that a patient is planning a mass murder, for example? Mr. Burns, who is dying of cancer, poses one version of the problem. He might well benefit from the effects of breaking confidence by disclosing to his children that he is dying. He would surely be made happy by the news of his youngest son's progress. Martha Spencer, the nurse in the case, is also concerned about the welfare of the younger son and the fact that he would be deprived of winning his father's approval before his father dies.

This concern for the son's welfare is admittedly not quite like the concern for the potential murder victims of someone planning a murder, but it is an important benefit to another party that would predictably come from breaking the confidence. Are there ways that Ms. Spencer could accomplish the good she is pursuing without disclosing Mr. Burns' condition?

Claire Temple's case, the case of the nurse in drug trouble, is different in that the potential beneficiaries of the disclosure (aside from Claire Temple herself) are not easily identified. It could be that no one would ever benefit. On the other hand, many people could receive substantial benefits in the form of being protected from a dangerously incapacitated nurse.

Claire Temple's case is different in another respect. The duty of confidentiality is, in effect, a promise made to the patient. A right is something that the patient may exercise or waive. If that is the case, the relationship between Claire Temple and her nursing colleague is not necessarily governed by the same moral rules as that between patient and professional. Presumably, there is some kind of promise implied between professional colleagues that generates an expectation of confidentiality, but it is not the explicit commitment made to patients in codes of ethics and professional conduct rules of various state licensing boards. Confidentiality with regard to communications from patients is justified, in part, by therapeutic necessity. Without an expectation of confidentiality, patients would be reluctant to disclose. This is not present in communications among colleagues, at least not in the same way.

The promise to the patient is present in the case of the patients who are being video-taped without their consent for the training of medical students. Moreover, in contrast with all of the previous cases in this chapter, the condition of the patient does not necessitate the concern about breaking confidence. In fact, nothing about these particular patients generates the invasion of privacy. Other patients would serve just as well. It is hard to see what moral reasons would be given for failing to ask permission for the video-taping. Whereas not every patient would approve, probably enough would consent to successfully fulfill the objective of helping students learn interviewing techniques.

One method of assessing the legitimacy of such practices is sometimes referred to as the "criterion of publicity." One asks, "Would we be willing to announce publicly the rule under which we are acting?" In this case, one would ask, "Would we be willing to announce that some patients in the emergency room are being taped for teaching purposes without their knowledge?" The physicians argued in defense of the taping that their hospital was a teaching institution and that patients should be willing to contribute to that goal through the taping. If, in fact, that is their position, they should at least be willing to announce the practice to patients entering the emergency room. That way, if patients would prefer not to receive care on those terms, they could go elsewhere or simply decline the care. Lack of willingness to announce the moral rule under which one is acting is a sign of a moral problem.

The issue is whether a commitment is made to the patient to protect privacy and confidentiality and, if so, under what circumstances. An exceptionless promise would commit the professional to withholding information even about anticipated major crimes and even when reporting is required by law. On the other hand, a promise that would permit breaking of confidence whenever the individual clinician believed it would benefit the patient or benefit some other party probably would not gain the support of either lay persons or health professionals. One plausible exception to the confidentiality promise occurs when the welfare of other parties is significantly threatened if the information is kept confidential. Some people limit the threat to others to "grave bodily harm." Others might include substantial psychological threats as well. Would breaking of confidence be justified under these criteria in the three cases in this section?

When Required by Law

In order to overcome the problems raised by having too many exceptions to the confidentiality requirement, the AMA Principles of Medical Ethics of 1980 appear to permit only one exception: when breaking confidence is required by law. Presumably, the writers had in mind such requirements as reporting gunshot wounds, venereal diseases, and infectious diseases. If the moral community has gathered together and passed a law requiring specifically that certain information be reported, then clearly any implied promise of confidentiality is overturned. Patients have no right to expect confidentiality when a public law requires that information be disclosed.

There may also be cases in which nurses are required to disclose information about a patient. The following case is one example.

Case 56: Minor Children of the Dying Cancer Patient Who Refuses Treatment

A 38-year-old divorced mother of two girls, ages 8 and 10 years, has refused further treatment for metastatic cancer of the larynx. She remains at home and manages quite well with occasional visits from the community health nurse to check on her medications and nutrition. Over a period of weeks, the nurse begins to notice that the patient is losing weight and seems to require more medication to relieve the almost constant pain. She begins to worry about the two daughters, particularly their supervision and their understanding of their mother's condition.

The older child tells the nurse that her mother's appearance and growing dependency on physical assistance frightens her. She also mentions that the school has contacted the home about her sister's poor work in school during recent weeks. Before their mother's illness, both girls were apparently good students. Could the nurse contact the school nurse and let them know about the situation at home? The nurse is not sure if the information she has learned about the patient, her daughters, and the home is confidential or not. She is aware that local law in her jurisdiction requires that health professionals (nurses, as well as physicians) report cases of suspected child abuse or neglect. She suspects that what she is witnessing amounts to child abuse or neglect.

Commentary

The community health nurse who visits this mother with two daughters sees what she fears may constitute child abuse. It is presumably not malicious; rather, it can be explained by the illness of the mother. Nevertheless, the daughters seem to be suffering. It may be that child protective agencies should be contacted. Health professionals have obligations to report child abuse in other contexts, as well. For example, the Baby Doe regulations, designed to protect disabled infants subject to parental nontreatment decisions, require that mechanisms for reporting child abuse be established.[10]

If there is a specific law requiring reporting of child abuse, the ethics of confidentiality is somewhat different from that applying in earlier cases. In those cases, a decision to break confidence was contemplated on the basis of the clinician's judgment that the patient or others would benefit substantially from the disclosure. Patients might have no reason to anticipate the clinician's judgment. In fact the clinician's judgment may be idiosyncratic, one that even colleagues would not share. When a specific law requires reporting, however, lay persons have reason to anticipate that confidences may have to be broken. Moreover, the judgment justifying the disclosure is made in public with due process. It cannot be idiosyncratic. This suggests that in cases where disclosure is required by law, the disclosure will be easier to justify than in the earlier cases.

This leaves the clinical professional with one remaining problem. What should happen in the case where the disclosure is required by law, but the nurse is convinced that it, nevertheless, violates the duties of the clinical relationship? For example, if the law requires reporting of child abuse and the nurse is convinced that reporting of abuse would be a deterrent to the parent's willingness to accept treatment and might result in removal of the child from his home, the nurse who believes that his or her duty is to the client rather than to society may be convinced that it would be immoral to report (thus deterring the parent from getting the treatment and removing the child from his home). The situation may be one in which the clinician is willing to promise confidentiality even though society does not approve of that promise. If a nurse makes such a promise, is it morally or legally binding? If confidentiality is rooted in the ethics of the principle of fidelity, the nurse may find herself occasionally in the bind of having made two contradictory promises: to protect confidential information and to obey the law that requires reporting. What should a nurse do when two contradictory promises are made?

References

1. Tate BL: The Nurse's Dilemma: Ethical Considerations in Nursing Practice, p 72. Geneva, International Council of Nurses, 1977
2. International Council of Nurses: Code for Nurses. 1973
3. American Nurses' Association: Code for Nurses with Interpretive Statements. Kansas City, American Nurses' Association, 1985

4. Edelstein L: The Hippocratic Oath: Text, translation and interpretation. In Temkin O, Temkin CL (eds): Ancient Medicine: Selected Papers of Ludwig Edelstein. p 6. Baltimore, The Johns Hopkins Press, 1967
5. American Medical Association: Judicial Council Opinions and Reports, p 53. Chicago, American Medical Association, 1971
6. American Medical Association: Current Opinions of the Judicial Council of the American Medical Association, p ix. Chicago, American Medical Association, 1984
7. Cited in: Britain Strengthens Confidentiality Clause. JAMA 216:2151, 1971
8. World Medical Association: International Code of Medical Ethics. In Reich WT (ed): Encyclopedia of Bioethics, vol 4, pp 1749–1750. New York, The Free Press, 1978
9. World Medical Association: Declaration of Geneva. World Med J 3(suppl):10-12, 1956; reprinted in Reich WT (ed): Encyclopedia of Bioethics, vol 4, p 1749. New York, The Free Press, 1978
10. US Department of Health and Human Services: Child Abuse and Neglect Prevention and Treatment Program: Final Rule: 45 CFR 1340. Federal Register: Rules and Regulations 50(72):14878–14892, 1985

Chapter 8

Avoiding Killing

In the Western tradition, especially as influenced by Judeo-Christianity, human life has often been viewed as sacred. Holders of this view maintain that human life, especially innocent human life, should not be taken even for noble motives. When life is taken in conditions of war or even serious crime, such action is often justified on the grounds that the people being killed are not innocent. In health care, the problem of taking life emerges in a number of contexts—in abortion, in suicide, and in the decisions about ending the lives of terminally ill or suffering patients. In these cases, however, the lives under consideration are innocent, and justifications for taking life are not easily made. For example, the person whose life is at stake may be pleading for death; in other cases, such as abortion, the individual is in no condition to plead. In some cases, such as suicide, the individual may be contemplating taking his or her own life.

The reasons for contemplation of killing in the health care sphere are usually related to mercy. Someone makes a judgment that the patient would be "better off dead," or perhaps other persons would be better off if the patient were dead. If it is the health professional's duty, at least in certain circumstances, to benefit patients and protect them from harm, can health professionals assist in putting a suffering patient out of misery by hastening a death? Can they actually kill patients who are incapable of making such decisions on their own? Can they withhold or withdraw treatments even knowing that these actions will surely hasten death?

Some people argue that these issues can be resolved by making use of the ethical principles already addressed in earlier chapters. The principles of beneficence and non-maleficence, of doing good and avoiding evil, provide ready arguments to support those who wish to defend merciful killing as well as decisions to withhold or withdraw treatment. In the case of patients who are competent and capable of making their own choices, the principle of autonomy also provides a moral basis for approving of or at least tolerating treatment-refusal decisions by patients. It also helps explain our great reluctance to approve of killing a person who does not want to be killed, even if we have good reason to believe that that person would be better off dead.

There are other arguments against killing for mercy, though, that do not require abandoning traditional intuitions about the morality of killing. Some will argue that the principles of doing good and avoiding evil themselves, if carefully applied, lead to policies prohibiting killing.[1] They point to the risk of well-intentioned persons making erroneous judgments about whether death would benefit the patient. They also point to the danger of malicious persons using such reasoning as a rationalization or excuse for killing the patient who is difficult to care for. These people who believe ethics is a matter of consequences nevertheless maintain that consequences should be used to judge rules of conduct involving killing rather than individual actions of killing. They argue that a rule against killing, even for mercy, will have better consequences than any other rule, including a rule that would permit killing when it is merciful. These people, then, believe they can explain the intuition against killing just on the basis of consequences.

There is one other possibility that might help explain the intuition that killing is wrong. Perhaps there is an ethical principle prohibiting killing of others. Analogous to the position that it is simply wrong to lie or break a promise, it might be that it is simply wrong to kill. This view would be congruent with certain religious traditions (Judaism, for example) that proscribe killing or limit it to special conditions demanded by retributive justice or self-protection.

If one accepts some moral reservations about killing, even in cases where it appears that the patient wants to be killed or when the patient would be benefited from being killed, a number of issues become important. Does the prohibition on killing apply only to active killing or does it also extend to decisions to let a person die? Is there a difference between actions and omissions? If so, do cases of withdrawal of treatment count as actions or omissions? Does a prohibition against killing proscribe behaviors for which the intent is not the death of the patient but in which it is known that death is a risk (risky surgery or research, for example)? And does the request or consent of the person who might be killed justify killing that would otherwise be proscribed? The cases in this chapter are designed to help clarify these issues.

ACTIONS AND OMISSIONS

One of the classical problems in biomedical ethics is that of whether there is a difference between actions and omissions, especially when the result would be the death of the patient. If a patient is inevitably dying (for example, a terminal patient in a coma) many people believe that it is morally preferable to withhold or withdraw treatment than to actively intervene to kill that patient. They would prefer simply omitting treatment to let the patient die, other things being equal. On the other hand, other things are not equal. The patient may not be in a coma. He may be suffering intractable pain. If he is inevitably dying, would it not be morally preferable, under these circumstances, to actively intervene to hasten the death and end the agony? The cases in this section help analyze these issues.

Case 57: Mercy Killing in the Newborn Nursery*

In 1985, Carol Frances Morris, a former nurse at Central Memorial Hospital, pleaded guilty to the 1983 murder of an infant in Central's neonatal intensive care unit. The infant had been born with anencephaly, or lack of cranial development. The infant's skull was an open sore that the nurses packed and layered with gauze to give his face a round appearance. After his birth, the infant was admitted to the neonatal intensive care unit and placed in a bassinet. He was reported to be kicking and breathing, and his heart was beating. The hospital issued him a "live birth" certificate.

Months after the infant's death, Ms. Morris was heard to say that she once "terminated" a dying infant at Central's neonatal unit. An investigation ensued. Following exhumation of the infant's body, an autopsy revealed a quarter-inch bruise over the infant's left chest. The autopsy report was changed to read "death by mechanical compression of the chest."

Central County prosecutors argued that Morris and another nurse, Tanya Jean Simmons, killed the infant. Ms. Morris admitted to compression of the infant's chest in order to stop his heart from beating. She pleaded guilty to manslaughter and faced a possible 20 years' imprisonment at sentencing. Prosecutors charged that Simmons assisted Morris by covering the infant's mouth and nose while Morris compressed her tiny chest. Simmons stood trial for murder and refused to plea bargain, testifying that she did *not* attempt to suffocate the child. She had apparently discussed the hopelessness of the child's condition with Morris and had expressed concern over the trauma and strain the infant was bringing to his family. Simmons, Morris, and other nurses had also apparently debated the morality of "mercy killing." Testimony in the case revolved around the state's definition of death and whether Simmons could reasonably be charged with murder when the infant in question did not have a brain and was, therefore, legally "brain dead" according to state law. At issue was whether or not Simmons' actions could be seen as active killing or simply helping the infant to complete the dying process.

After less than 2 hours of deliberation, the six-man, six-woman jury found Simmons not guilty of first-degree murder. Morris, however, by pleading guilty to voluntary manslaughter, was sentenced to 4 years' imprisonment. Additional legal proceedings involving Simmons are still pending.

Commentary

Increasingly, there is a consensus that not all severely afflicted infants must have all treatments provided that could preserve their lives. The federal regulations that took effect May 15, 1985, allow that infants need not receive life-prolonging medical treatment when

1. The infant is chronically and irreversibly comatose;
2. The provision of such treatment would merely prolong dying, not be effective

---

*The names of the nurses involved in this case have been changed to protect their privacy.

in ameliorating or correcting all of the infant's life-threatening conditions, or otherwise be futile in terms of the survival of the infant; or

3. The provision of such treatment would be virtually futile in terms of the survival of the infant and the treatment itself under such circumstances would be inhumane.

Presumably, the baby under the care of Carol Morris and Tanya Simmons would have qualified under either of the first two exceptions so that, if the parents had asked that treatment not be rendered, withdrawal of medical support would have been acceptable under those regulations. The infant with anencephaly was irreversibly comatose and inevitably dying. Nothing could have been done to preserve the life beyond some additional, apparently useless, extra hours. These nurses, however, were charged with choosing a different course. They actively intervened, and were later accused of manslaughter for their actions. Presumably, since the infant's brain had not developed, it felt nothing; it apparently did not suffer a painful death. One of the nurses pleaded guilty to an illegal death, however. In the United States, it is illegal to kill even if the motive is mercy. Was it ethically different, however, from simply stepping aside and letting the baby die?

Those defending the nurses argued that the baby was already dead because she had no brain function. In some 45 states brain criteria can be used for pronouncing death. If the infant were already dead, presumably the nurses could not be charged with murder. That approach raises several problems, however. First, most anencephalic infants, in fact, have lower brain function permitting them to carry out certain bodily functions. Thus, they would not meet the criteria for death based on brain activity. Second, even if there were no brain activity, this baby had apparently not been pronounced dead. No nurse can assume a patient is dead if death has not been pronounced. Finally, even if they were certain the infant were dead, it would be very hard to explain why nurses had compressed the chest of a dead infant.

The more puzzling problem is whether the nurses considered simply allowing the infant to die, and whether they believed such a course would be morally different from actively intervening in the dying process. If their position was that the infant would not suffer from the active killing, they might have considered showing mercy and hastening the process along. They might, for example, have even given emphasis to the ethical principle of beneficience—the principle that they should do good and avoid evil.

Of course, concluding that killing would do more good than simply letting the patient die would take some argument. It would, first of all, require the belief that killing the infant was itself not a harm (or at least not any more of a harm than if death resulted from simply stepping aside). It would also require an assessment of the benefits that would result from the rapid death. Often, mercy killings are defended because they would relieve the patient of suffering pain or agony. That would not apply in this case, assuming that the anencephalic infant felt no pain. The other possible consideration is benefit to other parties—the suffering parents, the other patients, who were not getting the attention of the nursing staff, or the nurses themselves, who might otherwise have to exert energies expending pointless care for the patient.

The first moral question, especially for a clinical professional, is whether the benefits to any of these other parties count. If they do not, then killing on those grounds would not be acceptable. If they do count (or if it were the patient who would benefit from the killing), we then would have to face the question of whether active killing is wrong when the justifiably considered benefits exceed the harms.

Two types of responses might be offered by critics who oppose the notion that patients can be killed morally when the justifiably considered benefits exceed the harms. Some critics would argue that benefit and harms are the right basis for the moral judgment, but that benefits and harms should be used to assess the moral rules for conduct rather than individual actions. They would say that the expected benefits and harms should be used to choose from alternative possible rules, but that the rules should then be applied without regard to benefit–harm calculations in every case. They might support this approach out of fear that if individuals did the calculations everytime they acted, they might make too many mistakes. Especially when the conditions are emotionally stressful and when the result is irreversible (as would be the case in a possible mercy killing), they conclude that following the rule that tends to produce the best consequences will result in more good overall than having fallible humans make their own judgments in individual cases. It is simply the nature of morality that people live by rules. Once the rules are established (based on the assessment of the consequences), then they should be followed even in cases where the conseuqences in the individual case might not be the best. Critics of the actions of Morris and Simmons might apply this type of reasoning.

Other critics might argue that there is a straightforward moral principle in opposition to killing another human being (even in cases where, hypothetically, it would result in more good than harm). Just as it is simply wrong to break a promise or tell a lie or distribute goods unjustly, so it might be wrong to kill human beings (or possibly even any living creature). Killing another human being simply has wrong-making characteristics. If that were the case, it might explain why many hold that it is wrong to kill.

This explanation would require, of course, that we reassess the alternative of simply letting the baby die rather than killing actively. If the moral principle also includes letting humans die as a wrong-making tendency, it would not explain our intuitive belief that killing is worse. It is hard to imagine that the prohibition could be extended to letting die, however. No human could possibly act on a principle that says it is always wrong to let people die. However, people could act on the principle that it is always wrong to kill people (at least innocent people) actively. If one holds that there is a principle that identifes killing as something that always ought to be avoided and that it does not extend to instances where people are allowed to die, that would help explain the widely held intuition that active killing is morally worse than letting die. The nurses in this case apparently believed that their criterion for action should be to do good, that the good of the family counted even when the patient's welfare was not at stake, and that no general rule or principle against killing prohibited their actions.

CRITERIA FOR JUSTIFIABLE OMISSIONS

Most cases confronting a nurse do not involve proposals for actively killing a patient. They involve treatments that the patient or others deem unacceptable. What is proposed is an omission. Presumably, not every possible treatment should be provided for every patient. What is needed is a set of criteria for justifiable treatment refusal by the patient or agent. From the standpoint of the nurse, the critical question is often, "Am I justified in going along with a decision to treat or omit treatment?" The problem is illustrated by the following case.

Case 58: The Patient Who Was Not Allowed to Die*

Mr. John Corbett was newly retired after 30 years of managing a small truck transport company. He had never married and had no children. His only brother had died the year before his own health problems began, and he did not have many friends. Originally hospitalized for resection of the colon and a colostomy following a bout with cancer of the colon, Mr. Corbett was readmitted several months later with pneumonia following a severe case of the flu. Adult-onset diabetes was also diagnosed on this admission, and he became hypertensive. Now, Mr. Corbett is being admitted again—he apparently tripped on his dog's leash and has suffered a broken hip.

Gretchen Kerns was assigned as Mr. Corbett's primary nurse. Over several weeks, they developed a bantering, congenial relationship. Mr. Corbett frequently referred to himself as "a disaster that found a place to happen," and commented that "Jolly Jack, the Grim Reaper, is coming to get me—the slow way. That is sure not the way I want to go." Soon he was well enough to return home. He did well at home for several weeks with a walker and occasional visits from a home health nurse. Then Mr. Corbett suffered a stroke and was readmitted to the hospital. This time, there were no jokes and bantering. When Ms. Kerns inserted the IV to provide antibiotics for a bladder infection (a three-nurse fight), Mr. Corbett made loud guttural noises, wept, and fought the familiar nurses with flailing arms. When he refused to eat, clenching his jaws and moving his head from side to side, he was force-fed a pureed diet from a syringe until a nasogastric tube was inserted (a four-nurse fight). When Mr. Corbett developed congestive heart failure, his hands were restrained so that nasal O_2 could be administered. It was almost a relief to the nursing staff when he became semicomatose.

Still, it took some juggling to keep Mr. Corbett going. Ms. Kerns regulated his blood sugar, fought multiple bladder infections from his indwelling Foley catheter, replaced infiltrated IVs, and packed pressure sores that multiplied despite turning and massages. His blood pressure dipped and soared, the liquid diet caused diarrhea, and his arthritis caused contractures. When he suffered a respiratory arrest, he was resuscitated. The staff were praised for their fine work. When Mr. Corbett suffered a second arrest 3 days later, some of the staff began to doubt the wisdom of their efforts. Yet Mr. Corbett improved, to the point where he could shout guttural sounds again and fight off Ms. Kerns and the other nurses with his fists. Then his kidneys began to fail, and he was dialyzed.

*Adapted from Huttman B: The bitter end. Am J Nurs 84: 1366–1367, 1984

Eventually, he "stabilized" with dialysis three times a week although his blood gases, electrolytes, cardiac enzymes, urine cultures, and whatever else was tested were always abnormal.

One day when his blood pressure dropped steadily, his physician indicated that they should "let nature take its course." A do not resuscitate (DNR) order was written, and the physician said "goodbye" to the patient. Ms. Kerns, however, refused to follow the order. "You can't do that. We've brought him back before—twice. We can pull him through again. Let's give him some dopamine," she said. She argued with the physician, the rest of the staff, and her supervisor, claiming that everyone deserves to be resuscitated and that she could not participate in euthanasia—"It is morally and legally wrong," she said. The physician obliged Ms. Kerns and rescinded the DNR order. Two days later, Mr. Corbett had a third arrest. Ms. Kerns and the resuscitation team performed expertly. "God gave us the technology to preserve the lives of our patients," she said.

Two months after the first arrest, the sixth resuscitation attempt failed, and Mr. Corbett died. "We did the best we could," Ms. Kerns said proudly. "We gave him the benefit of everything we had to offer." Other members of the nursing staff were bitter. One said, "When I get to heaven, I'll explain to God that I did the best I could for every patient. But who's going to explain to Mr. Corbett?"

Commentary

Ms. Kerns was clearly opposed to euthanasia. She apparently believed that withdrawal of treatment from Mr. Corbett constituted euthansia. The term *euthanasia*, however, is an ambiguous one. Sometimes it means (based on its Greek root) any good death. Sometimes its use is limited to decisions that hasten the death of a critically or terminally ill patient. At other times, its use is limited to active killing for mercy, whereas others use the term more broadly to include decisions to withhold or withdraw treatment such as was contemplated in Mr. Corbett's case.

Legally, there is a clear difference between active killing and simply letting a patient die.[2] Whether there is an ethical difference is a matter of debate.[1,3-5] That is the ethical question that Ms. Kerns ought to be addressing, however. It may be that although omissions are legal even though they can be predicted to hasten death, Ms. Kerns would nonetheless find them morally objectionable. If so, she is within her right to protest omissions and, if necessary, to withdraw from involvement in this patient's care. Should Ms. Kerns consider withholding or withdrawing treatment from Mr. Corbett unethical?

Several different treatments were being considered for Mr. Corbett: an IV for administration of antibiotics, force-feeding, a nasogastric tube, nasal O_2, an indwelling Foley catheter, CPR, and hemodialysis. Each might have to be assessed separately. Some people label treatments that are required *ordinary* and those that are expendable *extraordinary*. That terminology has increasingly been called into question because it is so ambiguous. Many clinicians have equated ordinary with *statistically common* and extraordinary with *unusual*, as the terms might apply in everyday usage. In the moral and legal debate over withholding and withdrawing treatment, however, that is not what the terms have meant.

Others have equated ordinary with *simple* and extraordinary with *complex*. Under that usage, the hemodialyis for Mr. Corbett might be expendable because it is accomplished with a complex machine, whereas the CPR and nasogastric tube might be viewed as more simple.

The President's Commission for the Study of Ethical Problems in Medicine and Biomedical and Behavioral Research considered the distinctions between usual and unusual and between simple and complex as bases for distinguishing between morally required and morally expendable treatments and rejected them.[6(p84)] Instead, it adopted a pair of criteria that were originally developed in Roman Catholic moral theology.[7,8] Treatments are expendable, according to the President's Commission, if they are useless or if the burdens exceed the benefits.[6(pp84-87)] This means that, logically, a very simple treatment such as Mr. Corbett's IV or nasogastric tube could be expendable, just as is his hemodialysis, if such treatment were burdensome to him. The ethics of withholding IVs and nasogastric tubes will be explored more fully in the cases at the end of this chapter. In any case, not everyone agrees that withholding and withdrawing treatment are the same, morally, as active killing. It is clear that in the American legal system they are not the same. It is for Ms. Kerns to determine whether she is willing to accept the morality of withholding or withdrawing treatment, at least in cases where the patient's wishes are that it be withdrawn. Were she to do so, she would be in agreement with the President's Commission and many, but not all, of our religious traditions. However, should she decide that withholding or withdrawing treatment is legal, she would still have to face the question of her own conscience. If her conscience tells her that withholding or withdrawing treatment is *not* moral, then she might decide that she must withdraw from the case. Should she make this choice and other provisions can be made for the nursing care of her patient, her rights need to be respected.

She might be particularly concerned about the fact that the nasogastric tube, the IV, and several other treatments being provided for Mr. Corbett are already in place, so that withdrawing them would appear to be more like actively killing him. The problem of withdrawing treatments already begun is the subject of the next case.

WITHHOLDING AND WITHDRAWING

If withholding certain treatments—those that are useless or disproportionately burdensome—is not considered by everyone to be the same as active killing and therefore might not be prohibited under a principle of avoiding killing, what about withdrawing a treatment once begun? In that case, the nurse or someone else must actively turn off a switch or remove a tube. If the critical distinction is based on whether someone actually makes a movement, then is withdrawing a treatment proscribed under a principle of avoiding killing?

Case 59: Is This Nurse a Killer?*

Mary Rose Robaczynski, a nurse at Maryland General Hospital in Baltimore, was charged with murder. She disconnected the respirator of a comatose patient, 48-

*Saperstein S: Unhooked system, nurse says. Washington Post, March 20, 1979, p C3; Nurse, on trial for murder, called compassionate. The New York Times, March 14, 1979, p A17

year-old Harry Gessner. Mr. Gessner, a former taxicab driver, had been hospitalized with bladder cancer, cirrhosis of the liver, and pneumonia. He suffered heart failure and had stopped breathing. It was claimed during the nurse's trial that he would have died in any case within hours. Asked during the trial if she disconnected the respirator, she said, "Yes, after I felt he had no pulse and no blood pressure." Later pressed on why she did it, she said, "I was trying to act in the best interest of the patient. I felt helpless. I don't know exactly why I did it." At another point, she was quoted as saying, "I only do it to GORKs (patients for whom 'God only really knows' whether they are alive)."

Others, commenting on Ms. Robaczynski's actions, observed that if they were Mr. Gessner with a terrible array of fatal conditions, they would not have wanted further treatment. They would have wanted their respirator disconnected. One critic, however, said, "She was not willing to just wait for him to die. She had to kill him. She murdered him." Testimony was introduced during the trial that Ms. Robaczynski had spoken in favor of mercy killing in cases of comatose patients who had little or no hope of recovery. Was disconnecting the machine a "mercy killing"? Was it morally different from simply failing to resuscitate Mr. Gessner when he had his next respiratory arrest?

Commentary

Something seems very wrong with Ms. Robaczynski's action. Was the problem here that Ms. Robaczynski had crossed the line between the decision to let the patient die and active killing? We have seen that even for reasons of mercy, active killing is illegal. It is morally condemned by many, but not all, who reflect on Ms. Robaczynski's actions. She disconnected a respirator, the result of which was the death of her patient. Should that be classified as killing?

Traditionally, many clinicians have thought of withdrawing treatment as a kind of action. If the withdrawal resulted in the death of the patient, it would then be considered active killing. Withdrawal of treatment requires an action. Switches must be thrown; tubes must be removed. Psychologically, the nurse or physician engaging in the withdrawal of an ongoing medical treatment might feel as if he or she is taking an action.

On the other hand, those outside the clinical setting have tended to classify withdrawing treatment as more akin to not starting treatment in the first place. Part of this argument is pragmatic. It suggests that ongoing treatments can be viewed as the continual repetition or administration of individual units of treatment. An indwelling IV supplying continuous medication is akin to repeated injections. A respirator is akin to continual compressions supplying air. Stopping a treatment is like deciding not to supply the next dose.

Moreover, if it is policy that treatments can be omitted, but once begun, they must be continued, there would be a strong incentive to refuse to start procedures. This would be true even if, as in Mr. Gessner's case, it would have been imprudent to have omitted them at the time they were begun.

Some of those who favor classifying withdrawing treatment as more akin to not starting it ask that we examine the moral basis of the right of refusal of treatment. It rests, in part, on the principle of autonomy, which gives people the right to consent or refuse consent to treatment. Omissions follow from the liberty right of persons to be left alone. The person with authority for Mr. Gessner's care would have the right to refuse treatment when that judgment is plausibly in Mr. Gessner's best interest. The authority to make that judgment, however, does not imply the right to have Mr. Gessner killed. The principle of autonomy could never authorize someone else to actively kill another person. Some people have concluded that if there is a moral principle prohibiting killing, it does not extend to all decisions to omit life-prolonging treatments. They are not considered proscribed active killings.

The President's Commission for the Study of Ethical Problems in Medicine and Biomedical and Behavioral Research reached a conclusion similar to this one. It says that, "Neither law nor public policy should mark a difference in moral seriousness between stopping and not starting treatment."[6(p77)]

Still, it appears that Ms. Robaczynski did something wrong. If she did not engage in an action that can be thought of as the same as actively killing Mr. Gessner, has she committed no moral offense? One possibility is that, even though she withdrew a respirator, and that withdrawal is morally akin to omitting treatment, there are circumstances when it is morally wrong to omit treatment. In some cases, omissions can even be the equivalent of murder. Withholding food from a starving child for whom one is responsible would be an example. If this were such a circumstance, Ms. Robaczynski might be guilty of murder by omission.

It is clearly wrong for health professionals (physicians or nurses) to omit treatment when there is a presumption in favor of treatment and the patient or agent for the patient has not decided to refuse treatment. The presumption in favor of treatment is present in Mr. Gessner's case. There is no evidence that he had refused the respirator. There is no evidence that he had a relative or anyone else speaking for him who had refused the treatment. Had there been such a refusal, the omission would have been plausible, but without it there is something akin to an abandonment. In this case, it was an abandonment that resulted in death. Those who follow this line or argument might conclude that even though withdrawing a respirator is an omission and, therefore, is morally as acceptable as other omissions, it is wrong to omit life-prolonging treatment when the patient or agent for the patient has not refused the treatment. The alternative way of accounting for our intuition that Ms. Robaczynski did wrong is simply to classify what she did as an active killing. That would mean, however, that withdrawals of treatment even upon the refusal of the patient would be so classified.

Case 60: The Patient Who Might Have a Living Will*

Jerry Packard was a staff nurse in the coronary care unit (CCU) of a large medical center. One morning he was informed that a patient from the recovery room (RR) would soon be admitted to the CCU. The new admission would be assigned to him. The patient, a 66-year-old man with known history of myocardial infarction (MI), also had cancer of the prostate. This hospital admission was for a transurethral resection (TUR), which had been aborted in the OR when the patient developed cardiac changes following spinal anesthesia. The patient had

*Case supplied by Albert L. Scheckterman, R.N. Used with permission

been transported to the RR with the diagnosis of possible MI and was to be transferred to the CCU for management and evaluation.

Mr. Packard went to the RR with a bed to pick up the patient. When he arrived, the patient was being coded. He had apparently gone into ventricular tachycardia/ventricular fibrillation (VT/VF) in the RR and had required countershock ×3, cardiopulmonary resuscitation (CPR), intubation, lidocaine, and vasopressors to maintain his blood pressure. A Swan-Ganz catheter was put in place. Recovery rhythm was sinus bradycardia to sinus tachycardia with occasional pauses. The patient was acidotic, in pulmonary edema by chest x-ray with a PaO_2 of 50–60, an FIO_2 of 100%.

During the events of the code, an attending cardiologist (Dr. Diamond) passed by, observed the code, and made the following statements to the RR staff and the CCU resident: "Say, that's Mr. Sawyer. I know him from his last hospitalization of 1 month ago when I was attending in CCU. I think he has a Living Will." While the patient was stabilized, Dr. Diamond called the patient's relative, who happened to work in another part of the medical center. The relative also expressed the belief that Mr. Sawyer had a Living Will and did not want to receive extraordinary support measures. Dr. Diamond relayed this information to the other physicians, and there was general agreement that conservative measures to ensure support were indicated while the Living Will was located.

The CCU resident and Mr. Packard transported Mr. Sawyer to the CCU. When admitted, the patient's systolic BP was in the 70s while on dobutamine, 8 micrograms per kg, and dopamine, 26 micrograms per kg. The patient ocassionally responded to verbal commands, opened his eyes, gripped Mr. Packard's hands, and responded to pain in the upper extremities (his lower extremities were still under the effects of the spinal anesthesia). Cardiac monitoring showed that the patient was still having sinus tachycardia (130), C.O.6.8, SVR800, PCWP28, temp. 35 5 core. Resp. ABG improving with 730/42/60 on 100%; IMV12, Peep5.

At this point, the CCU resident and an intern approached Mr. Packard and informed him that they believed that the present treatment of the patient was cruel. By reading the old medical record, they learned that the patient had been designated "do not resuscitate" (DNR) on his last admission and the patient was supposed to have a Living Will although it had not yet been located. They told Mr. Packard to slowly turn off the IV drip of dopamine and dobutamine. What should Mr. Packard do?

Commentary

Mr. Packard's situation is somewhat similar to that of Ms. Robaczynski. He also must contemplate withdrawing a treatment, and the treatment to be withdrawn is as basic and simple. Ms. Robaczynski withdrew a ventilator, whereas Mr. Packard would withdraw an IV. Some people might be inclined to say that the hospital team missed its chance when it failed to act decisively when it had a chance to omit the resuscitation. They might feel that now they would have to continue the supportive care that had been begun.

Two reasons for that position might be offered. First, it might be argued that aggressive resuscitation is "extraordinary," whereas an IV drip is "ordinary." We saw in the case in the previous section that these terms are ambiguous and that many people would make the judgments not on the basis of the complexity of the treatment, but rather on whether they fit with the patient's wishes. Then the question would become one of whether the patient saw the IV as serving a purpose any more than did the CPR. That is a question we shall address in cases later in this chapter.

The other possible explanation of the difference between omitting the CPR and stopping the IV drip is that one is an omission and the other would be a withdrawal. Just as in the Robaczynski case, we need to determine whether it makes a difference that a treatment is stopped or never started. Maintaining such a distinction might incline care givers to be reluctant to start treatments such as the IV drip. Defenders of the view that there is no legitimate moral distinction believe that it is better to start a treatment when there is doubt about the correctness of the course and then withdraw if the time comes when it is clear that the patient would not have wanted the treatment to continue.

Here, however, Mr. Packard is being told by the resident and intern to turn off the IV drip on the basis of an unconfirmed belief that the patient had a Living Will and the fact that he reportedly had been designated for nonresuscitation on his last hospital admission. Mr. Packard must face the question of whether that is sufficient reason to stop the treatment even with the apparent approval of Mr. Sawyer's relative.

It is likely that the next of kin's judgment would be sufficient in the case where the patient's wishes cannot be determined, but that does not seem to lead to a clear answer here. First, we are not even sure if the relative is Mr. Sawyer's next of kin. Moreover, even if it is, it seems possible that Mr. Sawyer has expressed his own wishes and those wishes would surely take precedence. While the rumor is that he has a Living Will, no one seems to know exactly what it says. Some Living Wills are even written today for the purpose of insisting that treatment continue. Unless Mr. Packard and the physicians know the content of the document and confirm that it, in fact, exists, they are taking considerable liberty. As for the existence of a nonresuscitation instruction during the previous admission, that does not provide definitive guidance for Mr. Packard either. First, even if Mr. Sawyer was willing not to be resuscitated at that time, it is not clear that those remain his wishes today under somewhat different medical and social circumstances. Second, Mr. Packard does not know whether the decision against resuscitation upon the previous admission was made by Mr. Sawyer or only by other parties. There are increasing incidents of physicians, on their own, writing nonresuscitation instructions without bothering to confirm that they are supported by the patient or the patient's surrogate. Deciding to let the patient die under such circumstances is morally controversial. It may be that Mr. Packard is being asked to omit treatment on the basis of a rumor that Mr. Sawyer has a Living Will and the purported fact that someone decided during a previous admission that Mr. Sawyer should not be resuscitated. Is either an adequate basis for Mr. Packard to withdraw treatment? If not, what are his options?

DIRECT AND INDIRECT KILLING

In trying to understand a principle that prohibits killing, there is another distinction that sometimes comes into play. Sometimes persons are killed although there is no intention to kill. Persons are killed in surgery because of anesthesia accidents. They are killed by risky research protocols where a feared, but undesired side effect occurs. In Catholic moral theology[9] and in some secular philosophical debate, as well,[10,11] a distinction is made between killings that are directly intended and those that are unintended.

The doctrine, sometimes referred to as the doctrine of double effect, holds that evil consequences of actions are morally permissible provided that four conditions are met[12(p7)]:

1. The action is good or indifferent in itself
2. The intention of the agent is upright; that is, the evil effect is sincerely not intended
3. The evil effect must be equally immediate causally with the good effect
4. There must be a proportionally grave reason for allowing the evil to occur

This doctrine, in effect, holds that evil consequences, even deaths, are morally tolerable provided the conditions are met.

Sometimes the direct–indirect distinction is confused with the commission–omission distinction. We have already seen, however, that sometimes omissions can result in deaths that are direct and intended. We shall now examine an action that results in a death, but one that is, arguably, not direct or intended.

Case 61: Sedating the Dying Patient*

Jennifer Lincoln was back to work on her oncology nursing unit after a week's vacation. As she received her report, she could hear the moans of pain coming from the room of Leonard Wilson, a 28-year-old man suffering the effects of metastatic bone cancer. This patient had been one of her favorites when he was hospitalized several months ago for chemotherapy. Now he was back to die. The metastatic growths in his spine were causing him excruciating pain, while brain stem metastases were threatening death.

The goal of Mr. Wilson's nursing care was to keep him as comfortable as possible. But as Ms. Lincoln checked his chart for his narcotic order, she stared in disbelief. She called over the head nurse: had Mr. Wilson really received 780 mg of morphine by continuous infusion during the last 8 hours, plus 20-mg boosters every 4 hours, prn? That was enough to cause respiratory depression, even in a 180-pound man.

The head nurse confirmed the dose and explained that Mr. Wilson's tolerance was extremely high, probably because he had been addicted to heroin as a teenager. "Give him another 20-mg booster," she told Ms. Lincoln. "We have to relieve his pain." Ms. Lincoln agreed that his pain should be relieved, but should she give him another dose on top of the amount of medication that he had already received? What if he arrested after she gave him the booster? What should she do?

*Adapted from A question of ethics: Sedating the dying (editorial). Nursing Life 1(Nov/Dec):41–43, 1981. Case used with permission

Commentary

Ms. Lincoln is concerned that she might kill her patient. She knows that a well recognized side effect of morphine is respiratory depression and that Mr. Wilson's dose is extremely high. She also knows that patients develop tolerances to morphine, which require increased dosages in order to produce the analgesic effect. But should she be willing to run the risk of killing her patient in order to get the desired analgesia? If she is governed solely out of a duty to benefit her patient, she will relieve his pain and give the injection. But if there is an independent moral principle that prohibits killing, she has a conflict.

In the previous case, a nurse might be able to avoid the implications of the principle of avoiding killing by arguing that withdrawing a respirator is not to be classified as an active killing. Ms. Lincoln's therapeutic mission, however, is giving an injection that may kill. It is not withdrawing a treatment.

It is impossible to escape the fact that many interventions in health care are somewhat dangerous. Administering a blood transfusion, weaning a patient from a respirator, even administering penicillin all have a risk of serious complications, including death. If it is always wrong to actively kill, then should physicians and nurses avoid all of these normally helpful interventions in order to avoid running the risk of killing the patient?

The doctrine of double effect provides one answer. If the death is not intended and is not a means to the good effect, it is tolerable provided it is for a proportionally good objective. The objective in this case is relieving severe pain, pain great enough that Ms. Lincoln can hear Mr. Wilson screaming down the hall. According to the doctrine of double effect, killings are wrong only if they are intended—and this one clearly would not be intended. The goal of the nursing care plan was to "keep him as comfortable as possible."

Some people question the adequacy of the doctrine of double effect when it establishes a qualification on the principle of avoiding killing. One question centers on the role of intention in determining whether an action is right or wrong. Some people maintain that the morality of an action can be distinguished from the blameworthiness of the actor. They hold that someone can do the right act out of a bad intention. The nurse who provides impeccable nursing care solely out of a desire to gain a promotion would be an example. Likewise, one can do the wrong thing out of a good motive. Someone who actively kills for mercy may be an example.

If that is the case, however, questioners ask whether intention is critical in deciding whether giving the pain-killing medication is wrong. In some cases, an actor may know with great certainty that death will result from an action, but still not intend the death. In the textbooks dealing with the doctrine of double effect, the example is sometimes given of a military officer who decides to bomb a munitions factory knowing that innocent children in a school yard next door will be killed. The intention might be only to destroy the munitions, but there is certain knowledge that the children will also be killed as an indirect effect. According to the doctrine of double effect, the bombing could be licit if the intention did not include killing the children (and there would be proportionally great good resulting from the bombing). Critics argue, however, that if it is known with certainty that the indirect evil will result, the good intention of the actor should not matter.

Applied to the health care sphere, giving a narcotic analgesic when death was a certainty would be as wrong an act as intending to kill the patient. The assessment of the moral character of the actor might be different, but the assessment of the act itself would be the same. In Ms. Lincoln's case, however, the death of her patient is not a certainty. Patients with tolerance can withstand very high doses of morphine. It is reasonable to give higher than normal dosages in order to relieve pain. If death is an unexpected and unintended side effect, it is acceptable. According to this view, active killings are acceptable only if they are not expected as well as not intended. By contrast, according to the double effect position, good intention makes such killings acceptable even if there is foreknowledge that death is a certainty. Thus, the critical question raised is whether good intention makes the killing morally a more acceptable action (*i.e.,* makes it more right, as the double effect position suggests) or whether it is wrong to act in such a way that death is known to be a likely result even if the intention is good. If there is an independent moral principle of avoiding killing, then there is a moral force pulling Ms. Lincoln in the direction against the injection to the extent that she believes it will kill her patient, even if her intention is a good one.

One of the groups that has expressed a view on this issue is the American Nurses' Association (ANA). The *Code for Nurses,* states that:

"Nursing care is directed toward the prevention and relief of suffering commonly associated with the dying process. The nurse may provide interventions to relieve symptoms in the dying client even when the interventions entail substantial risks of hastening death." [13(p4)]

Thus, the ANA appears to recognize the distinction between direct and indirect killing. While it apparently does not condone direct active killing, it explicitly recognizes that it is appropriate to take the risk of killing a patient provided one's intention is to prevent and relieve suffering associated with the dying process.

VOLUNTARY AND INVOLUNTARY KILLING

At this point we have explored several possible qualifications to the notion that life is "sacred" and that killing is prohibited. We have seen that some people limit the principle to active killing, permitting omissions and treatment refusals; some people include withdrawing of treatment as active killing, whereas others classify it as an omission; and some people exclude unintended killings that are the indirect result of an good action. There is another qualification to be explored. Some people argue that the prohibition on killing applies to the killing of others against their will. Since most people do not normally desire to be killed, this is not very important in most settings. However, in the care of critically ill patients, the question of the desire of the patient can be critical. The next pair of cases involves patients who may be ready to die and who may voluntarily undertake a course leading to their death. The question is whether the prohibition against killing ought to apply to patients who are voluntarily ready to end their lives.

Case 62: The Suicidal Patient Who Went Unrecognized*

Ralph Baxter, 52 years old, had chronic lymphocytic leukemia. He was weak and tired, and he lay listlessly in bed most of the time. However, despite his disorder, he maintained a good appetite and enjoyed the fresh fruit that his wife brought to the hospital every day. As the weeks passed, however, Mr. Baxter's condition declined. He was started on a series of chemotherapy treatments that soon left him nauseated. Even after the treatments ended, he was nauseated and would vomit whenever he tried to eat. His thin body became thinner, and his energy level fell. He became reconciled to the fact that everything that could be done for him had been done; he and his wife decided that it would be best if he were to spend his last few weeks at home.

Pamela Sorrenson was the nurse on the night shift the night before Mr. Baxter's scheduled discharge home. About 2:00 a.m., Ms. Sorrenson discovered Mr. Baxter walking slowly in the hall. He just seemed to want company and was talkative about his concerns for his family: whether he would be a burden to his family, whether his wife could care for him as he got weaker, whether he would be able to keep food down, and so on. She talked to Mr. Baxter, assuring him that her own impressions of his family led her to believe that they would never regard him as an encumbrance. In the course of the conversation, Mr. Baxter sounded depressed. He said that he was not sure that it was worth fighting any longer. After escorting him back to his room, she quickly went on to her other duties and the needs of other patients.

At 4:30 AM, the nursing assistant checked on Mr. Baxter and found him sitting on the toilet. She told him to ring the call light when he was through, and she would help him back to bed. When she went back to check on him 15 minutes later, she found him in the bathroom, slumped over the washbasin. She thought that he had fallen asleep, but as she approached him, she realized that he was dead. She quickly called Ms. Sorrenson. When the nurse straightened Mr. Baxter's shoulders, she noticed that he had cut his wrists with the little pocketknife that he usually used to cut up his fresh fruit. The pocketknife lay in the bloody washbasin. Ms. Sorrenson was at first shocked at what had happened, but the more she thought about it, the more she wondered whether Mr. Baxter's decision wasn't the best possible one for him under the circumstances. While at first she felt guilty for failing to intervene, she began to wonder whether the next time she encountered a terminally ill patient similarly depressed she should not purposely avoid intervening.

Case 63: The Quadraplegic Who Wants to Die

Albert Green is a 21-year-old man of normal intelligence who became quadriplegic as a result of a spinal cord injury sustained in an automobile accident 1 1/2 years ago. Albert was hospitalized for 9 months following his accident, first

---

*Adapted from Thielemann P: Suicide: Two views: A chilling encounter. Am J Nurs 84:597–598, 1984

in an acute care and later in a rehabilitative setting. During that time he suffered periodic bouts of depression that focused on his own significant physical losses and on his grief for his 15-year-old brother, who died in the same accident. He was able to discuss these issues with his physician, a psychiatrist who worked intensively with Albert throughout his admission and who judged his depression to be reactive and appropriate to the circumstances. By his discharge, 7 months ago, Albert was anxious about his return to home and the community college where he was a student, but he expressed confidence in his parents' support and that of two of his friends. He looked forward to a more normal life and to his education.

During his first semester at the community college, Albert started out well. By Thanksgiving, however, he expressed a growing disinterest in his classes, dissatisfaction with his dependence on his parents and some anger at his friends, who saw him less frequently because of their involvement with the school's soccer team. Albert refused to attend any social functions at the school and spent increasing amounts of time watching television. By Christmas, he had reduced his food intake significantly and had shown a marked weight loss. His parents cajoled, ordered, and begged him to eat. Albert insisted that he "wasn't hungry."

At his clinic visit, Albert confides to the clinic nurse, Caron O'Neill, that he intends to starve himself to death because "life isn't worth living if it has to be like this." He adamantly refuses to discuss any interventions and says that he will consider any recommendations by Ms. O'Neill to be a violation of his rights and his confidentiality. Ms. O'Neill feels quite sure that Albert's psychiatrist will continue to consider Albert to be competent both cognitively and emotionally and to be making an informed decision about the quality of his life. Should she remain silent about his intentions to starve himself to death?

Commentary

The case of Mr. Baxter, the man who committed suicide in the face of a lingering terminal illness with a bleak prognosis, raises the question of whether the prohibition on taking a human life includes taking one's own life on the basis of a rational decision that such action is the best alternative.

Suicide in the face of terminal illness raises some technical questions. First, was Mr. Baxter really competent? The argument that free, rational choice on the part of the individual himself justifies suicide or even homicide upon request rests on the premise that persons deciding that they should be killed can, in fact, be rational. Some persons who are suicidal clearly are not rational. They are not free agents making voluntary choice, and so any possible exception to the prohibition against killing based on voluntariness would not apply to them.

However, Mr. Baxter showed no obvious signs of mental incompetence. Some people now acknowledge that it is possible for people to make a rational choices that the best course for them is to end their lives. At least, persons should not be necessarily considered irrational when they make such a choice.

Second, could the nursing staff have proposed other alternatives for Mr. Baxter that would have made his remaining days more meaningful? They might have investi-gated home nursing care. They might have urged medical assessments to modify future chemotherapy, provided anti-nausea and anti-pain medication, and to explore anti-de-pressants. If a decision for suicide is based on an inadequate exploration of options or if modifications could have improved Mr. Baxter's life, then the suicide decision was questionable on its face.

Suppose, however, that all of those options had been explored and Mr. Baxter still felt that suicide was the best way out. Two arguments are given that would support an exception to a rule against killing in the case where the one being killed has consented (or does the killing himself). Some people might approach the problem strictly in terms of the consequences. Although killing normally has bad consequences, the cases where the individual voluntarily chooses to die might be the exception. David Hume has de-fended suicide on consequentialist grounds.[14,15] Alternatively, anyone committed to the priority of autonomy as a separate moral principle could argue that individuals have the right to dispose of their own bodies as they see fit even if the consequences of doing so are not the best.[16]

By contrast, there are arguments based on consequences against suicide. In some cases, the community will lose a valued member. Loved ones may be injured. These consequences, however, become less critical when applied to a terminally ill patient and compared with the suffering he may well suffer under any other course. The most im-portant argument against suicide may well be that it violates some moral obligation. St. Thomas has expressed this view in terms of the natural law and the duties the human owes to his God.[17] Secular persons may also hold that there is a duty to avoid killing that applies even to killing oneself.[18] If such a duty is recognized, it must be compared with the arguments in favor of self-killing. Mr. Baxter and Ms. Sorrenson may well conclude that there is something wrong with killing even if the patient consents to it and the pa-tient benefits more than under any other course of action.

Albert Green, the quadriplegic who has stopped eating, raises all of these issues in a somewhat more complex way. His nurse, Caron O'Neill, is aware of what he is doing and knows he is suicidal. Furthermore, he is not otherwise terminally ill and in danger of imminent death as was Mr. Baxter.

If Ms. O'Neill thinks her patient is doing the right thing, she is not likely to feel obliged to alert others at the hospital. But, if she thinks suicide is morally very wrong, a different course may be in order. Again, the first step may be to attempt to determine if Mr. Green is competent to make voluntary choices. His psychiatrist apparently has considered him competent in the past. If this judgment continues, then it is important to determine at what point voluntary choice on the part of the patient provides an exception to a principle prohibiting killing.

There is a further complication in Mr. Green's case. Whereas Mr. Baxter clearly killed himself (with a pocketknife), Mr. Green's course is really more of an omission than an active killing. If that distinction is critical, then maybe the prohibition on killing does not apply at all to Mr. Green.

We discovered, however, in the Robaczynski case that even some omissions are morally the equivalent of murder—when the omission comes in the face of a clear duty to act, for example, when the patient wants the treatment to continue.

Mr. Green obviously does not want the treatment (in this case, feeding) to continue. Does his refusal, together with the fact that he is merely omitting intervention, justify what he is doing? That is likely to depend on whether some interventions are so basic, so much a part of routine life-maintenance, that they are morally required. The next case helps clarify this issue.

IS WITHHOLDING FOOD AND WATER KILLING?

The most controversial decisions about withholding treatment are those involving very simple, routine treatments. We have already seen that some people consider any treatment that is simple or common to be morally required. This has generated controversy over withholding of antibiotics and other medications, CPR, and medically supplied nutrition and hydration. The following cases illustrate the controversy, first with a competent patient expressing her refusal and then with an incompetent patient, one of whose nurses objected to withholding an IV.

Case 64: Letting the Terminally Ill Patient Die*

Ms. Anderson was a frail, 80-year-old woman with severe kyphosis, who had recently been diagnosed with mycosis fungoides, or cutaneous T-cell lymphoma (CTCL), a malignancy that begins as a skin lesion and ends as a lymphoma with lymph and visceral involvement. Treatment for the disorder is palliative, and the life expectancy of the patient is only about 3 years from the time enlarged lymph nodes appear.

At the time she was admitted to Beth Reardon's oncology unit, Ms. Anderson had skin lesions on more than 10% of her body. Her pain was so extreme that she cried and moaned when Mrs. Reardon performed even the simplest procedure. Her nutritional status was very poor because even eating was an ordeal. Even when her pain appeared to be under control, she adamantly refused to eat. A nasogastric tube was inserted, despite Ms. Anderson's protests, and tube-feedings were instituted. But Ms. Anderson pulled the tube out, saying that she just wanted to die. After repeated attempts to replace the tube (and repeated removals by Ms. Anderson!) Mrs. Reardon and the other nurses assessed the situation. Clinically, Ms. Anderson was getting worse; her prognosis was extremely poor. Yet all of the nursing interventions seemed designed to make her uncomfortable and unhappy. If her comfort were established as the main nursing goal, then it seemed reasonable to not force the feeding tube on her. Clearly, Ms. Anderson wanted to die; her family did not want to continue watching her

*Adapted from Reiley PJ, Strecker L, Perna K, Burton C, Janeco D: Letting go. Am J Nurs 85:776, 1985

suffer. Yet the nurses hesitated to do nothing except comfort measures for Ms. Anderson. Wouldn't they be contributing to the hastening of death rather than the preservation of life?

Commentary

Ms. Anderson's agony presses us to the limits in determining what treatments may morally be refused. We have recognized that, at least at the level of law, competent persons have the right to refuse medical treatments being offered for their own good. Moreover, many individuals believe it is also morally right for them to refuse treatments that they find are serving no useful purpose or are gravely burdensome. It is evident that Ms. Anderson finds the nasogastric tube burdensome. Does the tube, like any other medical treatment, fall under the rules that permit treatment refusal or would removing it be "hastening death" as Mrs. Reardon asks?

It seems to be a matter of medical fact that removing the tube would hasten Ms. Anderson's death. That, of course, does not mean that her death would be intended or that removing the tube would constitute active killing. In fact, removing the tube would be a withdrawal of treatment. Of course, Ms. Anderson could refuse to have the tube reinserted at a time when it had been removed, in which case, she might be said to be refusing consent to treatment rather than withdrawing treatment. If withdrawing and withholding are not significantly different morally, it will make no difference anyway.

The real issue seems to be whether food and fluids are so basic that they must be provided even if they are serving no useful purpose or are gravely burdensome or, on the other hand, whether they are expendable on the same grounds as other treatments including ventilators and CPR.

Several philosophical commentators[19-21] and several legal cases[22-25] have come to the conclusion that nutrition and hydration can be withheld on the same grounds as other treatments. Once one acknowledges that it is not the complexity or the statistical commonness of the treatment that is morally critical, but whether the treatment is fitting for the patient, then even something as routine as medically administered food and fluids can sometimes be expendable when patients do not want them or when they would not be fitting for the patient in the eyes of the patient's surrogate.

Sometimes a comparison is made between the withholding of medically administered oxygen through a ventilator and medically administered nutrition through a nasogastric tube. Oxygen is as basic to life support as nutrition or hydration, as the argument goes, and so if one is expendable then the others should be as well.

Nevertheless, many critics are reluctant to accept the withholding of the basics of nutrition and hydration even upon the instruction of the patient, as appears to be the case with Ms. Anderson. Several state "natural death acts" explicitly exclude nutrition and hydration from the treatments that can be refused. The Baby Doe regulations require that infants receive "appropriate nutrition and hydration" even in cases where other treatments can be withheld.[26] Some scholars are beginning to express concern that provision of food and fluids is not really a medical procedure, but basic caring that should always be required.[27] Others are viewing provision of food and fluids as symbolic of our care of the hungry.[28] The question remains whether this would require provision of food and fluids even in cases where patients are not hungry or thirsty and, in fact, they suffer when nutrition and hydration are maintained.[29]

Case 65: The Nurse Who Blew the Whistle on the Clarence Herbert Case*

Sandy Bardenilla, nursing supervisor of the intensive care unit (ICU) at Kaiser Foundation Hospital, Harbor City, California, reviewed the chart of Clarence LeRoy Herbert, a 55-year-old racetrack security guard and father of eight children. Mr. Herbert, a familiar patient to the ICU staff, had been resuscitated in the recovery room 2 days ago (August 26, 1981) after he suffered respiratory arrest following the uneventful closure of an ileostomy. Upon admission to the ICU, Mr. Herbert's endotracheal tube had been connected to a Bennett MA-1 ventilator, and the previously placed nasogastric tube and intravenous lines were maintained. While his vital signs remained stable, Mr. Herbert had remained unconscious since his admission to the unit.

In reading Mr. Herbert's chart, Mrs. Bardenilla noticed that Mr. Herbert's physician had written a note that Herbert's wife had requested "no heroics" the day following his arrest. There had also been controversy over whether to remove Mr. Herbert's ventilator. However, the ventilator was withdrawn by Dr. Barber, and Mr. Herbert continued breathing on his own. His respirations improved and his vital signs restabilized with a normal sinus rhythm and a heart rate in the 70s. The physician in charge of the ICU subsequently wrote orders to withhold treatment for hypotension, hypertension, and arrhythmias and to give supportive care. As part of their supportive care, the nurses attached a misting device to Herbert's endotracheal tube to prevent the formation of mucous plugs.

On Monday, August 31, 5 days after Mr. Herbert arrested in the recovery room and also Mrs. Bardenilla's day off, Dr. Barber discontinued administration of all the patient's IV fluids and maintenance of the nasogastric tube. One of the nurses removed the IVs and the nasogastric tube, and the patient was transferred from the ICU to a room in the surgical unit. Dr. Barber also wrote an order to stop all blood work.

When Mrs. Bardenilla returned to work the following day, she found that all fluids had been discontinued on Mr. Herbert. Six days later, September 6, 1981, Mr. Herbert died. The preliminary autopsy report listed anoxia and dehydration as two of the causes of death. During subsequent weeks, Mrs. Bardenilla pursued her efforts to obtain written hospital guidelines defining "heroic"

*Adapted from Smith L: Zero intake. Nursing Life 3:18–25, 1983. Case used with permission; Annas GJ: Non-feeding: Lawful killing in CA, homicide in NJ. Hastings Center Report 13(Dec):19–20, 1983; also, Steinbock B: The removal of Mr. Herbert's feeding tube. Hastings Center Report 13(Oct):13-16, 1983. For the various legal actions see Superior Court of the State of California for the County of Los Angeles. People of the State of California v. Neil Barber and Robert Nejdl. Tentative Decision. May 5, 1983; Court of Appeal of the State of California. Second Appellate District, Division Two. Barber and Neijdl v. Sup. Ct., 2 Civil No. 69350, 69351, Ct. of App. 2d Dist., Div. 20 ct. 12, 1983. Barber v. Superior Court of California, 147 Cal. App. 3d 10006, 195 Cal. Rptr. 484 (1983).

and "supportive" care, as well as the criteria for deciding how much care a patient should get and whose decision it should be. She asked for guidelines that provided for peer review of the care given in ICU. Her efforts resulted in a sharp warning from her director of nursing. She was advised to adopt a more realistic attitude about the hospital system, and she was warned against taking her concerns outside the hospital. Several days later, Mrs. Bardenilla met with the chief of staff, who then promised to take her suggestions to the medical executive meeting. Several weeks later, Mrs. Bardenilla learned that her suggestions were never mentioned at the meeting and no action had been taken to discuss or implement the guidelines she sought.

By this time, Mrs. Bardenilla was thoroughly demoralized. She was undecided whether she ought to go "outside" to find anyone willing to investigate and evaluate the care and treatment that Mr. Herbert received. Also, what impact would going "outside" have on her employment and family? Her indecision ended, however, when she learned that two other patients had been removed from life-support systems under conditions as unclear as Mr. Herbert's situation. On September 23, she resigned her position at Kaiser Foundation Hospital. On September 25, she telephoned the county health department and made a formal complaint about the management of Mr. Herbert's care. After a year of investigation by the health department, police department, and the Los Angeles district attorney's office, Dr. Barber and Dr. Nejdl were charged with murder and conspiracy to commit murder. Following 6 weeks of testimony, municipal court judge B.D. Crahan decided that there was no evidence that Drs. Barber and Nejdl had acted in a "malicious, selfish, or foolhardy manner" in treating Mr. Herbert. The case was dropped without a trial. On appeal by the district attorney's office, Judge Crahan's decision was reversed and the original charges against Drs. Barber and Nedjl were reinstated, only to be dismissed again by the Court of Appeal. In the meantime, Clarence Herbert's widow filed a malpractice suit against the two doctors and the hospital. She claimed that she had been told by the doctors that her husband was brain dead; she would not have authorized the removal of life-support systems if she had known he was not brain dead.

Sandy Bardenilla is now working as a staff nurse in the cardiac unit of another California hospital. She still has questions about the care Mr. Herbert received and what a nurse should do when following a doctor's orders goes against the nurse's conscience.

Commentary

The decision to remove the ventilator and then the IV from Mr. Herbert raises all of the issues that emerged in the previous case plus many others. It is clouded by the clear tensions between Mrs. Bardenilla and the physicians. It is complicated by the absence of any clear sign of the patient's wishes. The problems of guardian deicsion-making will be addressed more fully in the cases in Chapter 14. The issue raised here, however, is whether there is any acceptable reason—beyond the patient's clearly expresssed wishes—to remove such basic treatments as ventilators, IVs, and nasogastric tubes.

A similar court case, involving a woman being maintained on a nasogastric tube led a New Jersey court to hold that such interventions could be removed under three conditions[30]:

1. It is clear the patient would have refused
2. There is some indication that the patient would have refused, and it would only prolong suffering
3. The burdens clearly and markedly outweigh the benefits

It is not clear that Mr. Herbert would meet any of these conditions. He never expressed himself explicitly on withdrawal of hydration. Even if it could be deduced that those would be his wishes, he is not suffering, since he is in a coma. Finally, since he is comatose, it is not clear that the burdens of the treatments clearly and markedly outweigh the benefits.

Of course, the fact that these are the conditions under which one court says that it is legal to remove such treatments does not necessarily resolve the complex ethical questions at stake. Several religious and philosophical commentators, for example, approach these issues applying exactly the same reasoning as in any other medical treatments; those treatments that are useless or gravely burdensome are expendable, whereas those where the burdens are proportional to the benefits are required.

Regardless of these legal and ethical complexities, Mrs. Bardenilla had strong objections to the decisions made. What other options were open to her under the circumstances? How do you assess the course she finally took?

References

1. Beauchamp TL: A Reply to Rachels on active and passive euthanasia. In Robison WL, Pritchard MS (eds): Medical Responsibility: Paternalism, Informed Consent, and Euthanasia, pp 181–194. Clifton, NJ, The Humana Press, 1979
2. Fletcher GP: Prolonging life. Washington Law Review 42:999–1016, 1967
3. Rachels J: Active and passive euthanasia. N Engl J Med 292:78–80, 1975
4. Menzel PJ: Are killing and letting die morally different in medical contexts? J Med and Philosophy 4:269–293, 1979
5. Thomson JJ: Killing, letting die and the trolley problem. The Monist 59:204–217, 1976
6. President's Commission for the Study of Ethical Problems in Medicine and Biomedical and Behavioral Research: Deciding to Forego Life-Sustaining Treatment: Ethical, Medical, and Legal Issues in Treatment Decisions. Washington, DC, U.S. Government Printing Office, 1983
7. Pope Pius XII: The prolongation of life: An address of Pope Pius XII to an International Congress of Anesthesiologists. The Pope Speaks 4:393-398, 1958
8. Congregation for The Doctrine of The Faith: Declaration On Euthanasia. Rome, The Sacred Congregation for the Doctrine of the Faith, May 5, 1980
9. McCormick RA, Ramsey P (eds): Doing Evil to Achieve Good: Moral Choice in Conflict Situations. Chicago, Loyola University Press, 1978
10. Graber GC: Some questions about double effect. Ethics in Science and Medicine 6(1):65–84, 1979

11. Foot P: The Problem of abortion and the doctrine of the double effect. Oxford Review 5:5–15, 1967

12. McCormick RA: Ambiguity in moral choice. In McCormick RA, Ramsey P (eds): Doing Evil to Achieve Good: Moral Choice in Conflict Situations, p 7. Chicago, Loyola University Press, 1978

13. American Nurses' Association: Code for Nurses with Interpretive Statements, p 4. Kansas City, American Nurses' Association, 1985

14. Hume D: On Suicide. Edinburgh, 1777

15. Brandt R: The morality and rationality of suicide. In Perlin S (ed): A Handbook for the Study of Suicide, pp 61–75. New York, Oxford University Press, 1975

16. Szasz T: The ethics of suicide. The Antioch Review 31(Spring):7–17, 1971

17. Aquinas T: Summa Theologica I-II, Q. 91. Art 2. The Dominican Fathers of the English Province (trans), Gilbey T (ed): Vol 28, pp 21–24. Cambridge, Blackfriars, 1966

18. Feinberg J: Voluntary euthanasia and the unalienable right to life. Philosophy and Public Affairs 7:93–123, 1978

19. Paris JJ, Fletcher AB: Infant Doe regulations and the absolute requirement to use nourishment and fluids for the dying infant. Law, Medicine and Health Care 11(5):210–213, 1983

20. Lynn J, Childress JF: Must patients always be given food and water? The Hastings Center Report 13(Oct):17–21, 1983

21. Micetich K, Steinecker P, Thomasma D: Are intravenous fluids morally required for a dying patient? Arch Intern Med 143:975–978, 1983

22. In Re Plaza Health and Rehabilitation Center, Sup. Ct., Onodaga County, New York, Feb. 2, 1984

23. In the Matter of Claire C. Conroy, Syllabus, Prepared by the Office of the Clerk, Supreme Court of New Jersey, A-108, September Term 1983

24. Court of Appeal of the State of California. Second Appellate District, Division Two. Neil Barber and Robert Nejdl v. Superior Court of the State of California for the County of Los Angeles. October 12, 1983

25. In the Matter of Mary Hier, 464 N.E. 2d Series 959, Mass. App. 1984.

26. U.S. Department of Health and Human Services. Child Abuse and Neglect Prevention and Treatment Program: Final Rule: 45 CFR 1340. Federal Register: Rules and Regulations 50 (No. 72, April 15, 1985):14878–14892.

27. Meilaender G: On removing food and water: Against the stream. The Hastings Center Report 14(6):11–13, 1984

28. Callahan D: On feeding the dying. The Hastings Center Report 13(5):22, 1983

29. Lynn J: The Choice to Forgo Life-Sustaining Food and Water: Medical, Ethical, and Legal Considerations. Bloomington, IN, Indiana University Press, 1986

30. In Re Conroy, No. A-108 (N.J. Sup. Ct. Jan. 17, 1985).

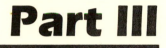
Part III

Special Problem Areas in Nursing Practice

The cases in Part I dealt with problems of identifying ethical and other values and gaining some understanding of how to adjudicate ethical disputes in nursing practice, including reflection on the role of codes in ethical decision-making. Those in Part II provided a framework of general ethical principles that can be applied to a wide range of dilemmas faced in nursing. There still remain some specific problem areas to which these general principles can be applied. The nurse readily recognizes certain kinds of problems that are likely to pose particularly difficult ethical issues: abortion, sterilization, contraception, genetics, psychiatry, experimentation, consent, and death and dying decisions. These areas have, in many cases, developed with certain concepts, analyses, and arguments. The cases in Part III pose these problems and provide an opportunity to apply the general principles to some of the most critical problems the nurse faces in day-to-day practice.

Chapter 9

Abortion, Sterilization, and Contraception

One of the classical areas in health care ethics deals with the set of problems of abortion, sterilization, and contraception. Whereas for some people some of the decisions surrounding these issues are not as critical as they once were, many important decisions remain for the nurse.

A woman's legal right to decide in favor of an abortion has not resolved many of the ethical issues of abortion. Every woman is now legally free to obtain an abortion, but exercising this legal freedom does not determine that abortion is ethically acceptable. The legal right does not necessarily imply the moral right. Even for those who decide that abortion is, in principle, acceptable in certain circumstances, the ethical decision must still be made to determine which circumstances. In addition, a nurse, if she is to be a responsible moral agent, must also decide what her role in abortion procedures ought to be. Even if a patient has decided in favor of an abortion, it remains an open question whether the health care personnel will and should choose to participate.

The cases in the first part of this chapter present mainly problems involving specific problematic abortion decisions: cultural and religious differences over abortion, the woman's right to make the decision on her own, the unmarried teenager, and abortion because the infant is not the sex the parents wanted.

The second section involves the related ethical issue of sterilization. While sterilization, like abortion, is not as controversial as it once was, many critical problems remain even for nurses who have no objection in principle. Serious problems of consent exist when a nurse believes a young patient has been sterilized while neither the patient nor her parents are informed.

The final case in this chapter involves contraception. Again, many newer, more subtle issues have emerged recently.

ABORTION

On January 22, 1973, the United States Supreme Court issued a ruling that, in effect, legalized most abortions.[1] Although the ruling resolved, at least for the time being, many legal controversies, it did not solve the ethical dilemmas faced by many women and many health care professionals who would still have to make critical choices about whether to interrupt pregnancies.

Abortion is a difficult moral problem, in part because so much of the decision rests on the moral status of the fetus, a question that is not easily resolved by appeals to ethical principles of the sort introduced in previous chapters. For example, the principle of avoiding killing seems clear enough in its implications, but at some point one needs to decide exactly to what the principle applies. Does it cover animals or only humans? Does it apply to all humans or only to those who possess what could be called "moral standing"?

The notion of moral standing is one used to convey who has moral claims on the rest of the community. Several positions are argued in the philosophical and religious literature.[2-6] Some individuals argue that the fact that living tissue is endowed with human genetic material is enough to make it the bearer of the rights that normally accrue to humans. Holders of such positions normally exclude human egg and sperm cells before conception, but they argue that with the combining of the genetic material of the two parents, a new life is created that bears full moral standing.[7,8] This position, sometimes referred to as the "biological" or "genetic" position, is based on what appears to be a biological fact: that a new individual with a new and fixed genetic endowment begins at conception.

Others disagree with this position because they disagree with the scientific claim on which it is based. Some biologists have pointed out that the genetic code is not always unchangeably fixed at conception. With twinning, some switching of genetic material might take place. These critics imply that the critical point at which moral standing accrues is more likely the second week after conception, the last time at which twinning can take place.[9,10] While adopting the genetic position, they simply disagree over when the genetic code is unchangeable.

Some individuals disagree on a more fundamental basis. They question whether the issue of moral standing can be determined solely on a biological, especially genetic, basis. There are many other events in fetal and postnatal development that might be seen as significant, including any of the following:

    The pumping of the heart
    Development of neurological activity of brain cells
    Spontaneous movement
    "Quickening"
    Development of circulatory system function
    Development of integrated neurological activity
    Viability
    Development of the capacity for consciousness
    Birth

Breathing of air
Development of speech
Development of capacity for rational thinking
Acceptance by others

This is a long and complicated list. More critical capacities could also be named. Some people might argue that certain social and cultural events are necessary for moral standing. Holders of these positions, sometimes referred to as "social" positions, claim that capacities for speech and rationality, as well as events involving the responses of other parties (quickening, the perception of movement by the pregnant woman) and acceptance by others, are required for moral standing. [11,12]

In addition to those who identify one biological, social, or cultural event as definitive for moral standing, a third group of individuals, called "incrementalists," hold that many of these events are important and that as the fetus develops its gains more and more of a moral claim on others. This position ends up requiring a much more rigorous justification of abortion of a fetus at 18 weeks than at 5 or 6 weeks because more and more of the purportedly critical events have taken place, giving the fetus more and more of a claim. Most people, whether incrementalists or committed to either the genetic or social position, hold that at some point "full standing of personhood" accrues. At that point, the organism with human genetic endowment has full moral claims including all of those based on the principles discussed in the cases in Part II.

The nurse faces many moral questions pertaining to abortion. In addition to facing them as a lay person making personal and public policy choices, he or she must face them as a clinically focused professional. For some, all abortion is morally unacceptable, no matter what the reason. Presumably, a nurse with this belief would face a serious ethical problem if asked to participate in an abortion. But for others who are open to at least some abortions, difficult choices may have to be made on a case-by-case basis. The nurse who is prepared to assess the reasons for abortion will face several types of abortions that may be problematic. The "hard case" abortions include those done for the health of the pregnant woman and in cases of rape, incest, and fetal deformity, as well as those where the woman simply does not want to carry a child for social or economic reasons. Abortions being considered by adolescents and others whose capacity to make well-thought-out choices are also controversial. Abortions for the health of the pregnant woman are, fortunately, a very rare occurrence these days. The other indications are all likely to be faced by any nurse working in an obstetrics unit in a hospital performing abortions. The first two cases in this section raise problems of possible fetal deformity and pregnancy in an adolescent. The third case involves what some would consider an abortion for trivial reasons.

Case 66: When Cultural Differences Limit the Patient's Choice of Health

Nao Vang Xiong, his wife Sheng, and their two small children, ages 1 and 2, were Southeast Asian refugees. Their settlement in the United States was being sponsored by an agency of the Catholic Church. After settling in their new community, the Xiongs visited the county health department for individual health evaluations. To their dismay, chest x-rays and other tests revealed that Mrs. Xiong had active tuberculosis. The clinic nurse, Miss Jane Murphy, explained with the help of an interpreter that Mrs. Xiong must take medications for an extended period of time and should have lots of rest and nutritious food. She was placed on isoniazid (INH), 300 mg once a day, rifampin, 600 mg once a day, and ethambutol hydrochloride (Myambutal), 800 mg once a day.

At a repeat visit to the clinic 2 months later, it was determined that Mrs. Xiong was approximately 6 weeks pregnant. Because of the risk of fetal abnormality from taking the antituberculosis drug during the first trimester of pregnancy, the clinic physician suggested that Mrs. Xiong consider an abortion. As Buddhists, she and her husband were not opposed to having an abortion. Arrangements for the procedure were easily made through the health department and the county hospital. The matter seem settled.

To Miss Murphy's surprise, the Xiongs and Mr. James Walsh, a representative of the church sponsored agency visited the clinic the very next day. The Xiongs appeared very upset and said, through the interpreter, that they had changed their minds about Sheng having an abortion. When Miss Murphy asked why they had changed their minds, Mr. Walsh pointed out that it was directly contrary to the sponsoring agency's religious viewpoint for Mrs. Xiong to have an abortion. He adamantly objected to the clinic's recommendation in this regard, since her life was not directly threatened by the pregnancy. Through the interpreter, Miss Murphy also learned that Mrs. Xiong was under the impression that she and her family would lose the agency's support if she underwent the abortion. Although Miss Murphy tried to reassure Mrs. Xiong and her husband that she had the right to make this decision regardless of the sponsoring agency's position on abortion, Mrs. Xiong was not convinced. The young family was completely dependent on the sponsoring agency and was very fearful of what might happen to them without this support.

Miss Murphy explained to Mr. Walsh why abortion was suggested in this case and supported Mrs. Xiong's right to make this choice without influence from the sponsoring agency. Mr. Walsh, however, insisted that abortion was morally unacceptable to the sponsoring agency. Since they were supporting the Xiongs, they could not permit them to make such a choice. He stated that he and his agency would arrange other health care follow-up for Mrs. Xiong and her family if the health department continued to suggest that Mrs. Xiong have an abortion. At this point, Miss Murphy was not sure what she should do. She could decide that the Xiongs' lack of proficiency in English and limited understanding of Mrs. Xiong's right to choose abortion were cultural problems beyond her expertise or intervention. On the other hand, she could decide to be an advocate for this patient by communicating with the International Refugee Service and requesting another sponsor for the Xiong family. This intervention could take many weeks, however, and Mrs. Xiong would be well into the second trimester of pregnancy before the abortion could be performed. Since Mrs. Xiong's general physical condition was not good, Miss Murphy wondered if this choice of action would, in the long run, be in her best interests.

Case 67: The Unmarried Teenager and Abortion

Mrs. Miriam Dwyer, team leader in family planning services at the county health department, was reviewing and coding the health records of patients seen for birth control counseling or pregnancy tests during the morning's clinic. With surprise, she noted that Karen Ferguson, the 16-year-old daughter of a longtime friend and neighbor, had visited the clinic for a pregnancy test. The test was positive, and, from personal history and physical findings, Karen was judged to be 10 to 12 weeks pregnant. The clinic record noted that Karen had specifically asked about available abortion services and that her parents did not know she was pregnant. In discussing all options open to Karen, the clinic nurse had advised that any decision for abortion would need to be made within 1 to 2 weeks. Her stage of pregnancy was at the upper limits of acceptable risk in elective abortion, and most abortion services would not perform a late abortion on someone of Karen's age without parental consent. Before she left the clinic, Karen was given the names, addresses, and costs of abortion services available throughout the state.

Mrs. Dwyer was faced with a dilemma. As a parent of teenage children, she was horrified that Karen must face this kind of choice at her age. Her concern took several forms: first, the physical hazards of an abortion this late in pregnancy; second, the moral and psychological hazards or potential sense of guilt that could harm Karen emotionally; and third, the fact that 16-year-old Karen—a minor—could make this kind of decision involving considerable risk without parental knowledge. As a friend of Karen's parents for over 15 years, she felt that they should know about Karen's pregnancy. They were understanding parents and were in the best position to counsel and support Karen in her decision. As a family-planning nurse, however, she knew that Karen had the right to make this decision herself and that she was obliged to keep Karen's pregnancy confidential. She struggled with the problem for several days and was still uncertain what she should do.

Case 68: When the Fetus is the Wrong Sex

Elena Hanchett is a team leader for a busy obstetrical unit in a well-known eastern medical center. Today she has decided to provide primary nursing care herself to a newly admitted patient, 37-year-old Mrs. Ostrum. She has decided to do this because Mrs. Ostrum is being admitted for an elective abortion, and two of Ms. Hanchett's team members have asked not to be assigned to this patient. Their reasons stem from the fact that Mrs. Ostrum and her husband have decided to abort her fetus because the fetus is not the sex that they want. Since they have several patients who have been on fertility drugs and are desperately attempting to become pregnant at great personal cost and marital stress, they feel that it is wrong for people like the Ostrums, who can afford children and are economically stable, to abort a fetus solely on the basis of sex. Ms. Hanchett seems to be the only member of her team who does not have any particular feelings about Mrs. Ostrum's elective abortion. Thus she thinks that she should do Mrs. Ostrum's admitting prep herself.

While completing the admission assessment and prepping her patient, Ms. Hanchett learns about the Ostrum's choice to discontinue this pregnancy. The Ostrums have three girls, 3, 5, and 9 years of age. They would like to have one more child if they could be assured of having a boy. Because of her age, Mrs. Ostrum does not feel that she wants to have any more pregnancies after this one. If the fetus is not a boy, both she and her husband would rather interrupt the pregnancy at an early stage and try again within a few months. A week ago, Mrs. Ostrum underwent chorionic villus testing, which demonstrated that her fetus is a girl. Deeply disappointed, the Ostrums have decided not to continue the pregnancy. Even though distressed by the thought of aborting the fetus, they simply do not want another female child.

While she does not usually question the reasons her patients choose abortion, Ms. Hanchett is becoming uncertain as to whether this particular abortion is morally right. Can parents decide not to continue a pregnancy that they have willingly initiated simply on the basis of the sex of the fetus? Would it make any difference in the nursing care she provided if it was morally wrong? Ms. Hanchett is not sure.

Commentary

These cases involve tragically difficult choices, but they are tragic for quite different reasons. Mrs. Xiong's pregnancy apparently was originally desired. Thus the substantive question is whether a pregnancy to which the prospective parents would otherwise be committed can be aborted because the fetus might be injured as a result of the effect of the drugs taken during early pregnancy.

One line of argument in the abortion debate holds that in order for a woman to be obligated to carry a fetus to term, she must have made some commitment to the pregnancy or at least to the risk of pregnancy.[13] This suggests that a woman who is pregnant, for example, as the result of a rape, would have no definitive obligation to the fetus even if abortion is otherwise a serious infringement—even if the fetus has what is sometimes called a "right to life." In such a circumstance, if the fetus could be saved without imposing on the mother, then perhaps society would have a right to save it. That, however, is impossible, and according to this line of argument, the woman would have no obligation to contribute against her will to bringing the fetus to term.

Conceivably, the same argument could be used for an adolescent (such as Karen Ferguson), a mentally retarded woman, or anyone else who had no real understanding of the risk of pregnancy. One moral factor in the abortion debate is whether the consent of the woman to the risk of pregnancy is relevant.

In Mrs. Xiong's case, however, this would not be the basis of accepting the patient's decision to abort. She apparently accepted the idea of pregnancy. While she did not accept the notion of carrying a possibly deformed fetus, she at least accepted the pregnancy. Then the question becomes one of whether the fact that the fetus may be deformed would justify her decision to abort.

Of course, for those who accept a very late event in fetal (or even postnatal) development as the basis for giving moral standing, this would not be an issue. Even a fetus that is definitely healthy could be aborted. Any sort of reason would do, for those adopting the genetic position, the fact that there is an injury would hardly justify killing the fetus (any more than it would justify killing a postnatal human who is handicapped). Of those who are incrementalists, however, some consider the risk of fetal deformity to be enough of a consideration that it will tip the balance. Is it the burden to the potential parents that justifies this reasoning? If so, would the abortion be less justified when competent institutional care givers were available to accept the deformed child or when other adults were standing by willing to adopt the handicapped child? On the other hand, is it presumed trauma to the fetus that justifies the abortion? In that case, an assessment of the likelihood of injury and suffering would be required. Abortion in this circumstance will involve the risk of aborting a normal, healthy infant. Does that make the abortion decision less acceptable?

Miss Murphy, the nurse in this situation, faces two questions. First, is she willing to participate in abortions for these reasons? Presumably, if she opposed all abortion, she could and should refuse assignment to nursing services performing abortions or at least seek assignment so that she would not have to participate. She might decide—if she is more of an incrementalist on abortion—that she can participate in certain abortions, but not others. Then she would have to seek elective exemption from nursing services where abortion was considered.

Second, she has the unique problem in this case of what her role should be in responding to the pressure that Mr. Walsh is exerting on Mrs. Xiong and her husband. If we accept the right of Mr. Walsh and his agency to adopt a moral position opposing all abortions, including those for fetal deformity, should they not also have the right to limit their aid to persons who are willing to follow such a policy judgment.

If so, what are Miss Murphy's options? Should she try to help the Xiongs find alternative sponsorship? Does a nurse's obligation really extend that far? Should she ask the hospital to assume the immediate medical costs with the hope of finding another sponsor in the future or persuading the existing sponsor to continue support? Should she turn to a hospital ethics committee for assistance? Should she propose to the obstetrician that they (falsely) announce that Mrs. Xiong's health requires the abortion? Should they rationalize such an announcement as truthful on the grounds that she would be upset if she delivered a deformed infant and so her health (*i.e.,* her mental health) required the abortion? What other options might Miss Murphy consider? Or should she simply stay out of the case altogether?

Miriam Dwyer faces similar questions. (She was the team leader in the family planning services who discovered that her teenage neighbor, Karen Ferguson, was being seen in her clinic and was planning an abortion.) She would first have to face the substantive question: Is abortion in these circumstances acceptable? If so, it would not be because of the compromised condition of the fetus. It would be acceptable either because Karen Ferguson really did not consent to the pregnancy or because, even if she did consent, she has the right to abort. If it is only because she did not consent to the pregnancy, that implies that Mrs. Dwyer is committed to the position that for older women who did consent to their pregnancies abortion would not be morally appropriate.

On the other hand, if her position is that essentially autonomous women have the right to abort in such circumstances, another set of problems emerge. If Mrs. Dwyer believes that the moral claims of the fetus can be compromised for good reason (or do not exist at all), then she would be willing to accept abortions chosen by women who are reasonably capable of making such choices autonomously. The problem then, however, is whether Karen Ferguson is in such a position. It cannot be denied that some 16 year olds are capable of making autonomous choices in even complex situations having long-term implications. On the other hand, it is not clear that all females capable of becoming pregnant are capable of making such decisions. As a society, we have made a policy judgment that adolescents under a certain age (usually 18) are to be presumed incapable of rational, autonomous actions. Although, in individual cases, minors may be capable of such actions, they may have to go to court to establish their competence. They are referred to in the legal literature as "mature minors."

For certain medical interventions, however, state laws permit minors to agree to treatment without parental involvement. Treatment of venereal disease and contraceptive and abortion services are frequently included in such laws. The state may simply take the position that adolescents are mature, competent persons in these areas while incompetent in other areas. However, the more likely explanation of these laws is that, for obvious reasons, adults (including parents) believe that the interests of minors are better served if they get treatment without parental supervision than if parental permission is required. In these areas of treatment, requiring parental permission might deter many adolescents from seeking any treatment. If that is the basis for the laws in this area, then it is a special case in which minors can be treated without real consent (that is, consent based on substantially autonomous, informed decisions).

Is that what is happening here? If so, how should Mrs. Dwyer respond if she remains convinced that, in this case, Karen Ferguson would be better off if her patients were involved? If the nurse is committed to doing what she thinks will benefit the patient, she might well inform the parents. If, however, she believes that minors are permitted to have access to abortion and other treatments because they are capable of making autonomous choices, and, furthermore, she believes that autonomy is a principle that takes priority, she will refrain from informing the parents. She might well still want to speak with Karen to see if she could be persuaded to involve her parents, but she would not infringe on her autonomy to choose abortion without consulting her parents. If she believes that Karen cannot be presumed to be autonomous, but that the law is written because it will generally do more good for minors than any other rule, then she has to face the question of whether she feels obliged to follow such rules. If she does, once again, she may try to persuade Karen to involve her parents, but she will not violate the rule simply because she believes that in this case it would be better for Karen if she did.

Similar analysis is appropriate for the dilemma faced by Elena Hanchett, the nurse confronted with the couple who want to abort because they have learned that the fetus they have produced is a girl. It is now possible, with great accuracy, to determine the health and sex of the unborn child using sophisticated prenatal diagnostic techniques.[14] The evidence is clear that many people have preference for a child of a particular sex, especially when, as in the case of Mr. and Mrs. Ostrum, they already have several children who are all of the same sex.[15] Is it acceptable, however, to ask health professionals to use their skills to bring this about by aborting an otherwise perfectly healthy fetus simply because it is of the sex not preferred?[16]

For those who grant full moral standing to fetuses at all stages of development, there is hardly any question. Likewise, for those who give no standing at all to unborn children, there is hardly a moral issue. A nurse such as Ms. Hanchett might still have reservations because she is diverting her attention from other patients, but she would not likely question the ethics of the abortion per se.

If Ms. Hanchett adopts a more incrementalist position, however, in which the fetus' claims are justifiably compared with other moral claims based on the stage of development of the fetus, then her decision is a more complex one. For one thing, by the time the amniocentesis is performed, the fetus is fairly far along in development. In the Ostrums' case, they are at the 18th week. For an incrementalist, that would suggest that a fairly strong argument would be needed to offset any claim of the fetus. The undesirability of the fetus' sex is not normally considered to be that strong a consideration. Is it appropriate for Ms. Hanchett to be an incrementalist in this matter, and, if so, does a late stage of fetal development, together with the relative weakness of the reason for the abortion, lead Ms. Hanchett to opposing the abortion? If so, would determination of fetal sex by chorionic villus biopsy, for example, at an earlier time make it easier for her to participate? Are there other circumstances where fetal sex determination would be more weighty in the abortion decision (such as when the fetus is at risk for carrying a sex-linked genetic disease)?

CONTRACEPTION

Closely linked to the ethics of abortion is contraception. Some of the same issues of sexual morality are raised, including the moral legitimacy of manipulation of the procreative process. In contrast to abortion, however, contraception does not raise the issue of conflict between two people with potential or actual moral standing.

Two basic moral arguments against contraception have existed historically. The classical argument, especially within the tradition of Roman Catholic moral theology, is that contraception is morally unacceptable because it artificially interrupts the natural process of conception. Those reasoning from natural law considerations hold that there are natural ends of bodily processes that cannot be disrupted with moral impunity.[17]

A second argument against contraception is that the tolerance of contraception will encourage illicit sexual activity. Some people who do not find the first argument convincing will nevertheless oppose contraception, especially for unmarried people, because they find that condoning contraception implies condoning unacceptable sexual contact. The following case suggests both of these themes.

Case 69: The Nurse as Contraceptive Salesperson

Rosetta Meeks had been admitted to the obstetrical service for her fourth abortion. She was 18, had dropped out of school, and was unmarried. To Donna Tallson, Rosetta Meeks was a walking set of paradoxes. She was a devout Catholic. She argued vociferously about the immorality of contraceptives, yet clearly made moral compromises with her church's teachings both with regard to premarital sexual activity and abortion.

Still, Rosetta would not listen to any suggestion that oral contraceptives would be better than abortion. She said she did not believe in birth control and would use abortion only as a last resort.

Ms. Tallson considered two approaches. She wanted to have a direct moral argument with the patient. She wanted try to convince her that oral contraceptives were morally acceptable, in fact morally obligatory, if she were to remain sexually active. On the other hand, she knew that such a confrontation far exceeded the traditional role of the nurse. She knew that some people still considered contraception ethically unacceptable. Nothing in her education as a nurse really prepared her to enter the role of moral advocate.

Commentary

A complex mixture of ethical and psychological issues is posed by this case. The nurse, Ms. Tallson, may be skeptical about the moral basis of Ms. Meeks' objection to contraceptives, since she is clearly engaging in other actions that are in violation of the moral tradition in which she claims to be standing. Perhaps there are deep psychological reasons why Ms. Meeks appears to object to contraception while she is willing to engage in premarital sexual activity and to have abortions when something goes wrong. There are psychiatrists who claim that some women, especially adolescents, willfully expose themselves to apparently unwanted pregnancies. On the other hand, such attempts to use psychology to rationalize apparently inconsistent behaviors are themselves morally questionable. It is as if the patient cannot be taken at her word. An abortion may become morally tolerable as an emergency measure, as a last resort. It is known that many persons standing in religious traditions opposing abortion will, in fact, have abortions in such emergencies. Perhaps that is an adequate explanation of Ms. Meeks' behavior.

Ms. Tallson's dilemma is somewhat different. She apparently has no moral objections to contraception herself, but faces a patient who, at least purportedly, refuses contraceptives on moral grounds. Convinced that contraception is at least acceptable, in fact probably morally required, for one in Ms. Meeks' position, does Ms. Tallson become a moral advocate of a controversial position in the name of patient welfare, or does she retreat to a more traditional professional role of accepting the patient's ethical stance as a given and work to further the patient's interests within that framework?

Ms. Tallson might consider some other options. For instance, she might attempt to recruit others to convince Ms. Meeks of the acceptability of contraception. If she knew a Catholic priest who supported birth control, would it be more acceptable for Ms. Tallson to ask the priest to discuss the matter with the patient? Could family or friends be recruited for this task? Does recruiting some other moral advocate for contraception leave Ms. Tallson in the more traditional nursing role or is she still indirectly being an advocate attempting to persuade Ms. Meeks to change her moral stance? Even if the nurse herself no longer has any moral problems with contraception, occasionally the patient may pose such a problem.

STERILIZATION

Sterilization raises all of the ethical questions of contraception and then some. Anyone who has objections to contraception will certainly object to sterilization. In addition, however, many people find sterilization particularly objectionable because it must be presumed irreversible. Thus many physicians who are committed to rational planning and "keeping one's options open" have traditionally been unwilling to participate in sterilizations even when they have no objections to contraception per se. In fact, they have been known to refuse to consider sterilization especially for younger women and women who have not borne many children.[18]

Even for those who generally approve of sterilization, certain situations pose particular problems. The sterilization of the retarded is an example that is illustrated in the following case.

Case 70: Sterilizing the Retarded Patient

Mary Ellen Thompson, a skilled maternal child nurse, has recently been employed by a public hospital in a large Southwestern city. Since she speaks fluent Spanish, she has been asked to serve as a translator for the scheduled cesarean delivery of a 14-year-old, mildly mentally retarded Hispanic teenager. The patient undergoes epidural anesthesia without incident and is delivered of a small but healthy 6-pound, 7-ounce girl. While the cesarean delivery is being completed, Mrs. Thompson suddenly realizes that the surgeon is going to perform a tubal ligation (TL). Checking the patient's chart, Mrs. Thompson finds no consent for the tubal ligation. She asks the physician if the procedure was anticipated and whether the patient was informed of the possibility of TL. The physician tells Mrs. Thompson that he believes that the procedure is "medically necessary" and he will record it as such in his operative report.

Several days later, Mrs. Thompson visits the patient and her parents. They are concerned about their daughter's ability to care for her child but have made a commitment to shoulder the responsibility for both mother and child. In talking to them, Mrs. Thompson realizes that they have no awareness of the fact that a tubal ligation was performed on their daughter. They are economically indigent and poorly educated. Yet Mrs. Thompson does not think that these circumstances warrant the involuntary sterilization of a mildly retarded individual without parental consent. What should she do?

Commentary

Sterilization of the low-income patient, the poorly educated, and the retarded has occurred in the past with less controversy than it now generates.[19-21] Several problems are worthy of discussion. First, one might question the ethics of sterilizing those who cannot consent, such as the retarded or any adolescent, even with parental approval. It is increasingly debated whether parents would have any legal or moral authority to approve a permanent blockade of fertility for an incompetent person such as a minor. The problem is particularly controversial when the incompetent is mentally retarded. In contrast with contraceptive methods such as the IUD, sterilization must be presumed to be irreversible. Is Mrs. Thompson on morally safe ground when she implies that the situation involving this 14 year old would have been different if the mother had given her approval? Some are arguing that the retarded have the right to retain their capacity to reproduce even if parents approve of sterilization.

The obligation of the parent is to do what he or she believes is in the child's interest. It is conceivable that parents in this particularly difficult set of circumstances would conclude that sterilization is in the child's best interest. On the other hand, there are limits to what parents can choose even if they sincerely believe that their choice is in the child's best interest. Is this one of those cases where a parent who opts for sterilization rather than some less permanent method of contraception should be prohibited from acting? Or, on the other hand, would the parent's choice be sufficiently reasonable that parental approval would make the procedure acceptable?

When the parent's approval was not sought, the case raises different issues. The physician has stated that he will record in the chart that the tubal ligation was "medically necessary." What would that mean in this case? There is one sense in which no procedure is medically necessary provided one is willing to accept the consequences. Even life-prolonging procedures cannot be termed "medically necessary" if ill patients are willing to accept rapid death as the alternative (as some terminally ill patients are willing to do when faced with heroic surgical interventions). Presumably, the physician must really mean that he believes that a terrible, unacceptable consequence will result if this 14 year old is not sterilized now. That seems very hard to justify given the fact that she could be placed on some other form of contraceptive until she had matured further. Alternatively, she could have been sterilized after her mother was asked. The physician could have discussed his plan with the mother if not the daughter prior to the delivery. It is not as if the physician could not have anticipated the problem before entering the delivery room.

More fundamentally, anyone contemplating this case must address the issue directly of whether it is acceptable to sterilize a nonconsenting mentally retarded person. Even if it makes no sense to label the sterilization as medically indicated, and even if the wishes of the mother are not definitive, are there reasons why the mentally retarded should be sterilized? Are there reasons why their reproductive capacity should be retained?

Mrs. Thompson seems to be on firm ground in questioning what has taken place. Her moral dilemma is, in part, one of deciding how to respond to what she is convinced is an unacceptable practice. How would you evaluate the following alternatives?

1. Ask the physician to inform the girl and her mother of what had happened.
2. Speak to the nursing staff about taking collective action against the physician.
3. Report to administrators that a surgical procedure was done without adequate consent or ask not to be assigned to work with that physician again.
4. Explain to the mother what took place.
5. Speak to a public advocacy group about the general problem of sterilizations without consent.

References

1. Roe v. Wade, 410 U.S. 113, 93 S.Ct. 705, 1973
2. Rosen H: Abortion in America: Medical, Psychiatric, Legal, and Anthropological, and Religious Considerations. Boston, Beacon Press, 1967
3. Callahan D: Abortion: Law, Choice and Morality. New York, Macmillan, 1970
4. Noonan JT: The Morality of Abortion: Legal and Historical Perspectives. Cambridge, MA, Harvard University Press, 1970
5. Feinberg J (ed): The Problem of Abortion. Belmont, CA, Wadsworth Publishing, 1973
6. Bayles MD: Reproductive Ethics, Englewood Cliffs, NJ, Prentice-Hall, 1984
7. Granfield D: The Abortion Decision. Garden City, NY, Doubleday, 1969
8. Grisez GC: Abortion: The Myths, The Realities, and the Arguments. New York, Corpus Books, 1970
9. Lejeune J: Wann beginnt das Leben des Menschen? Padiatrie und Padologie 16:11–18, 1981
10. Hellegers A: Fetal development. Theological Studies 31(Mar):3–9, 1970
11. Tooley M: Abortion and infanticide. Philosophy and Public Affairs 2:37–65, 1972
12. Fletcher J: Humanhood: Essays in Biomedical Ethics. Buffalo, New York, Prometheus, 1979
13. Thomson JJ: A defense of abortion. Philosophy and Public Affairs 1(1):47–66, 1971
14. Netwig MR: Technical aspects of sex preselection. In Holmes HB, Hoskins BB, Gross M (eds): The Custom-Made Child? Women Centered Perspectives, pp 181–186. Clifton, NJ, The Humana Press, 1981
15. Williamson NE: Boys or girls? Parents' preferences and sex control. Population Bulletin 33:3–35, 1978
16. Fletcher JC: The morality and ethics of prenatal diagnosis. In Milunsky A (ed): Genetic Disorders and the Fetus, pp 621–635. New York, Plenum Press, 1979
17. Noonan JT: Contraception. A History of Its Treatment by the Catholic Theologians and Canonists. Cambridge, MA, Harvard University Press, 1966
18. Scrimshaw SC, Pasquariella B: Obstacles to sterilization in one community. Family Planning Perspectives 2:40–42, 1970
19. Buck v Bell 274 U.S. 200(1927)
20. In re Grady 426 A 2d 467 (N.J. Sup. Ct., Feb. 18, 1981)
21. Relf v. Weinberger, 565 F.2d 722 (D.C. Circ. Sept. 13, 1977)

Chapter 10

Genetics, Birth, and the Biological Revolution

New developments in genetics and the growing potential for human intervention in the process of procreation and birth are truly on the cutting edge of the biological revolution. They pose a wide range of new value conflicts for nurses. The problems are as mundane as discussing a client's general fears that her baby may have a genetic problem and as exotic as contemplating the nurse's role in experimental efforts to manipulate the genetic endowment of an embryo conceived in the laboratory.

Genetic counseling is the oldest of these interventions. Nurses are often the first ones asked by patients about the risks of having a genetically abnormal child. At prenatal clinics and during neonatal clinical encounters, the nurse may be the one who must confront ethical dilemmas such as whether to alarm parents by discussing small but real risks of minor anomalies. The nurse may also be the one who discovers that a client is a carrier of a recessive gene and is refusing to disclose that fact to her brothers and sisters. Also in the realm of counseling, the nurse may have to deal with clients who make unpopular decisions such as deciding not to abort a seriously malformed fetus. The issues here tend to raise problems of the principles of autonomy and truth-telling, as well as terrible problems of how to decide what will benefit clients, whether they be the future parents or their offspring. These are the issues of genetic counseling presented in the cases in the first section of this chapter.

Historically, the next group of problems to emerge centered around mass genetic screening programs. Here the conflict between the welfare of the client and others within the society can be critical. The nurse may find herself pressured into the role of protector of society's interests rather than her traditional role of advocate for the client. The first case in this section—the pregnant patient in an alpha-fetoprotein screening program—begins to raise problems of whether the nurse has any business advocating a test in order to prevent the birth of a seriously afflicted infant, thereby saving society, as well as the parents, considerable money. The second case pushes the idea of mass genetic screening further into the future. It envisions the day when the nurse might be asked to cooperate in a systematic mass screening program to identify fetuses that may someday be the expendable members of the society.

The remaining cases in the chapter deal with the ethical problems of newer technologies of birth and the biological revolution. In vitro fertilization, the process of fertilizing a surgically removed human egg in a laboratory dish, has recently become not only technically possible, but also an attractive intervention of last resort for some of the millions of infertile couples throughout the world. The nurse participating in such a program faces a wide range of ethical problems from such basic questions as whether the entire process is an immoral tampering with nature to more specific ethical controversies of whether embryos fertilized in vitro can ethically be implanted for gestation in a woman who did not provide the egg cells. The process of multiple fertilizations also gives rise to the problem of leftover embryos—embryos that are of great interest both to researchers, who might want to attempt brief gestation for scientific investigation, and infertile couples, who either may not be physiologically capable of supplying their own egg and sperm cells or who simply may not wish to go to the inconvenience and expense of a pregnancy.

The next case grows out of another manifestation of newer birth technologies. Artificial insemination has been both technically feasible and ethically controversial for many years. Traditionally, however, artificial insemination has involved inseminating a wife with either her husband's or a donor's sperm. There has never been any technical barrier to using the technique to fertilize some woman other than a wife either because the wife was incapable of bearing a child or simply because she preferred not to do so. Recently, such surrogate motherhood procedures have been attempted. Our case study explores the role of the nurse in them.

A final case explores the ethics of the most dramatic and innovative birth technology. Until recently, all genetic and birth interventions simply manipulated the existing genetic material, providing the prospective parents with opportunities to refrain from conceiving, to abort if the woman did become pregnant, or to manipulate the fertilization process through in vitro fertilization and artificial insemination. Now, however, it is rapidly becoming possible to change the genetic material itself through what has come to be called genetic engineering. The first attempts have actually taken place although in the future they will certainly be considered quite crude. Nursing personnel will play a number of roles in such genetic manipulations from providing information to clinical nursing services. Our case poses the problems faced by a nurse asked to participate in an experimental effort to manipulate the human genetic code.

GENETIC COUNSELING

The problems of genetic counseling have been with us since people first recognized that some medical problems run in families. The rapid development of technologies for diagnosing genetic anomalies, however, has made this kind of counseling a much more significant and controversial enterprise. We now not only understand the science of genetics, but also can detect both carrier status and genetic disease in postnatal humans as well as fetuses. We can detect fetal problems with varying degrees of reliability through the use of amniocentesis (biochemical and chromosomal analysis of fetal cells obtained from the amnionic fluid), ultrasound, and analysis of fetal blood samples. We can detect disease or carrier status in postnatal humans through biochemical and chromosomal tests.

The importance of this field has increased as abortion became legal and potentially available to cope with detected fetal anomalies. That is not the only reason for parents wanting genetic information about their fetus, however. They might also want to know whether they are carrying a fetus afflicted with a genetic condition in order to plan for its birth or to put their minds at ease should the fetus not be affected. Genetic counseling also involves issues of the clarification of complex scientific problems, of encouraging discussion with family members who may also be at risk, and of learning to deal with the fact that our bodies carry the potential of harmful genetic information.[1-3]

Most nurses do not have primary responsibility for genetic counseling. Some may be educated especially for these responsibilities and work in departments of obstetrics, pediatrics, or genetics. Others, however, need to be able to recognize the issues of potential controversy so that they can refer patients for counseling, consult with other members of the health care team, and discuss issues with patients. The first case presented in this section reveals how a nurse may be called upon to initiate conversations about genetic counseling when other members of the health care team have not done so.

Case 71: When the Risk of Genetic Abnormality is Uncertain

Vivian Torrance works as the staff nurse in a busy obstetrics/gynecology clinic in an urban HMO. She has noticed that more women are delaying their pregnancies until their late 20s and early 30s. This is a childbearing trend well documented in the literature and evidenced particularly in urban areas and clinic settings servicing professional women. Ordinarily, this trend would pose no particular problem for Mrs. Torrance, but she is becoming increasingly concerned about the number of older women in the HMO who are bearing disabled or handicapped children. The problem is being studied, and discussion is underway concerning appropriate counseling for the older pregnant woman, the availability of prenatal diagnostic procedures, genetic testing, and so forth.

In the meantime, however, the clinic is continuing to monitor a number of older pregnant women who have not previously received any counseling about potential risks of having a genetically abnormal child. The problem becomes acute for Mrs. Torrance one day when Stacy Carmichael, a 37-year-old administrator, visits the clinic for her routine pregnancy checkup. It is Mrs. Carmichael's first pregnancy, and she and her husband have planned the pregnancy to coincide with their purchase of a townhouse in a restored part of the city. As Mrs. Carmichael leaves the clinic, Mrs. Torrance overhears a parting conversation between the patient and her obstetrician. Mrs. Carmichael asks the physician if she has any risk of bearing an abnormal child at her age. Her physician tells her, "Don't worry your pretty head about such matters—rest, eat well, and exercise every day—you and your baby will be just fine!" Mrs. Carmichael beams at her physician and leaves the clinic under the assumption that she has nothing to worry about.

Mrs. Torrance, however, feels that someone *should* discuss potential risks with Mrs. Carmichael and the availability of prenatal diagnostic procedures. Should she do this while making the appointment for Mrs. Carmichael's next visit? Is the risk great enough to cause alarm in Mrs. Carmichael and to create a problem with her physician? Mrs. Torrance is not sure.

Commentary

Because of her age, Mrs. Carmichael is at higher risk than younger women of bearing a child with a genetic abnormality, such as Down's syndrome. The nurse, Mrs. Torrance, is aware of this. Mrs. Carmichael apparently had some suspicion but has been reassured by her physician. The justification of that reassurance is suspect. It involves some complex ethical judgments that Mrs. Torrance and Mrs. Carmichael may not share.

The medical literature today generally recommends amniocentesis for woman over 35 years of age. The reason for that is controversial. When data relating maternal age to risk of Down's syndrome were first gathered, they were collected in 5-year intervals.[2] A substantial increase in risk was noted for woman in the 35 to 39 age-group in comparison with younger women. When the risks of the amniocentesis itself and the scarcity of the resources available to perform the tests were considered, many believed that age 35 was a reasonable cutoff. That judgment, however, involved controversial value issues. On one hand, someone who opposed abortion of a fetus with Down's syndrome might consider the expense and risks of the tests unjustifiable at any age. On the other hand, if someone had an extreme fear of carrying a Down's syndrome infant and desperately wanted a baby, they might be more than willing to bear the risks and the expense of the test even at a very young age. From the individual's point of view, deciding what level of risk of Down's syndrome justifies the test is an ethical and value call. From the point of view of a society concerned about scarce resources, it seems prudent to offer the tests more readily to those women at higher risk, but even then, some consideration might be given to the unusual concerns of younger pregnant women. More recent data make clear that the risk of Down's syndrome increases gradually with age, and there is no major change at age 35.[4]

This suggests that Mrs. Torrance would have a potential problem if she witnessed even a younger patient, say a 32 year old, being denied requested information about fetal risks and tests that might be performed. The problem is more acute with a 37-year-old patient such as Mrs. Carmichael. The physician is clearly deviating from standard practice. Such deviation might be justified if it could be shown that patients in general or Mrs. Carmichael in particular wanted the deviation. There is no such evidence in this case, however. In fact, the patient seems to have asked for a discussion of the issue. There may even be legal liability for the physician who fails to provide the information in these circumstances. Courts have supported the cutoff at age 35.[5]

This leaves Mrs. Torrance in the position of being forced to make a judgment. Even though she is not trained in genetic counseling and has not sought out the role of amniocentesis advocate, if she believes that Mrs. Carmichael has a right to the information in order to make an informed choice about her prenatal care and possibly in order to make a decision to change physicians, she will have to take some action. Preferably, she would discuss the matter with Mrs. Carmichael's physician. She might also discuss the matter with the patient directly or call the matter to the attention of other members of the health care team.

A more intriguing problem arises if Mrs. Torrance realizes all of this but believes that an abortion, the most probable outcome if the test is performed and the fetus is found to have Down's syndrome, is morally wrong. If she really believes that abortion is so wrong that it is murder, can she take action to alert Mrs. Carmichael of the increased risk and the possibility of amniocentesis to diagnose Down's syndrome? She might even believe that referring the patient to another practitioner would be aiding and abetting a murder. In fact, that may have been the stance of the physician who decided not to counsel Mrs. Carmichael. If Mrs. Torrance recognizes that the physician's behavior is atypical, in fact perhaps even illegal, but also does not want to contribute to what she believes to be a seriously immoral action, should she follow the same course of the physician and just avoid the entire discussion?

Case 72: Counseling the Pregnant Woman with Sickle Cell Disease

The County Hospital prenatal clinic, serving a largely black, inner-city population, does routine sickle cell preps on all its patients. Audrey Brown, a 17-year-old, unmarried, black patient, tested positive. She was at least 16 weeks pregnant, and she had sickle cell disease. Moreover, early in her pregnancy, she had taken antinausea medication that has been reported to be teratogenic.

Gail Siegler, the nurse–practitioner in the clinic, saw an array of troublesome problems. Since Audrey Brown was not just a carrier of sickle cell, but actually had the disease, the pregnancy could cause her some problems. The exposure to a known teratogen along with the risk of the pregnancy both led her to explore alternatives carefully with her patient. Ms. Brown was quite resistant to the discussion of abortion as an alternative. She seemed to want to have a baby. Moreover, she was a very involved Catholic, for whom abortion was morally suspect. While she did not rule out the possibility of an abortion, it was clear she would find it difficult.

The issues swirled in Ms. Siegler's head. Since Ms. Brown was already 16 weeks pregnant, Ms. Siegler realized an abortion would require admission to the problem pregnancy clinic for a saline abortion. Audrey Brown would go through labor and experience a delivery; the fetus would be delivered formed. She envisioned the trauma the young woman would suffer.

Then she considered the genetic issues. Since Ms. Brown had sickle cell disease, the infant would at least be a carrier. Since her boy friend was black, there was about one chance in ten that he was a carrier, in which case there would be one chance in four of the baby also having sickle cell disease. Do these probabilities increase the justification for an abortion? Should this possibility be raised for the young woman to consider? Should Ms. Siegler initiate action to have the boy friend screened for sickle cell carrier status?

Ms. Brown's baby will definitely at least be a sickle cell carrier. Although there are virtually no medical problems resulting from having carrier status, it would increase the chances of the infant's offspring having sickle cell. Is that at all relevant to the choices to be made? Should she raise this for Ms. Brown to take into account? What is the role of this genetic information in Ms. Siegler's approach to her patient?

Case 73: The Pregnant Teenager with a Genetic Problem

Melinda Eades was a 16-year-old woman diagnosed at an outpatient neurology clinic as having neurofibromatosis (also known as Elephant Man's disease) 2 months ago. At the time of diagnosis, genetic counseling was recommended to Melinda's mother, since any children born to Melinda would always have a 50% chance of also having neurofibromatosis. Mrs. Eades was very concerned about Melinda because her daughter had become quite depressed by her diagnosis. She decided to wait a few months before discussing this problem with Melinda and making the appointment with the genetic counselor. Since there was no reason to believe that Melinda was sexually active, it was agreed that Mrs. Eades would contact the clinic for the genetic counseling in a month or so.

Within a few weeks, however, Melinda went to an obstetrics/gynecology clinic on her own for problems with menstruation. Testing revealed that she was approximately 7 weeks pregnant. She was counseled by the clinic nurse about abortion options and was advised to discuss her pregnancy with her parents. When Melinda mentioned that she was recently diagnosed as having neurofibromatosis, the clinic nurse recommended that she return to the neurology clinic for follow-up and counseling. Melinda did not seem to understand that her disease was genetically transmissible to her offspring.

After several days of agonizing over her pregnancy, Melinda told her mother. Mrs. Eades was very upset with Melinda and immediately decided that Melinda should have an abortion. When Melinda seemed uncertain whether she wanted to abort the pregnancy, Mrs. Eades told her that any of her offspring would have a 50% chance of having neurofibromatosis. Melinda was astounded by this news but was still uncertain what she should do. She was also very upset that she had not been informed of this fact earlier.

When Melinda showed up for her appointment at the neurology clinic, she was frantic and confused about making the right decision. She asked Janice Goldstein, RN, the nurse Melinda originally saw in the clinic 2 months previously, why someone had not told her that she needed to be careful about becoming pregnant. When she realized that her mother had decided to withhold this information from her for a period of time, Melinda was angry and confused. Didn't she have a right to know this information, even though she was a minor? Also, why had the nurse conveyed this information to her mother and not to her? Could her mother control her in that manner, even to the point of forcing her to have an abortion, a course of action that Melinda would not likely choose under any circumstances?

Commentary

These two cases, like the first case in this section, both raise questions about whether genetic anomalies provide justifiable grounds for abortion. The case of Audrey Brown, the 17-year-old patient with sickle cell disease, suggests several links between genetic conditions and abortion. First, Ms. Brown is at special risk of her pregnancy because of her disease, regardless of the condition of the fetus. Is this a case of abortion justified by maternal health risk? Second, Ms. Brown was exposed to a known teratogen during her pregnancy. Teratogens, especially encountered early in pregnancy, cause genetic changes in some fetuses, some so serious that they produce serious genetic afflictions. The risks, however, are very difficult to assess. No precise risk figures are going to be available. Aborting on these grounds could avoid a serious genetic affliction, but it could also mean ending the life of what would be a normal child. Third, it is conceivable that someone would choose to abort because of what is known about the fetal genetic composition. The child will definitely be a sickle cell carrier. Someone might argue that the abortion should be performed in order to avoid passing the sickle cell gene along in the gene pool. The problems to the patient of possessing a single sickle cell gene (of being a carrier rather than actually having the disease) are extremely small, however. Few people would be so committed to the purity of the gene pool that they would advocate aborting a known carrier just to preserve the gene pool. The fact that the patient, like many sickle cell patients, is black could easily lead to racist implications if an abortion were suggested simply to eliminate a fetus with carrier status.

The possibility that the baby could get two sickle cell genes might also be considered. In that case, the baby would actually have the disease. Having sickle cell disease causes problems in life—pain from sickle cell crisis and even potentially life-threatening risks. Much of the time, however, patients with sickle cell disease live reasonably normal lives. Deciding to abort because a fetus actually has the disease could be controversial but not so much as aborting a baby with carrier status. In order to give Audrey Brown a chance to consider all of this it might be necessary to begin asking questions about the father of her child. Should the father be identified? Should he be screened to see if he is a sickle cell carrier? If he is black, there is about one chance in ten he is a carrier. If so, then one pregnancy in four would result in a fetus with two sickle cell genes, that is, with the actual disease. Tests are being developed to obtain a fetal blood sample. Because of the risks involved, they would be used only if both parents were carriers and the baby could have the disease. Should Gail Siegler become involved in all of these complexities? Especially if she is not trained in genetics, would it be better if she simply remained quiet, or should she take on the complex of scientific, ethical, and racial issues the case raises?

The case of Melinda Eades, the 17 year old with neurofibromatosis, is in some ways similar. It involves a pregnant teenager with a genetic problem. Yet Ms. Eades' case involves a disease that is transmitted by a single gene; hers is an autosomal dominant condition. That means that regardless of the absence of the gene in the father, each of Ms. Eades' offspring has a 50% chance of having the disease. Does the increased risk make the abortion easier to justify and therefore action by nurse Janice Goldstein easier to justify? Does the seriousness of the disease in comparison with sickle cell disease make intervention easier?

On the other hand, whereas sickle cell disease might potentially be diagnosed in utero, neurofibromatosis cannot be. This means that, if an abortion is pursued, it will be on the basis of the 50% chance of the fetus being affected. Does the fact that there is a 50% chance of the child being normal make action on Ms. Goldstein's part more difficult?

GENETIC SCREENING

Genetic screening raises all of the issues of genetic counseling and then some. Screening usually refers to preliminary genetic tests done routinely on large populations. Normally, a positive test leads to further, more careful assessment, including counseling of the sort possible on a one-to-one basis. Sometimes screening is done in the community as, for example, when a Jewish community organization organizes screening for Tay-Sachs carrier status, a condition occurring with increased frequency in the Jewish population. In such community-based screening, nurses may be the only health care professionals with direct contact with the people being screened.

The first case in this section the screening is conducted by a nurse to measure alpha-fetoprotein levels, a preliminary diagnostic test for neural tube defects and Down's syndrome.[6] The second case, one of the few purely hypothetical cases in this volume, anticipates future mass screening programs for a marker that correlates with low intelligence.

Case 74: The Pregnant Patient
in an Alpha-Fetoprotein Screening Program

Polly Barnes is a new graduate nurse in a community-based prenatal care program. She has just been informed that all new patients admitted to the program are to become part of the clinic's new maternal serum alpha-fetoprotein screening (MSAFP) project. Each patient will have a small amount of blood drawn by fingerstick at 6 to 7 weeks of pregnancy to determine her their serum level of alpha-fetoprotein (AFP). High levels of AFP suggest that the pregnant patient is at risk for bearing an infant affected by a neural tube defect. Low levels are being interpreted as a preliminary indication of possible Down's syndrome. Additional testing—repeat MSAFP levels, sonogram, amniocentesis—as well as genetic counseling will be provided for the patient who demonstrates abnormal levels of MSAFP.

When Ms. Barnes asks why this screening program is being performed on all patients, she is told that it is believed that most pregnant woman who know they are bearing a neural tube defect affected fetus will want to abort the fetus rather than risk bearing a child with the potential for long-term disability. The test is provided as a community service to help reduce the the public cost of supporting infants born with these defects. Since the initial cost of the MSAFP test is negligible, the potential cost-saving to the community is considerable, even if only one or two affected pregnancies per 1000 births are aborted. Thus the screening program is of considerable value to the community in terms of future costs required to support disabled children.

Ms. Barnes understands why the community might want to require the performance of this test on all pregnant women. However, she also realizes that the performance of the test might have false positives, particularly at the initial screening test levels. The results of the tests might cause mental trauma to patients who are already distressed by their pregnant condition. It is also possible that abnormal test results might alarm some patients to the extent that they even abort their otherwise normal pregnancy before concluding further testing. Since the nurse's primary goal is to serve the patient. Ms. Barnes is not certain that any nurse should participate in a MSAFP screening program. To do so seems to support the goals of society over that of the pregnant woman and the fetus. What is the nurse's obligation in this type of situation?

Case 75: Screening for the Expendables: Nursing in the 2000s

Mary Jane Taylor has been assigned to assist in a community-based mass screening program scheduled to begin in June, 2010. Based on alpha-fetoprotein screening techniques developed in the 1970s and 1980s, it is now known that tests performed on blood samples can predict not only neural tube defects and a range of conditions having impact on intelligence, but also can be used as a reasonably accurate predictor of significant mental function deficits. Although the tests are not 100% accurate, they are reliable enough that many parents use them to make procreation decisions, including abortion decisions. Moreover, since these deficits are now clearly linked to genetic anomalies, pressures are being generated to make the diagnostic tests mandatory and withdraw insurance funding for care for any children borne by parents in spite of test results indicating significant problems.

The goal is to prevent the suffering and expense generated by the birth of affected children and, secondarily, to decrease the frequency in the gene pool of the genes responsible.

Although social values have changed dramatically in the past 20 years, Ms. Taylor is not sure that nursing values have changed to the extent that she can participate in this type of screening program. The results of the screening will determine which fetuses will be viewed as expendable both for the good of the individuals involved and for the good of the community. The obligation to avoid killing is still strongly held by most members of the nursing profession, but it is increasingly recognized that the nurse has an obligation both to prevent suffering when it can be avoided and to serve the community. However, there is rumor that if members of the nursing profession do not reconcile some of their values with the changing needs of society, the government will create an entirely new type of nurse that will be responsive to social values and the needs of the community. Assuming the test is reasonably accurate, should Ms. Taylor participate in the project while it remains voluntary? Should she continue to participate if the tests become mandatory?

Commentary

Polly Barnes, the nurse working in the community-based prenatal care program, faces all of the ethical questions that she would face if she were working in a hospital-based genetic counseling program. She must decide whether she wants to be a part of a program that would almost certainly have as one of its major impacts an increase in the rate of abortions for neural tube defects and Down's syndrome. If she believes that abortion for these conditions is not justified, she may well have a hard time working in the program. She must also face the more subtle effects of any genetic counseling program. She is worried about anxiety produced in her patients, about false-positives, about precipitous abortions of normal fetuses, the obligation to relatives of the patient who may also be at risk, and so forth.

But beyond these, she faces additional difficulties because she is participating in a mass screening program. While she may have the most noble objectives and be committed to her patient's welfare, she will have only limited contact with the patients who test positively in the initial screening. She will have to rely on others in clinics or private offices, many of whom she may not even know, to carry out the followup counseling on a one-to-one basis. She may unwittingly be referring her patients into a network that could eventually lead to contact with some other practitioner who is unrealistically zealous in promoting abortion (or in keeping the implications of the tests from patients in order to forestall abortion).

The nurse working in mass screening is divorcing herself from the traditional clinical relationship and becoming a part of a larger, more bureaucratized delivery system. Realistically, the use that will eventually be made of the information she generates is pretty much outside her hands.

One example of how this information may be used in ways incompatible with traditional nursing ethics is seen in the agenda that the sponsors of the program imply. While Ms. Barnes may undertake the screening for the purpose of benefiting the individual client, it seems clear that the others who are sponsoring the program have a much more social objective: reducing the public costs of supporting infants born with these defects. Ms. Barnes is aware that nurses increasingly recognize that they have social as well as individual patient obligations. As long as the goals of the individual patient (avoiding the mental and physical suffering resulting from the birth of an afflicted child) and the society (cost-saving) converge, this is no problem. But would not a sponsoring agency with its announced agenda want Ms. Barnes actually to promote the abortion of the afflicted fetus? They might at least expect her to make the possibilities known and perhaps encourage the patient with positive tests to pursue this course.

The implications are projected into the future in the hypothetical case set in the year 2010, when the use of screening tests has been perfected to the point that deficiencies in mental functioning can be predicted with substantial accuracy. If deficits in intelligence can be predicted accurately and it is agreed that most rational people would prefer not to have a child with such a deficit, would it not make sense to make the diagnostic tests mandatory? And, if so, would not other implications follow, such as prohibition of the use of insurance funds for care of such children and perhaps even the mandatory avoidance of suffering in children by prohibition of their births?

Does Ms. Barnes, the nurse in the first case, have any responsibility to anticipate potential future uses of the technologies to which she is currently contributing? Could she justifiably say that the decision to use social controls to foster elimination of children with subnormal mental function is so much a violation of her understanding of morality that she should not even participate in the first stages? If she is willing to participate in the initial uses, but finds the later uses unacceptable, when should she stop participating? What aspects of the envisioned later use might give her pause? Is it the involvement of the government with social purposes? If so, that has already occurred in the earlier use of AFP screening. Is it the rejection of children with predictably subnormal mental function? If so, that also is implied in the earlier use. Is there anything morally different from the later use that is not implied in the earlier one?

IN VITRO FERTILIZATION AND ARTIFICIAL INSEMINATION

The ability to detect genetic status and use genetic information to make decisions about fertility is just the beginning of the birth technologies that are now becoming available. Many couples who are concerned about the birth process are not concerned about genetic problems, but about infertility or other problems with normal conception. It is now technically possible to deal with some of these problems by the technique of in vitro fertilization: the extracorporeal fertilization of a human egg surgically removed from a woman's ovary.

Once the process of fertilization is separated from the human body, it is technically possible to perform many new kinds of manipulations. The egg removed from a woman could, after being fertilized by her husband, be implanted in the womb of some other woman. A woman with an intact uterus but no ovaries could become pregnant after her husband's semen was used to fertilize an egg cell removed from some other woman, perhaps one undergoing the procedure so that she herself could become pregnant. Beyond these variations, it is now recognized that it is technically possible, in fact, technically preferable to fertilize several egg cells at once, storing the extras for later use if the first implantation is unsuccessful. These extras, however, are, for the first time, available for other potential uses, including research. Moreover, once the pregnancy is achieved, there may remain fertilized ova that the couple no longer wants to use. Nurses participating in programs involving birth technologies such as these will have to decide the extent to which they can participate in such programs and when they must speak out about practices they witness in their clinics and laboratories. The next case illustrates the problem.

Case 76: The Case of the Discarded Fertilized Ova

Central Medical Center has just received monies from a private donor to initiate an in vitro fertilization program. One of the first tasks of the medical director is to hire nurses to staff the clinic and a small six-bed unit where patients will rest after their fertilized ova are implanted.

Doris Nordstrum has heard about the impending opening of the clinic and the nursing positions available. Curious about the clinic and in vitro fertilization, Mrs. Nordstrum applies for a position. On interview, her responsibilities are explained, and she is given a tour of the almost completed laboratories and the unit. She is impressed but has some nagging questions about the moral issues involved with in vitro fertilization and the process itself. When she tries to discuss these questions with the medical director, he seems to brush away her concerns and focus on the novelty of the technology, the benefit of its use to childless couples, and the social demand for the service. Mrs. Nordstrum, however, is concerned about some very basic questions about fertilization of human ova, conception, and the values she has usually associated with these human events. She wonders whether she can work effectively in an environment that treats the traditional "mysteries of life" as simply scientific events that can be manipulated by human invention. She also wonders what guidelines the clinic will have for the treatment of fertilized ova that are not implanted in the prospective pregnant woman. Will they be used for other purposes? Or will they be discarded in the sink drain? If they are stored for any period of time, what policies will the clinic have for discarding them at a later date? These are issues of fundamental importance to Mrs. Nordstrum and impact on both her professional and personal values.

Commentary

The questions Mrs. Nordstrum is raising have been posed by others as well. Some of the early commentators on in vitro fertilization questioned the "demystification" of the birth process, taking what was once procreation and converting it into the "manufacture" of babies.[7-9] Some of these commentators grounded their objections in what amounts to natural law positions, that certain biological processes constitute the naturally appropriate way of procreating and that artificial manipulations of something as fundamental as human germ cells violate the natural order.

They also objected on the basis that in vitro fertilization constituted an experiment on a nonconsenting subject, exposing it to risks that technically cannot be for its own benefit. Since the being upon whom the experiment of in vitro manipulation would be conducted would not otherwise exist, it would be impossible for the intervention to be for the new being's own good.

In vitro fertilization is generally undertaken for the good of adults who perceive a child as beneficial to *them*. As in vitro fertilization has become more commonplace, the concern about possible risks has diminished. Evidence seems to show that babies born through in vitro fertilization are not at any greater risk than those conceived more traditionally. Still, the underlying ethical questions remain, the questions that seem to trouble Mrs. Nordstrum.

Whereas many ethics commentators have raised these questions, others have defended the process, some even calling it more ethical because it is a "more human" way to reproduce.[10] They argue that the human is a rational animal and that traditional reproduction simply left matters to chance. According to them, rational planning of a pregnancy—overcoming the limits of nature if necessary—is more human and therefore more ethical.

Mrs. Nordstrum may be struggling with these now traditional issues about the risks of in vitro fertilization and the morality of manipulating human embryos. On the other hand, she may be raising newer, more specific questions such as those about the disposal of leftover embryos. One approach to the problem is to view the extra embryos as essentially the property of the parents who produced them. Since they have the right to abort early fetuses far more developed than the embryos under question here, it can be reasoned that they should also have the right to control the embryos produced by in vitro fertilization.

Even if one grants the parents the right to destroy the embryos, however, it does not follow that they have the right to do other things with the embryos they produce. In particular, it does not give them the right to maintain them to the point that they live to be more mature. For this reason, many have held that either no research should be permitted on embryos or that such research should be limited to the very early stages of life, for example, the first 14 days.

Even if such research manipulations are prohibited, there is still a problem of what to do with the extra embryos. Should there be norms of proper disposal? Should other couples wanting to conceive but unable to supply ova be permitted access? If so, does the couple that was the original source of the embryo have to consent? Should they be compensated? The recipient couple is, after all, saving the expense, risk, and discomfort of the surgery to obtain an ovum.

Before Mrs. Nordstrum agrees to accept a position with the clinic, she should be prepared to answer these questions.

Case 77: Counseling the Surrogate Mother

Janice Collins has worked in the office of a private physician of obstetrics/gynecology for several years. In addition to routine care, Dr. Ellis specializes in artificial insemination. Over the years, Ms. Collins has seen the results of his work and has been delighted to participate in a service that brings such happiness to otherwise childless couples who truly want to have children.

Although the majority of Dr. Ellis' patients receive artificial insemination using the husband's sperm (AIH), some couples have, because of a variety of problems, chosen artificial insemination by donor sperm (AID). During the past year, Dr. Ellis has even employed the services of a surrogate mother for one of his female patients incapable of carrying a pregnancy to term. A recent patient, however, has requested the services of the surrogate mother because she does not want to take the time from her work to be pregnant. Both she and her infertile husband want a child and can afford to pay for the costs of surrogate motherhood. In fact, they would rather choose this method than wait to adopt a child through private agencies. They feel that they will have greater success in selecting a child to meet their intellectual and social needs through surrogate motherhood and AID than through adoption. They have asked Dr. Ellis to provide this service for them. Both Dr. Ellis and Ms. Collins, however, are not sure that they want to employ their surrogate mother for this situation. Somehow, it does not seem right.

Commentary

Ms. Collins and Dr. Ellis have apparently already answered some of the ethical questions to their satisfaction. They have confronted the traditional ethical questions about the artificiality of manipulating human germ cells that were discussed in conjunction with the previous case. They have no insurmountable ethical problem about the transfer of germ cells to someone outside of a marriage; they have previously accepted artificial gamete transfer by a donor when the donor was a male.

What they now confront is a newer variant on this theme. To be sure, the involvement of a female gamete donor is more substantial. She will serve as the host for the pregnancy in addition to supplying the ovum. In reflecting on the ethics involved, they might ask themselves whether there is a significant moral difference between a woman who simply supplies an ovum, perhaps during a sterilization procedure, and a woman who serves as a surrogate mother. In the latter case, the woman's involvement includes substantially more physical and emotional commitment. It will be much more difficult for the relationship to be anonymous than in the case of traditional artificial insemination. Some surrogate mothers have developed unanticipated attachments to the fetus that is part theirs biologically, but not socially.

Since the surrogate mother is necessarily involved for a long period of time, other problems might arise that would not appear in traditional artificial insemination. Would the prospective parents have the right to insist that the host mother maintain good prenatal practices: avoidance of alcohol and smoking, regular visits to the prenatal clinic, and so on? Would they have the right to insist on prenatal diagnosis to detect possible fetal anomalies? If so, would they have the right to insist on an abortion if some undesirable pattern of fetal development emerged? Would the parents be able to insist on abortion whenever a risk occurred that was unacceptable to them, or would it have to be a risk unacceptable to the host mother or to a "reasonable person?" Would the husband of the host mother have any rights: the right to consent to the involvement of his wife in what would seriously disrupt the traditional marital relationship or the right to veto an abortion if he were willing to accept responsibility for the child? All of these questions needed to be answered before Dr. Ellis and Ms. Collins agreed to participate in any surrogate motherhood procedures at all.

Now they face still another moral twist. Is there any moral difference between a surrogate mother serving as a substitute for a woman unable to carry a child to term and one who simply would rather not do so? Is surrogate motherhood a last resort procedure to be limited to those incapable of bearing a child, or should it be an arrangement that is acceptable as long as all parties consent? In some sense, condoning surrogate motherhood when it is not necessitated by inability to bear a child requires a judgment about the legitimacy of the priorities of the woman who will eventually have the nurturing responsibilities for the child. With an increasing acceptance of nontraditional roles for women, some women are bound to want parenthood without pregnancy. There is no technical barrier. Are we prepared to say that there should be a moral barrier, or are we willing to let the marketplace and the compassion of potential host mothers dictate the practice?

GENETIC ENGINEERING

The newest and, in many ways, the most controversial birth technology that the nurse may encounter is what is often referred to as genetic engineering. Genetic counseling and screening focus on determining the existence of genetic conditions and helping the patient accommodate to them through psychological interventions, support systems, and abortion. It has taken the actual genetic endowment as a given. Since the 1970s, the ability to make actual changes in the genetic makeup of an individual has been on the horizon. While isolated attempts have been made to change genetic endowment in humans, they have not received the support of either the scientific community or the general public. As far as we know, these attempts have all been failures.

The technical knowledge to attempt changes in genetic endowment is developing rapidly. Further attempts will surely be made. In fact, some leading research centers are already at the point of planning such interventions. Nursing personnel will be called upon to provide clinical and research support for these attempts. The following case, based on the current state of the field, is hypothetical but is constructed on the basis of the experiences of persons in such research environments.

Case 78: The Nurse in Experimental Genetic Engineering*

Louise McHenry is a staff nurse at the Clinical Research Center at University Hospital, a major research center affiliated with a leading medical school. Two of the major lines of research that have been going on at the center are converging toward a bold experiment. The molecular biology group under the direction of Dr. Horrace Windover has for years been conducting research on the basic processes of gene manipulation. Using techniques involving recombinant DNA, they have become proficient in the basic science and laboratory techniques that are now known to make possible the introduction of additional genetic material into living cells. Using partially inactivated retroviruses as vectors, bits of genetic material can be carried into cells and become incorporated into them.

Collaborating in the proposed research is the group that has conducted a long line of studies of metabolic processes under the direction of Dr. Todd Walsh. The Windover team is aware that one of the first attempts at genetic manipulation in humans is likely to be for the treatment of adenosine deaminase (ADA) deficiency, a serious, otherwise untreatable metabolic disorder. Some months ago, Dr. Windover approached Dr. Walsh about the possibility of collaborating in an attempt to become the first laboratory to provide a formally approved method to treat a human disease through gene therapy.

*This case was constructed with the assistance of LeRoy Walters, the Chairman of the Working Group on Human Gene Therapy of the NIH Recombinant DNA Advisory Committee.

The approach would be one of removing bone marrow from an affected individual and exposing it to gene splicing techniques developed by Dr. Windover's group and others working on recombinant DNA worldwide. If all goes well, the treated bone marrow would take up the missing genetic material, and the corrected bone marrow would be reintroduced into the patient. That patient would then have a newfound capacity to produce the needed adenosine deaminase.

Louise McHenry, as a nurse in the clinical center, would be called upon to provide the now standard nursing services involved in bone marrow transplantation. She and the other personnel in the center have attended several meetings where the new project was explained. She would be asked to do nothing different from what she has done for patients receiving bone marrow transplants in a protocol in oncology on which she had worked for the past 2 years. The bone marrow in this case, however, would be reimplanted in the patient from which it was taken rather than being given to a different patient. It would be reintroduced with new genetic material incorporated, presumably the genetic material needed by the patient.

The researchers were blunt in addressing the potential staff for the project. This is new and potentially controversial. The same technologies could be used to make other changes in the basic genetic structure in human beings. Moreover, once fairly simple genetic manipulations proved successful for critically ill patients such as those with ADA deficiency and Lesch-Nyhan syndrome, the way would be cleared for more controversial interventions. Whereas these first attempts at gene therapy would involve only attempts to modify somatic cells, eventually efforts would be made to modify germ cells and to make it possible to transmit from one generation to the next new genetic material introduced into the species. Ms. McHenry is being asked whether she is willing to agree to be part of the team for this research. She has had experience in assessing these features of research protocols in the past, and she is familiar with both the national standards and the local standards used by their institutional review board (IRB). She knows that their IRB will review the proposed research and that, since part of the work will be supported by National Institutes of Health (NIH) funds, a national level panel will also review the work. She has no doubts that the proposed research will meet the highest technical standards and that the investigators are acting in good conscience. She still needs to decide whether, ethically, she can be a part of the proposed project.

Commentary

In making a decision, Ms. McHenry will have to take into account all of the now standard questions of the ethics of research involving patients. The Working Group on Human Gene Therapy, which is part of the NIH Recombinant DNA Advisory Committee, has published a set of questions entitled *Points to Consider in the Design and Submission of Human Somatic-Cell Gene Therapy Protocols*. It calls for an assessment of (1) the objectives and rationale of the proposed research, (2) research design, anticipated risks and benefits, (3) selection of patients, (4) informed consent, and (5) privacy and confidentiality.[11] Ms. McHenry is used to making these assessments based on her past involvement in other research projects.

Still, questions remain to be answered.[11] In the assessment of risks, several are unique to genetic engineering. Animal studies are less informative in this area than in many other kinds of medical research. There are no known animal models for some of the enzyme deficiency diseases likely to be the targets of gene therapy. Even where animal models are available, it is unlikely that clinical outcomes can be assessed clearly until trials are attempted in humans. It is possible that the retroviruses will recombine with other DNA material to produce deleterious effects, disrupting other genes or producing carcinogenic effects.

It is conceivable that the viruses will affect other persons, either workers in the laboratory or members of the public, although steps are taken to minimize these risks.

The most fundamental question Ms. McHenry will face is whether there is something that, in principle, is morally suspect about human efforts to manipulate genetic material and incorporate new genes into the cells of human beings. Genetic engineering has been compared to manipulation of the atom. These two 20th-century scientific efforts have the capacity to change the nature of the universe in ways that some people find of an order of magnitude more dramatic than other scientific and medical endeavors. It is now generally recognized that DNA, the genetic material, makes individual living species what they are. Until now all medical efforts have, by and large, left the nature of the species intact. To be sure, over extremely long periods, medical interventions might evolutionarily make infinitesimal, incremental changes in the nature of the human, but by and large, the species itself would remain constant. Now we are on the verge of developing the capacity to make wholesale changes in the genetic composition of the species. Nurses like Ms. McHenry and laboratories like the one described in this case will be making choices to participate or refuse to participate in that change.

The initial project, quite possibly the adenosine deaminase deficiency experiment, will be what is referred to as gene therapy—attempts to correct a medical genetic defect. In early cases, this will be by attempting to add missing genetic material. Some people distinguish gene therapy from other efforts at genetic engineering in which efforts would be made to improve upon the already normal human genetic endowment.

Another distinction that Ms. McHenry will have to consider is whether it is important to limit such experiments to changes in somatic cells. Such changes, such as the one contemplated in the proposed research, would have their impact only in the individual patient. The patient's reproductive cells would remain as before, without the gene responsible for producing adenosine deaminase. This has two implications. First, if the subjects of this experiment are treated successfully, they will survive to produce offspring who also lack the critical gene. But, on the other hand, if something unexpected were to happen, if some harmful genetic material were incorporated, the effect would be limited.

Ms. McHenry should realize that these first experiments involve not only decisions to treat individual patients having a particular disease, but also policies having long-term impacts. The same technologies, those using retroviruses and techniques of gene transfer, that are developed in this experiment will also be available for use by others in other settings to transfer other genetic material. Ms. McHenry must decide not only whether she is willing to participate in the first formally sanctioned attempt to change the human genetic endowment. She must also decide whether she is willing to participate in starting what is likely to be a long line of experiments with impacts far more dramatic than those involving a few adenosine deaminase deficiency patients. Her question is whether humans are rational agents with the right and responsibility for reshaping their very nature or, alternatively, whether they ought not to be tampering with matters so fundamental.

References

1. Veatch RM: Ethical issues in genetics. In Steinberg AG, Bearn AG (eds): Progress and Medical Genetics, vol 10, pp 223–264. New York, Grune & Stratton, 1974
2. President's Commission for the Study of Ethical Problems in Medicine and Biomedical and Behavioral Research: Screening and Counseling for Genetic Conditions: The Ethical, Social, and Legal Implications of Genetic Screening, Counseling, and Education Programs. Washington, DC, U.S. Government Printing Office, 1983
3. Mulinsky A, Annas GJ (eds): Genetics and the Law II. New York, Plenum Press, 1980
4. National Institute of Child Health and Human Development: Antenatal Diagnosis: Report of a Consensus Development Conference. Department of Health, Education, and Welfare, Washington (1979) at I-49, cited in President's Commission for the Study of Ethical Problems in Medicine and Biomedical and Behavioral Research. Screening and Counseling for Genetic Conditions: The Ethical, Social, and Legal Implications of Genetic Screening, Counseling, and Education Programs. Washington, DC, U.S. Government Printing Office, 1983
5. Werth v. Paroly, No. 74025162NM (Wayne CO., Mich Ct.. verdict, Jan. 12, 1979); Call v. Kezirian, 185 Cal. Rptr. 103 [1982].
6. Gastel B, Haddow JE, Fletcher JC, Neale A (eds): Maternal Serum Alpha-fetoprotein: Issues in the Prenatal Screening and Diagnosis of Neural Tube Defects. Washington, DC, U.S. Government Printing Office, 1980
7. Kass LR: Making babies—The new biology and the "old" morality. The Public Interest pp 18–56, Winter 1972
8. Ramsey P: Shall we "reproduce?" JAMA 220(June 5 and June 12):1346–1350, 1480–1485, 1972
9. Kass LR: "Making babies" revisited. The Public Interest pp 32–60, Winter 1979
10. Fletcher J: The Ethics of Genetic Control: Ending Reproductive Roulette. Garden City, NY, Anchor Books, 1974
11. Working Group on Human Gene Therapy: Points to consider in the design and submission of human somatic-cell gene therapy protocols. Recombinant DNA Technical Bulletin 8:116–122, 1985
12. Walters L: The ethics of human gene therapy. Nature 320:225–227, 1986

Chapter 11

Psychiatry and the Control of Human Behavior

A third area of health care practice that presents ethical problems for the nurse is that of psychiatric nursing and the control of human behavior.[1-3] The problems of the meaning and justification of ethical claims—such as an argument over whether homosexuality or aggressive violence is an immoral behavior rather than a manifestation of an illness—arise here with great regularity. Serious conceptual problems are at stake in deciding whether a generally unacceptable behavior should be considered the result of mental illness rather than some moral deviance. The second problem raised in Part One of this book—what the source of these moral judgments is—also arises in cases involving psychiatry and other forms of behavior control. Should experts, for example, be the ones who decide for society whether a behavior such as drug addiction is a crime, an immorality, a disease, or acceptable behavior? If so, which ones? What should happen if psychiatrists claim that aggressive violence is a mental illness, while prosecuting attorneys claim it is a crime, moral philosophers claim it is an unethical voluntary behavior, and the clergy claim it is a sin? Just as intriguingly, what should happen if each of these groups of experts insists that whatever a particular act of aggressive violence is, it is not a manifestation of the type of behavior about which they claim expertise—psychiatrists saying it is not mental illness, prosecutors saying it is not a crime, and so forth? The first case in this chapter provides an opportunity to examine these issues.

These cases also raise some of the most basic conflicts among the ethical principles introduced in the second part of this volume. Often the initial problem in cases involving psychiatry and other forms of behavior control is not an ethical one at all. It is one of determining the extent to which the behavior in question should be thought of as voluntary or autonomous. As we saw in the cases in Chapter 4, deciding whether the patient is to be thought of as autonomous may make a great deal of difference in determining whether a particular ethical principle applies. For example, it is often argued that the principle of autonomy should dominate in evaluating behaviors that may involve harm to the individual but no risk to other parties, especially when the person engaging in the behavior is thought to be substantially autonomous. If the client engaging in the behavior is not substantially autonomous, then the principle of beneficence—benefiting the client—should prevail in some way. The case of the nurse dealing with the suicidal patient raises these problems in a particularly dramatic way.

After looking at several cases involving psychiatry and psychology, we look at two cases involving other mental health interventions—psychosurgery and psychopharmacology. The same range of ethical principles applies to these cases, but several conceptual issues basic to the ethics of behavior control are also presented. The cases involve questions such as whether a physical intervention—surgery—is more controversial than "merely talking with the patient." They asked whether the fact that an intervention is presumably permanent—as psychosurgery may be—makes it more suspect than one that is reversible—such as a pharmacological intervention. If this factor of permanency is morally relevant, the next question to consider is an empirical one: Just how reversible are various interventions? Some have argued that psychological interventions, particularly those at an early age, may leave impressions that are just as irreversible as psychosurgery.

Still another question raised by the use of behavior-controlling interventions is whether finding identifiable physical evidence of pathology—a lesion or an abnormal electroencephalogram (EEG) pattern, for example—makes intervention more justifiable. Is it more acceptable to do pinpoint destruction of brain tissue when it is known that tissue is generating abnormal EEG patterns than when there is documented evidence of a positive behavioral change with such ablation but no evidence of abnormal electrical activity? The cases in the last section of this chapter provide a chance for the nurse to struggle with these problems and his or her role in treating patients when they are raised.

PSYCHOTHERAPY

Many of the philosophical problems faced by the nurse related to human behavior arise in the context of psychotherapy. In order for psychotherapy to be appropriate, there must be a judgment made that the behavior is morally undesirable. One does not try to change behavior or experience if it is good. Even if the experience is undesirable, however, there are a number of interpretations to explain why the behavior exists and why it is undesirable. When the nurse participates in psychotherapy, he or she is making judgments involving these issues. Other problems also emerge in the psychotherapeutic context, including the conflicts between patient welfare and the interests of others (examined in Chapters 3 and 4) and between patient welfare and autonomy (examined in Chapter 5).

The Concept of Mental Health

The first case in this section demonstrates how the nurse must make conceptual distinctions in deciding whether a patient has a problem within the health sphere.[4,5] First, the judgment that there is a problem must be made; second, the judgment that the problem is one that lends itself to the mental health model must also be made.

Case 79: The Psychotherapist Confronted by Different Values

Lorna Shettler had 15 years' experience working with patients with various psychological disorders. In addition to undergraduate and graduate degrees in nursing with a focus on mental health nursing, she had advanced degrees and experience in clinical psychology. She was now a partner in a private, community mental health clinic and carried a full case load of outpatients requesting therapy for behavioral disorders. Recently, however, a patient challenged her expertise and experience to a far greater degree than any other patient.

The patient was Rosalind Torrance, a successful executive in sales merchandising. Ms. Torrance was a lesbian deeply troubled by her sexual orientation and her present life-style. Ms. Torrance described her life as extremely lonely and isolated. Having lived in a small but prosperous Southern city for 4 years, she wanted to initiate a relationship with another woman but was afraid to do so. She was afraid of discovery, of losing her job in a conservative business operation, and of being rejected. She had had one brief lesbian relationship immediately after finishing her college education, but it had ended when her partner started dating a man and eventually married him. Her own dating experience with men had been limited, painfully embarrassing, and stressful. She liked the company of women much better but had not attempted to form a sexual relationship until after college. Having lost that relationship and moved to another city, she was uncertain whether she had the emotional energy and psychological fortitude to initiate another relationship. Since her own experience as a lesbian was so limited, she was even wondering if she could overcome her sexual orientation. The strain of trying to conceal her orientation was becoming very troublesome; yet, she was very reluctant to visit singles bars and sports clubs to find a lesbian partner. Could Dr. Shettler help her? She would try anything—shock therapy, behavior therapy, anything—if she could be helped to overcome her anxieties.

Dr. Shettler knew that she could follow several strategies in trying to help Ms. Torrance. One strategy often used by behavioral therapists was popularly called a "hetero-strategy." It enjoyed a high rate of success if the patient really wanted to change her sexual orientation. It included instruction on heterosocial and heterosexual techniques, and covert sensitization, an aversive conditioning procedure whereby the client imagines lesbian situations while at the same time being induced to feelings of nausea and disgust.

A second strategy often used by behavior therapists was a "homo-strategy." This strategy assumed that sexual preferences probably cannot be eliminated, that the patient can be better helped by raising her self-esteem and reducing her social anxiety, that the patient can be helped to find support systems like gay liberation groups, and that there is nothing inherently wrong with sexual fulfillment between consenting adults, in any form, as long as it does not generate self-hate, or psychological or physical injury. Dr. Shettler was uncertain which strategy she would employ with Ms. Torrance. Since she was the first lesbian that Dr. Shettler had ever treated, either strategy seemed to create value conflicts that Dr. Shettler had not experienced before.

Commentary

Dr. Shettler's first task is to determine whether there is, in fact, a problem, and if so, what it is. She is aware that some homosexuals are able to function quite well and that they take offense at being labeled "sick" or "pathological."[6] On the other hand, some people, like Ms. Torrance, are suffering with their homosexuality. Does the decision about whether there is a problem reduce to the question of whether the patient is suffering? Does the fact that one does not suffer mean there is no problem? Does the fact that one is suffering mean there is a problem?

It is always possible that persons may have problems and yet not be aware of them. If the problem is related to health, it may be a problem because it is likely to lead to something the individual will find undesirable in the future. Undiagnosed hypertension could be an example. By analogy, there may be unperceived problems in other spheres. People could have conditions that do not trouble them, but nevertheless ought to be perceived as troubling.

In Ms. Torrance's case, she clearly perceives a problem. Does Dr. Shettler automatically accept the patient's definition of the problem, or does the real difficulty remain an open question? In this case, the problem can be defined in at least two very different ways. It can be defined as engaging in a behavior that is morally unacceptable. Formulating it that way makes it a problem in the sphere of morality. To do so would require several assumptions on Dr. Shettler's part. First, she would have to view the homosexuality as in some sense voluntary. It makes no sense to make use of moral categories if the behavior is totally beyond human control. This assumption is supported by the fact that both she and her roommate had engaged in heterosexual experiences although, in her case, they were not particularly satisfactory. Second, even if it is a voluntary choice on Ms. Torrance's part, in order for the homosexuality to be a moral *problem* a judgment needs to be made about the morality of the behavior. It could be viewed as voluntary, but praiseworthy. More plausibly, it could be viewed as voluntary, but neutral. In either case, it would not be a moral problem because it is not viewed as morally wrong.

If the behavior is not voluntary, then some other model might be invoked. Dr. Shettler might view the behavior as caused by social, organic, or psychological forces beyond Ms. Torrance's control. Again, it would only be a problem if the behavior is evaluated negatively. One difficulty in dealing with complex psychosocial situations such as this is that professionals in various fields are likely to vary systematically in the way they formulate the situation. Priests might view the lesbian behavior as sin; law enforcement officers might view it as illegal behavior; ethicists as moral behavior; psychologists as psychological behavior; and organic medical specialists as physically determined behavior. Clearly, the fact that a specialist in psychology interprets the situation psychologically cannot settle the matter.

Dr. Shettler appears to interpret the problem psychologically; she sees it as open to psychological intervention. She perceives two strategies of intervention. One assumes there is nothing wrong with the behavior. The only problem is Ms. Torrance's psychological response that has become attached to the behavior. That may lead to the "homo-strategy." The other strategy could be based on the assumption that homosexuality is wrong, leading to the "hetero-strategy." The hetero-strategy could also be adopted on strictly pragmatic grounds, however. If the only problem is the anxiety attached to the behavior, Dr. Shettler could either remove the anxiety, leaving the behavior without the anxiety, or she could change the behavior thereby removing the cause of the anxiety.

What Dr. Shettler will choose to do depends first on some assumption she will make about the voluntariness of the behavior, then on what she perceives to be the nature of the problem. She cannot help making evaluative judgments about what types of outcomes will be desirable, as well as what types of outcomes are most easily achievable.

Mental Illness and Autonomous Behavior

Even if the nurse successfully determines that the problem presented is in the health care sphere and is amenable to nursing intervention, problems still remain. One is determining if the patient is autonomous and, if so, whether the therapeutic strategy for reducing the problem will be employed at the expense of overriding that autonomy. The ethical tension is one between the principles of autonomy and patient welfare. The next two cases illustrate this tension.

Case 80: Force-Feeding the Psychiatric Patient

Rosalind Jacuzek was newly employed on the psychiatric ward of a large county hospital. One of her patients was Daniel Forester, a 47-year-old man admitted for severe depression. A once successful owner of a small business, Mr. Forester had became depressed following the failure of his business and a messy divorce from his wife of 18 years. His wife and children now lived in another city. His only visitor was a younger sister, who seemed concerned about her brother's condition out of a sense of family obligation rather than genuine concern for him. His depression was complicated by the recent diagnosis of a rare form of leukemia for which there was only palliative treatment and no demonstrated cure. Burdened by the loss of his business and family and by his illness, Mr. Forester's depression had progressed to the point where he was refusing all medications, food, and water in the hope that he would die.

Intravenous (IV) therapy had been instituted, and he was receiving his antidepression medications per IV. His depression was so severe, however, that the antidepression medications were not noticeably effective. It was hoped that Mr. Forester's nutrition could be maintained by forced feedings and his hydration maintained by the IV until the antidepression medications had the opportunity to effect some change in his alarming state of depression and his desire to die.

Force-feeding Mr. Forester, however, was a distasteful act to Ms. Jacuzek. Whenever she attempted to put food into Mr. Forester's mouth, he spit it out and moved his head away from the food offered on a spoon. A nasogastric (NG) tube was finally passed and a liquid supplement given to Mr. Forester. Despite the fact that his hands were tied and he was restrained in bed, he always managed to dislodge the NG tube, necessitating that the NG tube be passed anew each time he was fed. This procedure was a real nuisance to the nurses and required additional sedating of the patient. Each time food was offered to him,

Ms. Jacuzek tried to force the food into his mouth but eventually wound up passing the NG tube in order to get some nutrition into his body. The ordeal usually required the assistance of three or four people to hold Mr. Forester while the NG tube was passed and he was fed. After a few days of this procedure, Ms. Jacuzek noticed that Mr. Forester's face, jaw, neck, and arms were bruised from the manner in which the nurses were gripping him while trying to force feed him. Sickened by the treatment of Mr. Forester and the marks on his body, Ms. Jacuzek discussed the situation with her supervisor. An experienced psychiatric nurse, the nurse supervisor acknowledged the difficulty of feeding a severely depressed patient like Mr. Forester. But she urged Ms. Jacuzek to cooperate in the feeding plan developed by the nurses. She assured the younger nurse that Mr. Forester would thank her and the other nurses when he got over his depression. The bruises were inconsequential considering the necessary nutrition that was being supplied. Ms. Jacuzek was not sure this was adequate moral justification for physical coercion of a very sick psychiatric patient.

Case 81: Must Suicide Always be Stopped?

Cynthia Morgan was an attractive, 26-year-old woman admitted to a psychiatric floor following an unsuccessful attempt at suicide. She had made the attempt several weeks after radical neck surgery to remove a highly malignant tumor from her lower jaw. Disfigured and faced with months of therapy and reconstructive surgery, she had decided that her life was no longer meaningful or worth living. Unmarried and with no living family that seemed to care about her, she was extremely depressed about her future, the cost of her medical bills, and her ability to become gainfully employed again. She had been an advertising agent for a growing cosmetic company and would not be able to return to employment that placed her in the public eye, given the results of the disfiguring surgery. She simply felt that it was better to die than live with her disabilities.

One of her nurses, Beth Amos, tended to sympathize with Ms. Morgan. Although Ms. Amos was obligated to prevent the patient from attempting to commit suicide again, she thought that Ms. Morgan was making a rational choice *for her* and that it was wrong to interfere in this choice. Yet, Ms. Amos did interfere in this choice by searching Ms. Morgan for any implements with which she could harm herself and by not allowing her to wear belts, stockings, a bra, or a slip. She also made Ms. Morgan open her mouth following the administration of each medication, limited the types of objects that could be taken into her room, and forced her to take tranquilizing medications that she did not want to take. Yet she wondered why it was "wrong" for a patient to end his or her life when no other parties would be affected and the patient would avoid the unpleasantness and pain that continued life created. Why can't a patient make this choice?

Commentary

One solution to each of these cases would be to find each of the patients incompetent or lacking in autonomy to make choices about their own care. Both are suffering from conditions that are traditionally associated with incompetency: depression in the case of Mr. Forester and suicidal behavior in the case of Cynthia Morgan. If they are not substantially autonomous agents, there can be no conflict between patient autonomy and doing what is in the patient's interest. The problem would seem to disappear.

However, the solution may actually not be quite that easy. For one thing, if the nurses, Rosalind Jacuzek and Beth Amos, really believe that these patients are so compromised by their mental problems that they are not substantially autonomous agents, then they should not rely on the patients' own refusal of treatment.

Even if Mr. Forester and Ms. Morgan are not autonomous, the nurses in these cases (or the patients' physicians) do not necessarily have the right to treat these patients in ways that they perceive as beneficial to the patients. If the patients are believed to be incompetent, then someone ought to be designated as the patients' agents for purposes of accepting or refusing treatment. The problems that can arise if guardians make what appear to be unreasonable choices will be discussed in the cases in Chapters 13 and 14. The judgment that these patients are incompetent, however, may simply put the nurses in the position of having to look to someone else as a decision-maker for them.

The other alternative is that Ms. Jacuzek and Ms. Amos conclude that Mr. Forester and Ms. Morgan are substantially autonomous agents. Especially in Ms. Morgan's case, she seems to understand the nature of the situation and has made a choice about whether it is worth continuing life. Her nurse, Ms. Amos, seems to believe that Ms. Morgan's judgment is quite rational. Then the ethical problem reduces to one of how the principle of autonomy should relate to promotion of the patient's welfare.

There are other variables beside the fact that Ms. Morgan's judgment seems more rational than Mr. Forester's. For one, Ms. Morgan's condition is not necessarily terminal, whereas Mr. Forester's is apparently irreversible. For another, the interventions in Ms. Morgan's case (forced tranquilization and constraints placed on normal living, dressing, and privacy) seem less invasive than the physical restraints, force-feeding, and bruising in Mr. Forester's case. Are these adequate differences to justify a different moral judgment about the interventions in the two cases assuming that each was substantially autonomous?

Mental Illness and Third-Party Interests

Sometimes patients with psychiatric problems may pose not only problems of the conflict between autonomy and patient welfare, but also conflicts between the welfare of patients and the welfare of third parties. The next two cases pose these problems.

Case 82: Sedating and Restraining the Disturbed Patient

Percival Guthrie was a 58-year-old man with a history of organic brain syndrome. In good physical health, Mr. Guthrie had been admitted to a nursing home by his family. Because of his forgetfulness, wandering behavior, sleep pattern disturbances, and inability to care for himself, his family wanted him to be placed in a care center that would meet his growing needs for supervision and personal care. The family had tried to care for him themselves for the past year but were exhausted from all the supervision that Mr. Guthrie needed. Despite the expense, they hoped that their relative would be happy in the nursing home and that he would receive the care that they could no longer give him.

Sandra Mooney was the day nursing supervisor of the nursing home selected by Mr. Guthrie's family. Recognizing the type of care that Mr. Guthrie would need, she agreed to place his room near the nurses' station and observe him while he adjusted to the routine of the nursing home. Adjustment, however, seemed an impossibility for Mr. Guthrie. It soon became apparent that his wandering into other patients' rooms was disturbing to them. During meals, he talked loudly and frequently called for his relatives. When sedated with a mild tranquilizer, Mr. Guthrie became more agitated and spent all night roaming the halls, wandering into the rooms of sleeping patients, and generally engaging in loud and boisterous behavior, much to the dismay of the nursing staff. Within a few days, it became apparent that mild medication was not going to affect Mr. Guthrie's behavior. He was also becoming very dirty and refused to change his clothes. Once he sat in his armchair all night and failed to use the bathroom to urinate. His clothes and the chair were soaked with urine, and this became a daily occurrence. Faced with the odor constantly emanating from Mr. Guthrie's room, his wandering behavior, his unkempt appearance, and his loud talking, Mrs. Mooney considered restraining the patient for considerable parts of the day and night. She discussed the problem with the nursing staff, and they decided to use a combination of chemical and physical restraints, since their one attempt at physically restraining the patient had resulted in loud, yelling behavior that disturbed the other patients, the staff, and that alarmed visitors. It was a course of action that Mrs. Mooney chose reluctantly, given Mr. Guthrie's good physical condition. Yet it seemed that his liberty would have to be restrained if the staff and the other patients were to have a satisfying nursing home atmosphere.

Case 83: Choosing a "Better" Patient than the Chronic Schizophrenic

Shannon McFee, a student nurse in her final year of undergraduate study, was starting a new clinical rotation with a focus on psychiatric/mental health nursing. She and five of her classmates were assigned to a small unit housing female patients at a state mental health facility. On her first day of clinical, Miss McFee was encouraged to talk with all the patients in the day room and to select two patients with whom she would like to work during her 7-week clinical rotation. After spending most of the morning talking with various patients, playing cards with a few of the more out-going patients, and even accompanying two patients to occupational therapy, she realized that a few of the patients on the unit did not seem to participate in the unit activities. On the pretense of checking to see if these patients had received their mid-morning snack, she visited their rooms.

In one room, she found a well-groomed 48-year-old woman, Willie Mae Chisholm, rocking in her chair and humming to herself. Miss McFee attempted to start a conversation with the woman but soon realized that this patient was quite paranoid, since she kept referring to secret microphones concealed on her body that were recording her thoughts and her speech. In checking the patient's chart, Miss McFee learned that Ms. Chisholm had lived in mental institutions for over 16 years. Her diagnosis was chronic paranoid schizophrenia. She had been released to her family 2 years ago but had been readmitted after only 2 months. The patient was fairly likable but easily slipped into her paranoia whenever Miss McFee tried to converse with her.

In checking another patient's room, Miss McFee discovered Ella Peacham, a 56-year-old woman admitted 2 days ago, completely wrapped up in her bedsheet, including her head, and lying across the bed. Miss McFee talked to the enshrouded patient for a few moments until Mrs. Peacham slowly removed the sheet from her head and cautiously began to glance at Miss McFee. After being coaxed into talking for a half hour, Mrs. Peacham agreed to accompany Miss McFee to the day room where she sat watching television, but would not interact with other patients.

In checking this patient's chart, Miss McFee found that Mrs. Peacham had been hospitalized for a "nervous breakdown" over 30 years ago but had returned home after 6 years of institutionalization. She had four children, most of whom were reared by her husband and her sister. She had been rehospitalized for a short period of time 8 years ago, following the death of her husband. Since that time, she had lived in a trailer next to her youngest son's house. She had been able to take care of herself with minimal supervision until just recently, when she became reclusive, failing to eat, bathe, and care for herself or her trailer. When she began to complain to her son of hearing "voices" outside her trailer all the time, he contacted the state facility and admitted her for treatment. Her diagnosis was chronic undifferentiated schizophrenia.

At the end of the day, Miss McFee and her classmates met with their nursing instructor. As they talked about their experiences of the day and the unit's patients, the instructor asked the students if they had decided which patients they would follow during the clinical rotation. Miss McFee indicated that she would like to follow Miss Chisholm and Mrs. Peacham. The instructor asked Miss McFee why she had picked those particular patients. Miss McFee was not sure why she had picked them except for the fact that she was interested in their histories and the diagnosis of chronic schizophrenia. After the post-conference, the instructor privately advised Miss McFee to select other patients. There were quite a few patients diagnosed as having adolescent adjustment problems on the unit; also, there were other patients with disorders that would rapidly respond to medication and therapy. She advised Miss McFee to invest her time in these patients because they had greater potential of returning to the community. Both Miss Chisholm and Mrs. Peacham were chronically ill individuals, and it was unlikely that they would ever leave the hospital setting and live productive lives apart from it. While Miss McFee saw the wisdom of selecting patients in whom she could observe the results of psychopharmacology and therapy, because she was a student and could herself benefit from the experiences, she was not sure that the nurse should selectively distribute herself, as a resource, to those who would benefit the most. She was especially troubled by the fact that chronically mentally ill patients did not seem as deserving of nursing time and energy as other patients. Was she obligated to invest her time in those patients who could obviously benefit the most from her attention and services?

Commentary

Percival Guthrie, the man with organic brain syndrome who was sedated and restrained by nurse Sandra Mooney, is in some ways like the patients in the previous section. Like them, Mr. Guthrie's autonomy is in question. In such situations nurses often decide to restrain patients in possible violation of their autonomy but for what appears to be the production of the greater good. Mr. Guthrie may well be less autonomous than the earlier patients. That is one possible difference in the cases. But there is another important difference. Mrs. Mooney decided in favor of physical and chemical restraints not primarily for Mr. Guthrie's benefit but for the benefit of other patients who were being disturbed by Mr. Guthrie's wandering and his eratic life-style.

We saw in Chapters 3 and 4 that even those who believe that patients have an autonomy-based right to make treatment choices (even when such choices appear to be contrary to their own interests) tend to agree that there are some instances in which the welfare of third parties justifies interventions against the patient's wishes. In Mr. Guthrie's case, Mrs. Mooney might have sought to intervene against Mr. Guthrie's wishes to benefit him. In that case she would be acting on grounds of patient welfare. She also, however, might intervene to protect others, such as the other patients in the center.

However, this poses a problem for Mrs. Mooney. Clinicians, including nurses, are traditionally committed to the welfare of their patients, *not* to promoting the overall greatest good. Mrs. Mooney might avoid this problem by considering all of the patients in the facility *her patients*, thus maintaining her clinical perspective. She might also conclude that the interventions serve not only other patients, but also Mr. Guthrie himself, thus turning the case back into one of purely patient welfare.

Many nurses, however, are increasingly willing to take at least certain third-party interests into account, as we saw in the cases in Chapters 3 and 4. Mrs. Mooney's problem is whether just any benefits to others justify constraining Mr. Guthrie with physical and chemical restraints or, if only certain benefits justify constraint, whether such benefits are present in this case.

The second case, that in which student nurse Shannon McFee is asked to choose patients for her clinical experience, may help shed light on the problem. She chose two chronic schizophrenics, patients whom her instructor believed would not improve dramatically during the 7-week rotation.

It is not clear exactly what the reasoning of the instructor was when she recommended that Miss McFee choose patients other than Ms. Chisholm and Mrs. Peacham. She may have been expressing the goals of nursing education. She may have been advising Miss McFee that she would learn more if she chose other patients. That alternative seems to be grounded in the ethical assumption that the student nurse should choose her patients on the basis of how much she will learn. While that seems to make sense insofar as the objective is student education, it is debatable whether it is compatible with the moral mandate of nurses to benefit their patients.

It sounds, however, as if the nursing instructor were applying a moral calculus to the choice, based on which patients would benefit the most. She may be saying that, at least when choosing among those who are one's patients (or from among those who are candidates to be patients), the nurse should choose the ones who will gain the most benefit from nursing interventions.

That is not her only option, however. As we saw in the cases in Chapter 4, Miss McFee might have decided to devote her time to those whom she thought were the worst off. Ms. Chisholm and Mrs. Peacham may well qualify as being worst off, at least worse off than the other patients with more acute and reversible disorders. Both Mrs. Mooney and Miss McFee must decide when, if ever, the welfare of others justifies a decision not to maximize the welfare of the individual patient. Mrs. Mooney and Miss McFee will have to decide whether the amount of good they could do to other patients justifies sacrificing patients or whether how well off other patients are is decisive for the distribution of nursing expertise.

OTHER BEHAVIOR-CONTROLLING THERAPIES

While many of the ethical issues faced by the nurse in the area of psychiatry and the control of behavior will arise around psychotherapy and psychoactive drug interventions, other emergent technologies may raise somewhat different issues. These involve surgical interventions, electroshock, electrical stimulation of the brain, and unconventional therapies such as orthomolecular therapy.[7] A nurse in a unit dealing with these therapies will have to face questions such as whether physical interventions in the brain are morally any different from psychotherapeutic interventions and whether irreversible procedures are more controversial. The first case involves possible psychosurgical intervention.

Case 84: Psychosurgery for the Wealthy Demented Patient

Gail Conover was a staff nurse on a surgical unit of a small private hospital in the South. One of her patients was Regina Dinsworth, a 49-year-old woman admitted for treatment of minor injuries sustained in a fall. Miss Dinsworth was the sister of Rex Dinsworth, a local wealthy philanthropist and the president of the Dinsworth Foundation. The Dinsworth Foundation had contributed a great deal of money to develop social and cultural resources in the city over the years, and many of the results of these investments bore the Dinsworth family name: Dinsworth Park, The Dinsworth Museum of Modern Art, Frances Dinsworth High School, and so on.

Regina Dinsworth, however, was apparently sheltered by the family because of mental illness and many previous hospitalizations. She lived in the Dinsworth's spacious family home in the middle of the city and was cared for at home by a private nurse. In recent months, however, she had become very difficult to manage at home. She wandered away from the house on several occasions, was in near-constant physical activity, and rarely slept. Her family was being exhausted by her activity and was increasingly embarrassed by her escapes from the house to areas of the city. During her latest escape, she had apparently wandered into a high-crime neighborhood of the city and had been attacked by two men. She was saved from more serious injury by an off-duty policeman, but she did sustain several broken ribs, cuts, and bruises.

The Dinsworths were considering psychosurgery for their relative as an alternative to permanent hospitalization. It seemed to be the easiest way for them to control Regina Dinsworth and solve the problem of caring for her. The family realized that the psychosurgery would alter her personality and would probably make her dependent on the family for the rest of her life. But this seemed a small price to pay for relief of the continued worry and embarrassment that her mental illness caused the family. Mrs. Conover, however, did not agree that this might be the best alternative for Miss Dinsworth. Surely there were important considerations here other than the family's comfort and ease of custodianship.

Commentary

The proposed treatment of Regina Dinsworth is controversial on several grounds. It is no wonder that the nurse, Gail Conover, would have doubts. The case report, however, does not tell us why she has concluded that the psychosurgical intervention is not the best treatment for Miss Dinsworth.

One major problem in this case is the apparent motivation of the family. They appear to be more concerned about the disruption and embarrassment Miss Dinsworth is causing than about her welfare. On the other hand, Miss Dinsworth's life does not appear to be very pleasant. Continued agitation, wandering, sleeplessness, and physical assault are not much to look forward to—nor is permanent hospitalization. Is it possible that, in spite of the family's motivation, the surgical intervention is in Miss Dinsworth's interest? If so, should a nurse or any other caring professional object simply because the family is not well-motivated?

If Mrs. Conover is not objecting solely on the basis of the family's motivation, that is, if she really believes some other treatment is better for Miss Dinsworth, what is the basis of her belief? Does she believe that there are other techniques available that can relieve Miss Dinsworth's symptoms more effectively? Is that the sort of issue about which a nurse should appropriately object, or is that a more technical question better left to other authorities?

It is possible that Mrs. Conover objects not so much on technical grounds as on moral grounds. Cutting into the human brain is an unusually controversial thing to do.[8] It conjures up prefrontal lobotomies of earlier decades. It suggests blunting of the human personality, irreversible physical change, and dehumanization. Is it valid for Mrs. Conover to object on these grounds? Some people hold that physical interventions such as psychosurgery should be avoided, at least when psychotherapies such as counseling and behavior-modification efforts could be used. Is there a moral basis for such a preference?

One possible basis for this difference is that psychosurgery is believed to be irreversible, whereas other psychotherapeutic interventions are not. That is an empirical claim worthy of exploration. Some counseling interventions may also prove irreversible;

surgery may actually be reversed in some cases, such as by having other brain tissues take on some of the functions originally performed by the excised tissue. Beyond the empirical question, is there any valid reason for reversible procedures to be morally preferable to irreversible procedures? Is it only because we may make mistakes that we would then want to reverse? If Miss Dinsworth's behavior is as debilitating as it appears to be, would it not be preferable if the change were irrevocable?

Mrs. Conover needs to be clear on why she objects to the proposed surgery even if the procedure seems intuitively revolting to her. Obviously, there might be a number of reasons for her to object, and different reasons may have different implications for her. If, after sorting out her reasons, she still is convinced that this psychosurgery could not be in Miss Dinsworth's interest, how should Mrs. Conover respond?

Case 85: Coercive Treatment in the Name of Science*

The head nurse of a 150-bed private psychiatric facility observed the coercive and abusive treatment of patients admitted to an orthomolecular program. Based on the belief that psychiatric illness is due to cerebral allergies, patients admitted to the program had their intake of food and medication restricted and were given only bottled water for 4 to 7 days. As foods were slowly reintroduced, vital signs were checked to help determine if the patient was allergic to the food substance. Patients were not allowed to smoke or leave the unit. One patient who was a drug addict was mistakenly admitted to the program. She dived through a plate glass window within hours of being admitted. Another patient with "cerebral allergy" turned out to be an alcoholic who went into withdrawal, then becoming very agitated and combative. She was institutionalized in another setting. A third patient went berserk when the physician in charge of the program ate an apple in the presence of the fasting patient. The patient was put in restraints and started with vitamin therapy per IV.

The final blow came when a wealthy 34-year-old chronically disturbed man was admitted by his exasperated family to the orthomolecular program. After his psychotropic medications were discontinued, he became agitated, confused, and combative. Several staff members were hurt in trying to restrain him. When restrained, he begged the physician for his medications to calm him down. The physician refused, and the man was kept in restraints for 8 days and nights—screaming continually and urinating all over himself.

At about this time, the orthomolecular physician claimed that he was curing nine of ten "last resort" cases with his starvation treatment. He published an article on his "successes," and a large number of patients from gullible, weary families looking for the "last resort cure" were admitted to the unit. The nurse realized that something was very wrong with this approach but found it hard to challenge a "noted authority" in the field.

*Adapted from Witt P: Notes of a whistleblower. Am J Nurs 83:1649–1651, 1983

Commentary

Patients with psychiatric illnesses generate more than their share of unorthodox therapies. Since many patients are seriously afflicted and standard treatment regimens have failed them, sometimes these unorthodox therapies are quite invasive or traumatic. Sometimes the therapeutic strategy may even be intentionally traumatic so that the patient will be changed by it. The head nurse in the orthomolecular program appears to be confronting such a traumatic intervention.

She might consider approaching her dilemma as a consent problem.[9] For any treatment to be undertaken (as we shall see in more detail in Chapter 13) there must be an effective consent. When possible, this should come from the patient. When the patient is not competent to give that consent, it should come from the legally authorized surrogate, presumably often the next of kin. The nurse might be able to stimulate a review of the orthomolecular program by questioning the adequacy of patient consent to be treated in the program. Such questions may trigger legal as well as ethical concerns that could provide assistance in ensuring that the case is reviewed carefully.

Some patients referred to the orthomolecular program may actually be willing to consent (or may have legally effective consents from authorized surrogates). The surrogates, unlike the family in the previous case, may even be well-motivated. In spite of such legally effective, well-motivated consent, the nurse may still have questions about the justification of the orthomolecular therapy.

She might consider whether the program constitutes research on human subjects. If it is not a well-established therapy, it is possible that it is (or should be) considered research. It is at least nonconventional therapy. Most institutions have policies requiring special review of research. Some include nonconventional therapies in such review. This might include requiring a formal protocol, approval by a department chairperson, and formal, institutional review board procedure. In this case, perhaps, the nurse ought to call the orthomolecular program to the attention of the institutional review board or its nursing member. The ethical problems associated with participation in research and nonconventional therapy (which this nurse may well be doing) are the subject of the cases in the following chapter.

If the consent for the orthomolecular therapy is adequate and if the treatment does not constitute research or innovative, nonconventional therapy, then perhaps the nurse must face the question of patient welfare directly. Even if the surrogate has consented and even if it is established that the therapy satisfies the requirements of the institutional review board, it is still possible for any health care professional to ask whether the patient's interests are being served. In cases where there is a serious abridgment of patient interest, other interventions are possible, including appeal to hospital authorities, family members, and, ultimately, government authorities charged with protecting incompetent patients. Does the orthomolecular therapy constitute such an abuse of a patient that the nurse should pursue one of these routes?

References

1. Bloch S, Chodoff P (eds): Psychiatric Ethics. New York, Oxford University Press, 1981
2. Rosenbaum M (ed): Ethics and Value in Psychotherapy: A Guidebook. New York, The Free Press, 1982

3. Engelhardt HT, McCullough LB: Ethics in psychiatry. In: American Handbook of Psychiatry, 2nd ed, vol 7, pp 795–818. New York, Basic Books, 1981

4. Flew A: Disease and mental illness. In: Crime or Disease? pp 26–94. London, Macmillan, 1973

5. Caplan AL, Engelhardt HT, McCartney JJ: Concepts of Health and Disease: Interdisciplinary Perspectives. Reading, MA, Addison-Wesley, 1981

6. Bayer R: Homosexuality and American Psychology: The Politics of Diagnosis. New York, Basic Books, 1980

7. Physical manipulation of the brain. Hastings Center Report, special supplement, May, 1973

8. Gaylin W, Meister JS, Neville RC: Operating on the Mind. New York, Basic Books, 1975

9. Lidz CW, Meisel A, Zerubavel E, Carter M, Sestak RM, Roth LH: Informed Consent: A Study of Decisionmaking in Psychiatry. New York, The Guilford Press, 1984

Chapter 12

Experimentation on Human Beings

The nurse often participates in medical and behavioral research involving human subjects—sometimes as a principal investigator and at other times as a research team member or advocate for the research subject. Systematic research designed to test hypotheses and generate statistically significant, generalizable results is quite a modern phenomenon. Traditionally, the primary objective of trying new interventions was to provide benefits for a particular patient, especially when the usual remedies were not producing satisfactory results. Since about the middle of the 19th century, however, we have seen a change, with health care professionals attempting to conduct systematically designed studies for the purpose of gaining knowledge to benefit society or specific groups within society, as well as the individual subjects of the investigation.

When this new purpose is added to the agenda, a new group of moral problems arises. The most conspicuous is the potential conflict between the health care professional's traditional duty to serve the individual patient—to benefit the patient or, as holders of newer, more rights-oriented biomedical ethical positions would say, to protect the rights of the patient—and the newer interest in benefiting others. Since the Nuremberg trials, soon after World War II, researchers, potential subjects, and the society at large have been concerned about the possibility that research agendas might conflict with traditional patient-centered obligations. At Nuremberg, after all, it became conspicuously clear that any investigator who approaches a human being as a subject for the purpose of gaining generalizable knowledge abandons, at least partially, the traditional focus on the welfare and rights of the patient. After Nuremberg, there were two major options: return to the ethic that required the health care professional to work only out of concern for the patient or develop an ethic of research that would permit a limited shift of attention and, at the same time, protect the rights and interests of the potential subject.

At Nuremberg, the second option was chosen. The primary strategy for protecting subjects was a strong, apparently exceptionless, requirement that subjects give voluntary consent to participation. As the Nuremberg Code states in its first provision:

> The voluntary consent of the human subject is absolutely essential. This means that the person involved should have legal capacity to give consent; should be so situated as to be able to exercise free power of choice, without the intervention of any element of force, fraud, deceit, duress, overreaching or other ulterior form of constraint or coercion; and should have sufficient knowledge and comprehension of the elements of the subject matter involved as to enable him to make an understanding and enlightened decision. This latter element requires that before the acceptance of an affirmative decision by the experimental subject there should be made known to him the nature, duration, and purpose of the experiment; the method and means by which it is to be conducted; all inconveniences and hazards reasonably to be expected; and the effects upon his health or person which may possibly come from his participation in the experiments.[1]

While this made possible research interventions that were not primarily for the benefit of the subject, it was soon discovered that it made impossible many kinds of research that were considered important: Research involving children, the mentally incompetent, and anyone else who could not exercise voluntary consent; research on emergency care where there was no possibility of getting a consent; and psychological studies involving deception were just a few of the types of research that could not possibly conform to the Nuremberg requirement.

In the mid-1960s, the United States government began to express concern for the protection of subjects of research conducted at major government research centers or research conducted with government funds. The result has been a system of institutional review boards (IRBs) that reviews all research to see that it conforms with a set of regulations established nationally, as well as any additional state, local, and hospital requirements.[2,3] It is not uncommon to have one or more nurses serving on these IRBs.

The current regulations require that seven criteria be met before any research be approved under the regulations:

(1) Risks to subjects are minimized: (i) By using procedures which are consistent with sound research design and which do not unnecessarily expose subjects to risk and (ii) whenever appropriate, by using procedures already being performed on the subjects for diagnostic or treatment purposes.

(2) Risks to subjects are reasonable in relation to anticipated benefits, if any, to subjects, and the importance of the knowledge that may reasonably be expected to result. In evaluating risks and benefits, the IRB should consider only those risks and benefits that may result from the research (as distinguished from risks and benefits of therapies subjects would receive even if not participating in the research). The IRB should not consider possible long-range effects of applying knowledge gained in the research (for example, the possible effects of the research on public policy) as among those research risks that fall within the purview of responsibility.

(3) Selection of subjects is equitable. In making this assessment the IRB should take into account the purposes of the research and the setting in which the research will be conducted.

(4) Informed consent will be sought from each prospective subject or the subject's

legally authorized representative, in accordance with, and to the extent required by section 46.116.

(5) Informed consent will be appropriately documented, in accordance with, and to the extent required by section 46.117.

(6) Where appropriate, the research plan makes adequate provision for monitoring the data collected to insure the safety of subjects.

(7) Where appropriate, there are adequate provisions to protect the privacy of subjects and to maintain the confidentiality of data.[2(p8389)]

These seven criteria can be seen as falling into four groups. The first, most obvious requirement of any ethically acceptable research is derived from the principles of beneficence and nonmaleficence. Any investigator, research team member, IRB member, or nurse concerned about the protection of patients must make sure that the risks to the subjects are minimized and that the benefits anticipated are reasonable in proportion to those risks. This requires sound research design and an assessment of the importance of the knowledge expected to result. It also calls for an assessment of risks and benefits specific to the research subject. The criterion calling for adequate provision for monitoring of data to ensure subject safety can also be seen as stemming from the ethical principles of beneficence and nonmaleficence.

One of the critical ethical problems in research is whether risk can justifiably be increased proportionally to the importance of the knowledge to be gained so that extreme risk—even certain death—might be justified if the expected benefits of the knowledge to be gained were great enough. A pure ethic of benefits and harms in which the ethical goal was to maximize the aggregate good would seem to permit, even require, such high risk–high gain experiments. Yet many IRBs and many philosophers object to this possibility. The alternative is to impose additional ethical requirements. One such requirement would be that, in addition to expected benefits to society proportional to the risks to the subject, there must also be a reasonable balance between the benefits and risks to the subject. Sometimes, especially with subjects who cannot consent, such as children, this requirement is expressed as the insistence that the risks to the subject be minimal regardless of the anticipated social benefits. The federal regulations dealing with research on children permit risks slightly beyond minimal under special cases, but under no circumstances can the risks exceed those limits even if the benefits to society would be enormous.[4] The cases in the first section of this chapter present situations in which the nurse will be required to assess the relation of subject risks to the anticipated benefits to the society and subject.

In addition to requiring that subject risks be compared specifically to the potential benefits to that particular subject, several more ethical criteria are imposed on research under Department of Health and Human Services (DHHS) regulations. In addition to considerations of benefit and harm, there must be adequate provision to protect subject privacy and ensure confidentiality of data. This means that even if great benefit could come from conducting a study in a manner that required violating privacy or breaking confidentiality, that will not be sufficient to override the privacy requirement. Subjects may, under normal circumstances, waive their rights to privacy and confidentiality, but the promise of confidentiality generates an independent moral requirement of research, not capable of being overridden simply because great good would come of it. The cases in the second section of this chapter present the problems of privacy and confidentiality in research.

Another independent requirement for research to be approved by DHHS is that the selection of subjects be equitable. We have known for some time that a disproportionate number of research subjects have come from oppressed groups—the poor, the institutionalized, and clinic patients. The principle of justice is now taken by many as having direct implications for research. The most obvious impact is going to be on subject selection. Although at this time the regulations apply the criterion of equity only to subject selection, there is concern that other aspects of research, such as experimental design, may likewise be affected by interpretations of justice. The widely held opinion that burdens to subjects must be reasonable in proportion to the expected benefits to the subject is evidence of this concern. Justice requires that benefits and burdens be distributed fairly. That means that even if great benefit could come to others it may be unjust to impose serious risks to subjects, at least without their consent. The cases in the third section of this chapter present these problems of equity.

The remaining criteria for research under the DHHS regulations all deal in one way or another with this notion of consent. While, as we saw, the Nuremberg Code makes voluntary consent an absolute requirement, the DHHS regulations are more complex. According to these regulations, the consent can come from the subject's legally authorized representative, as well as the subject himself. In either case, the consent must be documented appropriately, and special safeguards must be established when some or all of the subjects are likely to be vulnerable to coercion or undue influence.

The ethical basis of the consent requirement has been the subject of considerable debate. In some cases it may function to protect the subject, thus being an application of the principle of beneficence—benefiting the subject.[5-7] This is especially true in cases where a proxy consent is obtained. Often, however, the real basis for the consent requirement is not protection of the subject from risks, but rather protection of the subject's autonomy. Especially with competent subjects, the ethical goal is to preserve the subject's self-determination even if it does not maximize his welfare according to an outsider's assessment of it. Some of the most interesting cases are those where preserving the autonomy of the subject conflicts with doing what will most reasonably promote the subject's welfare. In this chapter two cases involving consent issues are presented. These cases raise issues that are unique to experimental medicine. They will set the stage for a larger group of cases involving consent that is presented in the next chapter.

In these cases it is important to keep the research separate from various interventions that are justified solely on the grounds of the welfare of the patient. While some people designate research "therapeutic" and "nontherapeutic," we, following Robert Levine and the National Commission for the Protection of Human Subjects,[8] will speak of interventions justified for research and interventions justified on grounds of patient welfare. Research interventions would include anything done to normal persons for the purpose of gathering systematic data but would also include some things done to patients while undergoing therapy (such as an extra interview, drawing a blood sample that would not be drawn except to obtain research data, or a formal randomization to determine which of two treatments the patient will receive).

When, and only when, two treatments are approximately equal in value might the patient reasonably choose either. In such circumstances, random choice sometimes makes sense. In such cases, as well as in cases where no recognized treatment is available, patients may receive what is now being referred to as "innovative therapy," that is, therapy that is not well accepted as standard practice (such as a new surgical procedure). With such innovative therapy, it is often reasonable to gather information about the impact of the treatment. Some would argue that gathering such information is, in fact, morally required. When actions are taken to gather the data (rather than simply to treat the patient), those actions are research as we are using the term.

CALCULATING RISKS AND BENEFITS

The first and most obvious task in assessing the ethics of research on human subjects is to ensure that the risks are justified by the potential benefits. The DHHS mandate for IRBs requires that they determine that the "risks to subjects are reasonable in relation to anticipated benefits, if any, to subjects, and the importance of the knowledge that may reasonably be expected to risks." Determining the risks and benefits is only the first problem. The decision-maker must also judge how the impact on the subject is to be related to the impact on others. Presumably, if all the risks taken together (considering both their magnitude and likelihood of occurring) exceed the anticipated benefits, then the intervention is not justified.

Often, however, the projected harms to the subject are at least as great as the projected benefits, but the projected total benefits—including the benefits to others of the knowledge to be gained—tip the balance so that benefits reasonably outweigh harms. The following cases pose questions of assessing benefits and harms, including the question of what should be done when benefits to the society are potentially great, whereas harms to the subject possibly outweigh his or her benefits.

Case 86: When a Parent says "No!"

Charles Sutter was born with a large lumbar meningomyelocele, kyphosis, and bilateral dislocated hips. Shortly after his birth, his parents were told that there was little hope for Charles and that they should be prepared to "let him go." They took him home from the hospital when he was five days old and were determined to care for him themselves. Within a few weeks, Mr. Sutter contacted another physician who told him about a new treatment for meningomyelocele being performed at a university research medical center in a nearby state. Mr. Sutter called Dr. H. Kron, the surgeon performing the treatment, and was invited to bring Charles to the medical center for examination and potential admission to the treatment program.

Becky Paxton, a pediatric nurse–practitioner, admitted Charles to the research unit and conducted the initial assessment. She was impressed by Charles' physical condition, despite his deformities, and the positive outlook of his parents. After a few days of examinations and testing, Charles was offered admission to the treatment program. His parents were fully informed about the experimental nature of the treatment, including both risks and benefits. Since there was limited hope for Charles with conventional treatment and no hope without any treatment, the Sutters agreed to Charles' participation in the treatment program.

Within a few days, Charles' meningomyelocele was closed and a partial kyphectomy was performed. Complications developed, however, when cerebrospinal fluid (CSF) started to leak through the closure site, Charles developed a high fever, and his CSF cultures showed *Staphylococcus aureus* ventriculitis. Before the infection was brought under control, Charles suffered frequent convulsive episodes. While receiving treatment for the infection, Charles began to experience disturbing spells of apnea, requiring constant monitoring and tactile stimulation. Since his condition did not improve over several weeks of continued treatment, Charles' parents began to doubt the wisdom of the treatment program for their son. They became further discouraged after a new infection and repeated seizures. The Sutters decided to withdraw him from the treatment program, saying that they thought he had suffered enough pain and discomfort for his young life. They would take him home and care for him the best they could.

Dr. Kron and Ms. Paxton tried to persuade the Sutters to keep Charles in the treatment program for a while longer. They felt that all of Charles' present problems were expected and treatable. Furthermore, once Charles was withdrawn from the program, they could no longer provide treatment or follow-up for him. The Sutters realized that the loss of continued treatment and follow-up might be damaging to Charles, but they were adamant about their wishes. Ms. Paxton wondered if parents could make this kind of choice for their ill child. Without continued treatment, Charles' prognosis was very guarded. With continued treatment, there was a chance that he would survive and receive benefit from the surgical technique and treatment. Yet his parents said, "No."

Case 87: Finding Out the Relative Benefits and Harms of Self-Care Treatment

Samantha Long is a cardiovascular clinical nurse specialist. During the past 2 years, she and her colleagues have been studying the physiological and psychological effects of self-care activities in patients recovering from myocardial infarctions. Patients admitted to the studies have been carefully screened and selected according to the amount of myocardial damage suffered, the absence of known cardiovascular disease prior to their present illness, and the overall prognosis of the patient. To date, the results of the studies have indicated a significant positive correlation between self-care activities and psychological status. No relationship has been found between self-care activities and physiological effects.

Ms. Long and her colleagues would like to extend their research to the use of self-care activities with patients having more extensive myocardial damage and those with known cardiovascular disease prior to this hospital admission. Other studies have demonstrated that this type of patient has a higher incidence of depression, other pyschological problems, and noncompliance to follow-up treatment. She is uncertain, however, whether including these patients in the study would be ethical. Although she has reason to believe that self-care activities will have a beneficial effect on the pyschological status of these patients, she does not know what effects self-care might have on their physiological status. She is aware that the use of self-care in the recovery of these patients poses some risks, but it is not known how serious these risks might be. Should she extend her study to include these patients?

Case 88: Taking Care of Baby Fae*

Marie Whisman, a neonatal nurse–specialist, once cared for a very special baby. This baby, known to the public as Baby Fae, was born on October 14, 1984, with hypoplastic left heart syndrome, a normally fatal cardiac abnormality. The recommended treatment was a heart transplant. Since a human heart was not believed available for Baby Fae, her physicians considered performing an xenograft—a procedure replacing her heart with that of a baboon. The procedure was explained to her parents, their consent was obtained, and the surgery was performed on October 26, 1984. Baby Fae survived for 21 days but died of complications from rejection of the xenograft.

Marie Whisman was Baby Fae's primary nurse. At the infant's funeral, Ms. Whisman read a statement about the nursing care that this special infant received. Unstated, however, were many questions about the role that nurses play in the care of patients undergoing innovative therapies that can also be described as research. Of what benefit to Baby Fae was this particular procedure? What obligation did Ms. Whisman have to Baby Fae's parents to inform them of the special risks and limited benefits of the planned procedure? Was the planned procedure of such great benefit to society that the risk to Baby Fae's life was justified? How does a nurse caring for a patient assess the risks and benefits of innovative procedures and decide whether or not he or she wants to continue to participate in care involving innovative treatment? Ms. Whisman was the human being who touched and cared most for Baby Fae during her short life and was a participant in every procedure that was performed on the infant. What obligations does a nurse have in this situation to the infant? To the parents? To the research team?

Commentary

In all three of these cases the first task is to determine what counts as research and what as therapy, and what difference it makes. The treatment of Charles Sutter, the baby born with a meningomyelocele and other problems, poses the problem well. The first ethical

*Mathews J: Baby with baboon's heart making steady progress. Washington Post, p 2, October 30, 1984; Mathews J: Head nurse shares memories of Fae. Washington Post, p 14, November 18, 1984; Cummings J: Memorial service held for Baby Fae. New York Times, p L-30, November 18, 1984; Altman LK: Learning from Baby Fae. New York Times, pp L-1, L-30, November 18, 1984

question raised is whether the parents made the right choice when they decided to take him home from the hospital rather than decide for the standard surgical treatment. Assuming Dr. Kron's new treatment were not in the picture, some would argue that there is a moral, if not legal, duty on the part of the parents to have Charles treated using conventional therapeutic measures. That is not in itself a problem in research or innovative therapy, but rather one of the limits on parental judgments made in the name of promoting their child's welfare. That is a problem to be addressed in the cases in Chapter 14.

Assuming, however, that the parents have decided against the conventional therapy and that Dr. Kron is prepared to offer the innovative treatment, a new set of ethical problems arise for the parents, the physician, and the nurse, Becky Paxton. It appears that the parents and health professionals were willing to accept the conclusion that, on balance, the risks were justified, considering the potential benefits. If that is so, the treatment itself, in one sense, is not research. It is therapy, innovative therapy, but therapy nonetheless. It is justified by the judgment that the benefits to Charles himself outweigh the risks. Just as when the conventional therapy was rejected, this judgment is controversial. In either case, society could require that the judgment made by the individual practitioners and the individual parents be reviewed by some sort of committee. Society has not seen fit to have such review of conventional therapeutic decisions (even when the judgment is controversial). It might do so in the future, using ethics committees or some other mechanism to monitor certain kinds of problematic therapy decisions.

Society has seen fit to ask for such review in cases involving innovative therapy. Part of the reason is that some of the parties—the surgeon, for example—may have interests other than those of Charles on his agenda. He may be uniquely partial to a technique he is developing. He may want to have several cases, so that he can publish an article on the procedure. It is now common for such innovative therapies to be reviewed by institutional review boards. Normally, in addition to the fact that the therapy is innovative, Dr. Kron and Becky Paxton would be gathering data about the procedure. They might photograph the operation, do extra tests to monitor the effectiveness, or special follow-up studies. These would be research. They would have moved from innovative therapy to data gathering. Possibly, when Ms. Paxton and Dr. Kron tried to persuade the Sutters to keep Charles in the treatment program a while longer, they were not motivated solely out of a commitment to Charles' welfare. They may have been afraid of losing one of the patients in their series. Those are the special agendas that many people believe call for additional monitoring of innovative therapies.

With that background, it is still important to determine whether the risks to Charles are justified by the potential benefits. We shall see in the cases in Chapter 14 that these are inherently subjective calls. Deciding the benefits and the harms depends not only on guesses about the probabilities of various outcomes, but also qualitative assessments of how bad or how good the outcomes will be. They need to decide whether preserving life with fever, infections, and convulsions is good or bad, on balance. They need to decide whether the pain and dysfunctions are justified. In principle, medical science cannot answer these questions.

In addition to these problems, Dr. Kron and Becky Paxton need to decide whether they should be taking into account the potential benefits to other children if Charles continues to suffer. Some would argue that only the potential benefits to this patient can count in justifying the burdens to him.[9] Others, however, including the National Commission for the Protection of Human Subjects, permit some exceptions. They would permit research on children when the interventions for research purposes that involve, at most, minimal risk or, under special conditions, "a minor increase over minimal risk."[10] The same language was incorporated into the DHHS regulations governing research on children.[4] In either case, the commentators seem to agree that even substantial potential benefits to society cannot justify unlimited risks to a child or some other nonconsenting subject of research. At most a minor increase above minimal risk is acceptable. That, of course, is taking into account the risks done for research, not those justified by benefits of the proposed therapy for the patient. Dr Kron, Becky Paxton, and the Sutters need to assess whether they will be asking more than this of Charles.

Marie Whisman, the neonatal nurse specialist caring for Baby Fae, had to face similar problems. It is possible that Baby Fae's transplant received from a baboon could be viewed in strictly therapeutic terms. Her parents evidently made the decision—rightly or wrongly—that the transplant was in her interest and was more reasonable than any alternative available. Ms. Whisman may have had a perspective on the risks and benefits different from that of Dr. Bailey, the surgeon who performed the procedure. If she does, then does she have a duty to make sure that her interpretation is presented along with the others that the parents receive?

It is possible that Ms. Whisman had a very low estimate of the possible benefits and a high estimate of the potential pain and suffering in store for the baby. In that case, she might face the question of whether it is moral to perform innovative surgical treatment. In her judgment, it could be a case of greater than minor increase above minimal risk, the standard called for by DHHS regulations. In that case, she might have to consider withdrawing and taking other actions to protect the baby's welfare.

Samantha Long's study of self-care with myocardial infarction patients poses a somewhat different problem. Some of those patients may be substantially nonautonomous. They may be senile or mentally incapacitated. Those patients would presumably have to meet standards for risks and benefits similar to those involving children. Ms. Long and the IRB that would eventually have to approve of her study could adopt the conservative standard, permitting no risks for research, tolerating risks only when justified for the patient's own welfare. Or she could adopt the more liberal standard permitting minimal risks for proportionally great benefits.

Many of her patients, however, are going to be adults capable of consenting to the risks of the self-care approach. Some may even find the approach so attractive that they would opt for it taking the risks even if they were not in a study. Others could be asked to agree to take the risk of physiological harm in order to make a contribution to science. Even if they thought the risks exceeded the benefits somewhat, they might be willing to assume the risks for the good of science.

That does not solve Ms. Long's problem, however. Even if she can recruit willing patients, she still needs to decide if it is moral for her to make an offer that will expose the patients to risks. If she takes the stance that she has a strict duty to avoid harm, a duty based in the principle of nonmaleficence, she would not be able to proceed. If, however, she is willing to trade off benefits and harms, she might be able to proceed if the benefits exceed the harms.[11] Her critical question is whether other conditions will also have to be met. For example, if she is to avoid the ethical problem of being committed to exposing subjects to extreme harm in cases where even greater benefit is predicted, she will have to set some limits on the amount of harm she is ready to let willing volunteers accept. She may do this for paternalistic reasons; she may simply want to protect the patients from harm. She may also do it for nonpaternalistic reasons. She may reason that she can not in good conscience be part of placing patients, even willing patients, in jeopardy simply because it would not be fitting with her own character. In that case, she could say that others may want to do the study, but she cannot.

Ms. Long's task at this point is to estimate what the risks will be and then decide whether she can, in good conscience, offer the self-care protocol to her patients.

PROTECTING PRIVACY

Ensuring that the benefits of research exceed the harms and that the welfare of the patient is not compromised severely for the benefit of society are not the only criteria for ethically and legally acceptable research. The DHHS regulations also call for "adequate provisions to protect the privacy of subjects and to maintain the confidentiality of data." In some cases, these privacy-violation risks can be incorporated into the calculations of benefits and harms. If a nurse discloses sensitive information from research files and that disclosure causes harm to subjects, then that would count as one of the harms. However, we saw in the cases in Chapter 7 that promises to protect confidentiality of medical information may not be based solely on concern for the harm that disclosure may cause.

Sometimes this concern is expressed in terms of a "right to privacy," a right to have information about oneself kept from public scrutiny even if that information would not necessarily cause harm. In other cases, the concern rests on an implied or explicit promise made by the one gathering the data that it will not be disclosed without the authorization of the one supplying it. This would be based in a principle of fidelity or promise-keeping.

A duty to keep research data private or confidential is widely recognized, but it is also recognized that there are some limits. The following case deals with disclosures of data for research purposes when the disclosure has not been authorized.

Case 89: Finding Out About Baby and Baby's Mother*

Kevin Oberman is a child health nurse in a public health agency in a large metropolitan area. Mr. Oberman is responsible for assisting new parents in their application for a Certificate of Live Birth in their state. In addition to the usual birth information, the state asks additional information that will be used in research studies related to newborn morbidity and mortality and parental health.

One day an angry group of women stormed into his office and questioned

*The names in this case are fictitious, but the case is based on actual events cited in Osonoff D, Osonoff VV: Registering baby: Data base or private record? Hastings Center Report 9(Dec):7–9, 1979

the state's right to ask for personal information about pregnancy history and maternal drug and alcohol use on the state's newly revised Certificate of Live Birth. Mr. Oberman explained the use of the information, but he was unable to explain how the state kept this information confidential and how the information might be used in the future.

Several months later, he learned that the women had sought legal counsel and were being supported by civil rights advocates in questioning the state's right to ask for personal information concerning pregnancy history and maternal drug and alcohol use during pregnancy on a public document. Their claims were presented in the state legislature and legislation was passed that limited the type of questions that could be asked on public documents such as birth registration forms. Soon Mr. Oberman received directions to inform his clients about the use of the information requested on the birth registration forms, the confidentiality protection of the information, and the perceived public benefit of the data collected from the answered questions. Other workers in his health agency, however, strongly protested the legislation. They felt that the overall restrictions on public health research that collected necessary data on such illnesses as fetal alcohol syndrome and fetal drug addiction were ultimately harmful to public health and obstructed the conduct of public health science. Mr. Oberman was sympathetic to the requirements of scientific inquiry, but he was also supportive of his clients' rights to privacy and their need to know the use of this information, now and in the future. When he was asked to join in his agency's protest of the new legislation, he was not sure what he should do.

Commentary

Without knowing it, Kevin Oberman has been employed as a field worker gathering data for research that the state or others may eventually undertake. The problem is more complex because the nurse is not even directly involved with those who will eventually do the research using the data. Still he must struggle with the ethical dilemma posed by patients who object to providing potentially sensitive information to a public data file.

If Mr. Oberman analyzed the problem strictly on risk–benefit grounds, it is not clear how he would decide. The problems potentially addressed by such data—fetal alcohol syndrome, sudden infant death syndrome, and other neonatal morbidity and mortality—are important. On the other hand, Mr. Oberman has clear data showing that some patients are distressed at having to provide it. It is also clear that some of the women could be at risk to legal and psychological problems if the information about drug and alcohol use were made public. If Mr. Oberman sees it as his duty to benefit his patient and if he considers the birth mother to be his patient, he may well consider that more harm would be done to her than good if the data were reported. Even if he considers the newborns as well as the mothers his patient, he may well reach the same conclusion. The actual infants Mr. Oberman is caring for probably will not benefit from the studies, only future infants can benefit. If, however, Mr. Oberman sees it as his responsibility to produce maximum net benefits in toto, then he may well conclude that much more good than harm will result from the reporting of the data.

He may be faced with an argument from the women that they simply have a "right to privacy" regardless of the amount of good for others that can be done with the data. Then he must determine what the status of such a purported right might be. To what extent do people have a right to keep private information that could realistically be expected to help others? Some precautions could be taken with the data. It could be reported in such a way that it could not be connected with specific women. On the other hand, the state may want the data in a connectible form. For example, it might want to monitor cases where infants are thought to be a great risk in the future because of the mother's behavior. The state might claim a concern for the welfare of either these or future children that overrides the women's purported right of privacy.

Mr. Oberman might also determine that the basis for the women's claim is not a right of privacy, but that confidentiality has been promised. He may find that the hospital has made such a promise or even that the state has. More critically, he may discover that he, himself, has made such a promise, at least implicitly. If he subscribes to the ANA *Code for Nurses*, he will have promised to "safeguard the client's right to privacy by judiciously protecting information of a confidential nature."[12] That, of course, raises the question of whether the information the state is requesting is "information of a confidential nature." Assuming the state has established its new Certificate of Live Birth form with due process (by law or by administrative decision), then perhaps one could argue that this is information that no one has promised will be kept confidential. In fact, it could be argued that, when the state requires disclosure by law, there is not even a right of privacy.

Mr. Oberman may find himself in an awkward position. He may be sympathetic with the women at least to the extent of wanting to insist that the data be stored in a way that will protect their privacy, but he may also be in no position to change state law or regulation that calls for the data. If he concludes that the law is justified, his project will be one of attempting to explain to the women why he has reached that conclusion. If, however, he thinks the law is not justified or that procedures must be established to better protect the data, then he will have to develop leverage for challenging the existing practice. This might mean anything from requesting assurances about the storage of the data to refusing to be part of the process in which the data are collected.

EQUITY IN RESEARCH

In addition to consideration of benefits and harms and of confidentiality, the DHHS regulations also require determination that the "selection of subjects is equitable." There are often times when it will be easier or cheaper to use special groups of subjects—prisoners, residents in a state school, or clinic patients. If efficiency in research were the only objective, researchers ought to use the most convenient subjects. However, people are increasingly concerned that the poor, the institutionalized or incarcerated not be singled out to make disproportional contributions to science as research subjects.[3(p8-10),13] The path of least resistance could easily lead to having persons in these groups contributing overwhelmingly as subjects.

The commentators recognize that for certain studies it is impossible to use any subjects other than those who are members of these groups. A sociological study of two different ways of housing or teaching the institutionalized retarded would be an example. Experiments in medical vouchers with which the poor could buy health insurance on the private market would be another. For this reason, the DHHS regulations ask that IRBs take into account the purpose of the research and the setting in which the research will be conducted.

These concerns are driven by the principle of justice or equity. In many of these cases, justice in subject selection may be in direct conflict with the requirements of the principle of beneficence. Doing the most good with limited research dollars could conflict with selecting subjects equitably. It may be that with the same budget twice as many subjects could be studied if the investigator limits recruitment to institutionalized populations.

The regulations limit their concern about the implications of the principle of justice to subject selection. Others are extending their concern to matters of actual research design.[14] They ask what should happen if the investigator designing a research project realizes that there are two different designs that could be used. One will efficiently and eloquently obtain the answer to the research question. It is an ideal design. It places considerable burden on some very sick patients, however. The alternative places much less burden on the patients, but sacrifices some of the efficiency in the design. If justice requires arranging things so that those who are least well off receive the benefits, justice would seem to require the second design, whereas beneficence—maximizing net benefits—would require the first. Equity is a problem not only in subject selection, but also in design and execution of research. The next two cases illustrate these problems.

Case 90: When the Subject Group of Choice Is Prisoners

Gail Lassiter was a doctoral student in a program in nursing when she encountered some difficult questions about research design. Miss Lassiter was studying violent behaviors and personality variables associated with violent behaviors. She was particularly interested in this topic because she was employed in the clinic of a large city jail and often witnessed the effects of violent behavior on unsuspecting inmates and guards in the jail. She hoped that the results of her research would ultimately help nurses to identify inmates with a tendency toward violent behavior, during the initial health assessment, before they harmed other inmates and guards.

Since Ms. Lassiter works in the clinic of a large city jail, it would be much easier and more efficient for her to recruit her subjects there. If she had to find a sample of persons prone to violence by going to the general population, she would either have to study very large numbers of persons picked at random or select subpopulations that she believes would be likely to be violent. The latter strategy might cloud the quality of the data, and the former approach would be practically impossible. Should she do this type of research using a prisoner population, and could prisoners in her own place of employment be part of the study?

Case 91: Inconveniencing the Dying

Martha Ward is the nurse coordinator for the clinical center of a large tertiary care unit. That unit is responsible for clinical trials involving budgets of several million dollars a year. She works directly on one project involving monitoring of patients in a multi-center trial for carcinoma of the prostate. The patients are randomized into three arms, each receiving a chemotherapy regimen involving at least four drugs. The patients are all seriously ill. They have received conventional treatments, but their disease has progressed. Most of the men in the study are quite elderly, and many have difficulty getting around.

Ms. Ward is responsible for maintaining records for the study and also for taking routine blood samples, blood pressure readings, weights, and so on. The protocol calls for taking these measurements weekly, at which time the patients are expected to come to the hospital. Ms. Ward is accustomed to such procedures. She has worked on research protocols for several years. Many of them have involved patients receiving medications on an out-patient basis who have come to the hospital regularly for data monitoring.

She is particularly troubled by the present protocol, however. She knows how difficult it is for her patients to come to the hospital. She realizes that they have to make the trip weekly and that most of the visits are solely for the purpose of the research. She knows that Dr. Hanson, the principal investigator for the study, has never considered any variations in the protocol that would ease the burden on these men. She wonders how much the study would be compromised if the data were gathered only when the men needed to come to the hospital for therapeutic reasons. Alternatively, she wonders whether nurses could visit the men in their homes to get the blood samples and data.

She has been involved in other protocols where patients were inconvenienced for the purpose of the study and that has not troubled her, but these men have such a difficult time getting to the hospital and are in such poor health that she wonders whether she should press for a modification in the study. Would it be ethical to compromise the quality of the data or to increase the costs? Is it ethical to ask these men to come to the hospital weekly in order to get slightly better data or to save the project money?

Commentary

Both of the two previous cases raise, in different ways, the question of whether we ought to be as efficient as possible in gathering data even if it means placing disproportionate burdens on certain classes of potential subjects. The principle of justice, discussed in Chapter 4, focuses on what is fair or equitable in the distribution of burdens and benefits. We saw that some people hold that the fair way to distribute benefits is simply the way that produces the most good on balance. That would mean that in these cases Gail Lassiter would use her prisoners as subjects because they can most efficiently give her the data about persons displaying violent behavior. It would mean that Martha Ward should forget about raising questions about the burden to the prostate cancer victims unless she can show that the burden to these men is greater in value than the benefits of the data obtained from having them come to the hospital.

The alternative position is that justice requires distributing benefits and burdens fairly. For some, that means making sure that the least well off would have their position improved. For others, it would mean trying to arrange things so that people have equal opportunity for well-being. For Miss Lassiter, it could mean that she would choose a more difficult, less efficient method of study in order to avoid asking that prisoners carry an undue portion of the burden of the study. In order to make this judgment, she will have to determine what kind of claim prisoners have. Are they among the least well off, who therefore have special claims not to be burdened further, or are they people who have voluntarily engaged in antisocial behavior, surrendering any claims they would have to be considered among the least well off?

The elderly, critically ill men for whom mobility is difficult would be just the kind who would have special claims under this interpretation of justice. In the protocol as designed, they are asked to make a sacrifice for the benefit of society. They are asked to bear the added inconvenience of trips to the hospital beyond what is necessary for therapy. Ms. Ward is willing to make such requests for patients who are better off. It is not as inconvenient for them, and so on benefit/harm grounds she has asked less of patients in previous studies. In this study, however, the patients are probably among the least well off of any of the people affected. When they are compared with who would be hurt by changing the protocol, Ms. Ward appears to recognize that it is particularly hard to ask the worst off persons of the community to make sacrifices, even relatively small sacrifices, for the benefit of others who are better off. If Ms. Ward is guided by a principle of justice she might be more inclined to ask for one of the changes in the protocol, either reducing slightly the quality of the data in order to make it easier on these patients or increasing slightly the budget for the project by asking that a nurse be hired to collect the data from the men at home when possible.

INFORMED CONSENT IN RESEARCH

A final major area of ethical assessment of research involving human subjects involves informed consent. The DHHS regulations call for ensuring that informed consent be sought from each prospective subject or the subject's authorized representative and that the consent be appropriately documented. These regulations speak of the "elements" of an appropriately informed consent, that is, the kinds of information that must be included. Those elements are summarized in Table 12-1. While the major problems of informed consent will be explored in the next chapter, which deals with consent in the therapeutic setting, consent is also a major issue in research. Some problems, consent for the use of health records for research, for example, are unique to the research context. The following cases raise these special research questions.

Table 12-1. Department of Health and Human Services Basic Elements of Consent

1. A statement that the study involves research, an explanation of the purposes of the research and the expected duration of the subject's participation, a description of the procedures to be followed, and identification of any procedures which are experimental;
2. A description of any reasonably forseeable risks or discomforts to the subject;
3. A description of any benefits to the subject or to others which may reasonably be expected from the research;
4. A disclosure of appropriate alternative procedures or courses of treatment, if any, that might be advantageous to the subject;
5. A statement describing the extent, if any, to which confidentiality of records identifying the subject will be maintained;
6. For research involving more than minimal risk, an explanation as to whether any compensation and explanation as to whether any medical treatments are available if injury occurs and, if so, what they consist of, or where further information may be obtained;
7. An explanation of whom to contact for answers to pertinent questions about the research and research subjects' rights, and whom to contact in the event of research-related injury to the subject; and
8. A statement that participation is voluntary, refusal to participate will involve no penalty or loss of benefits to which the subject is otherwise entitled, and the subject may discontinue participation at any time without penalty or loss of benefits to which the subject is otherwise entitled.

The regulations also contain several additional elements that should be included when appropriate. These include:

1. A statement that the particular treatment or procedure may involve risks to the subject [or to the embryo or fetus, if the subject is or may become pregnant] which are currently unforeseeable;
2. Anticipated circumstances under which the subject's participation may be terminated by the investigator without regard to the subject's consent;
3. Any additional costs to the subject that may result from participation in the research;
4. The consequences of a subject's decision to withdraw from the research and procedures for orderly termination of participation by the subject;
5. A statement that significant new findings developed during the course of the research which may relate to the subject's willingness to continue participation will be provided to the subject;
6. The approximate number of subjects involved in the study.

Case 92: Research Without Consent: What Do You Do with the Results?*

Between 1976 and 1983, Carmen Amato, a maternal/child health nurse, participated in the collection of data for a research study designed to identify major

*This case is adapted from the results of a study published by Ewing N, Powers D, Hilburn J, Schroeder WA: Newborn diagnosis of abnormal hemoglobins from a large municipal hospital in Los Angeles. Am J Public Health 71:629–631, 1981; see also, Wyatt PR: Issues surrounding genetic screening programs (letter). Am J Public Health 71:1411, 1981; also, Ewing N: Dr. Nadia Ewing responds (letter). Am J Public Health 71:1411, 1981

hemoglobinopathies in newborn infants. Ms. Amato's role was to collect samples of cord blood, label them, send them to the laboratory for testing for Rh type, Coombs, serology, bilirubin and hemoglobin type, PKU, and thyroid scan. On admission to the labor and delivery suite, pregnant women were informed that their infants' blood would undergo this examination, and consents forms were signed.

Collected from over 29,000 infants over the 7-year period, the blood samples were also examined for incidental information of genetic carrier states in the neonates. No consent was ever sought for these tests, and Ms. Amato did not know that these data were being collected in the study. She did know that when infants were found to have a major hemoglobinopathy, the study results, along with psychological support, education, and genetic counseling, were offered to the parents of the child. Apparently, when other genetic information was found, particularly the finding of genetic carrier states, no information was relayed to the parents. The results were simply forwarded to the referring physician and included in the infant's hospital record. Since no consent for the additional testing had been sought, the researchers assumed that the physician would be the appropriate person to assess the situation and to choose the most appropriate timing for conveyance of the information to the parents.

Like many of her colleagues, Ms. Amato read about the results of the research study in published reports in several professional journals. She became deeply concerned when she realized that 637 infants had been identified as having non-AA hemoglobin genotypes in the additional testing. She knew that under certain systemic disease conditions, these children were at risk of demonstrating complications of their genotype. Yet disclosure of the testing results had not been offered to those parents whose children were discovered to have these genotypes. When she voiced her concern to officials in her department and to the hospital's IRB, she was told that there were no federal guidelines for the use and communication of incidentally obtained genetic carrier state information. What should she do about this information and what could she do to prevent being involved in future research efforts that failed to disclose the results of incidental testing?

Commentary

It could first be asked what constitutes research and what constitutes therapy in the scenario described. It is reasonable that blood would be drawn from newborns for laboratory tests even if there were no study being conducted at all. This case raises important ethical questions even if all of the work being done were undertaken solely for therapeutic purposes. For example, the fact that certain information was being withheld from the parents raises questions of withholding information of the kind addressed in Chapter 6. The fact that some parents might conceivably have an interest in and conceivably could make reasonable use of the carrier status information adds to these moral problems.

Moreover, even if there were no research being undertaken, there would appear to be questions about the adequacy of the consent for the blood drawing and tests. It can be imagined that a clinician might ask for tests for hemoglobinopathy carrier state or that that information would be an inevitable by-product of the tests being performed. Even if there were no study being conducted, one might ask whether the mothers should have been asked to consent (or refuse consent) for the generation of that information. We shall see in the cases in the next chapter that the answer will depend, in part, on whether one emphasizes beneficence or autonomy as the central ethical principle underlying consent requirements. If beneficence (doing good and avoiding evil) is the key, then the clinician might argue that the patient was at absolutely no risk when this information was generated. (The blood was being drawn anyway.) Moreover, telling the mothers about carrier status could unnecessarily result in their developing a mindset that their children were "unhealthy," creating psychological problems for the children. On benefit–harm grounds, maybe the mothers should not have been told about the tests if they were performed for therapeutic purposes. On the other hand, if autonomy is the underlying ethical concern, then the patients may have a right to consent to diagnostic procedures even if there is no further risk to them. They may have reasons of their own for not wanting the tests performed. They may fear that they, or their physicians, may find out about the results and be influenced in undesirable ways. Hemoglobinopathy studies have racial implications that some parents may object to in principle. For whatever reason, a person committed to autonomy as the basis of consent would favor disclosing information about the tests that the patients would reasonably want to know.

These samples were being analyzed, however, as part of a study specifically to gain information about the patterns of major hemoglobinopathies. As such, the parents apparently were asked to consent to having the information about their children used for research purposes. In addition, if additional tests were performed, the question would arise of whether the women should have been asked to agree. This question would arise even if the tests performed were on a blood sample drawn for clinical purposes. Once again, if the driving ethical principle is beneficence, then deciding whether to disclose the fact that the data were also being used for research or that additional tests were being performed will be on the basis of whether the disclosure does any good. However, if autonomy is the basis of consent, then these decisions will be based on whether the disclosure increases the capacity of the patient to make an autonomous choice. In research, one of the elements of disclosure is normally the purpose of the study. Presumably, this helps subjects decide whether they wish to contribute to the objective of the investigation. Some women might, for example, not want to contribute to studies of hemoglobinopathy carrier status (perhaps because of racial implications) even though in doing so they are not at any risk of harm. Ms. Amato appears to be a party to both controversial therapeutic practice and the practice of research without informed consent. The question is whether either of those practices is ethically unacceptable.

Case 93: Selecting a Candidate for the First Artificial Heart in Humans*

Beth Vaughan-Cole was on the Institutional Review Board that approved Barney Clark as the first artificial heart recipient. An associate professor of nursing at the

*Vaughan-Cole B, Kee HK: Dilemmas in practice: A heart decision. Am J Nurs 85:535–536, 1985; also Eichwald EJ, Woolley FR, Cole B, Beamer V: Insertion of the total artificial heart. IRB: A Review of Human Subjects Research 3(7):4–5, 1981

University of Utah, she had a unique role on the IRB. She was a researcher with a definite interest in the conduct of scientific inquiry. For more than 10 years, she had closely followed the development of mechanical heart devices and their implantation in calves or sheep. As a nurse, however, she was concerned about the manner in which informed consent would be obtained for the first artificial heart implantation in a human. Areas of concern included the criteria for patient selection, the adequacy of informed consent, and the prediction of costs and its relation to informed consent. Of special concern to the University of Utah Medical Center's IRB were the means and adequacy of informed consent. After several revisions, the research protocol selected subjects from a group of patients whose cardiac condition could not be ameliorated by any other treatment. The subjects would be in the New York Heart Association class 4 stage of cardiac dysfunction (significant cardiac symptoms at bed rest) for a minimum of 8 weeks. The life expectancy of such a subject was estimated at several weeks to several months.

Yet, there were many questions associated with informed consent and this protocol. Would such severely debilitated subjects falsely perceive the impending implantation as the key to survival? Furthermore, could any patient (or family), aware of their loved one's impending death, accurately assess the research project for risks and benefits? Since this procedure had never been done in a human before, how could anyone assess the life-style changes that would inevitably occur? Most of all, how could the limitations of the procedure be assessed when the subject to be selected had no options but death in the near future? All of these questions were paramount to Dr. Vaughan-Cole and the other members of the IRB. Despite the 11-page consent form, no one was certain what "informed consent" really meant in this procedure and for the particular patient to be selected.

Commentary

As in the previous case, the first questions raised by the first artificial heart implant are whether this is therapy or research and what difference it makes. It is possible that Dr. Clark could have made the decision to have the implant solely on the grounds of risks and benefits. Although the risks were great, he appeared to have few alternatives. He might have concluded that volunteering for the surgery was in his interest in comparison to the alternatives. If so, he was a candidate for innovative therapy. As with conventional therapy, innovative therapy requires consent.

There were also research elements in Dr. Clark's implant, however. Data would be gathered and journal articles would be written. Some interventions and tests might be undertaken in order to gather data for publication that would not have been performed if the objectives were strictly therapy, even innovative therapy.

Beth Vaughan-Cole must make some choices because she is a member of the IRB charged with reviewing research at the University of Utah. It is an open question whether innovative therapy, as well as research, must be reviewed by the IRB. Most innovative therapy, however, ought to have a research component, and so the question may not be critical. It is reasonable that a committee review any procedures that are ethically problematic. Society has reached a consensus that these include all research involving human subjects. Logically, this includes innovative therapy as well. Whether some or all conventional therapeutic consents should have such scrutiny is open to question.

Aside from the question of whether Dr. Vaughan-Cole's IRB should review the case, the most serious question raised by this case is whether Dr. Clark was de facto coerced into consenting. This question is also raised by the following case.

Case 94: When the Patient Does Not Remember Giving Consent

Mr. Timmons was a 48-year-old unemployed laborer who sustained minor injuries when he walked in front of a slowly moving car. He was intoxicated at the time and had, in fact, been known to have a long-standing alcohol addiction problem. Treated in the emergency room of a well-known medical center, he was offered the opportunity for treatment of his alcoholism if he agreed to participate in a study on alcoholic encephalopathy. Dr. Wiseman, the PI of the study, and Mrs. Barnsworth, the head nurse of the alcohol research unit, explained to Mr. Timmons that the purpose of the study was to determine if a certain medication administered over a period of time would decrease encephalopathic symptoms and improve liver function in alcoholic patients. Mr. Timmons would be required to receive the medication via constant intravenous infusion 24 hours per day for 30 days. He would also be required to take multi-vitamins, eat three meals per day and other snacks, and take other medications as required (*i.e.*, antihypertensives for hypertension). Potential side effects of the experimental medication were explained, and the risks and benefits of the study were discussed. Mr. Timmons signed the consent form and was admitted to the research unit.

During the first 15 days of hospitalization, Mr. Timmons gradually regained his strength and began to increase his activity levels. He was cooperative with the nursing staff, was attentive to discussions about alcohol rehabilitation, and seemed content. By the 20th day, he began to be agitated and depressed, claiming that he was going "stir crazy." Since he felt better than when he was admitted, he especially wanted to go home. He was obviously better nourished and had few signs of alcohol encephalopathy by laboratory testing. When reminded that he had signed a consent form and had agreed to participate for a full 30 days, he claimed that he did not remember signing a consent form. He informed the nurses that he was going home whether they liked it or not.

When Mrs. Barnsworth checked the signed consent form, she noticed that it had been signed with an scribbled "X" and was almost illegible. The admission notes showed that he had been in DTs for the first 24 hours after admission, but that he was not hallucinating, he knew his name, and he knew he was in the hospital. Was Mr. Timmons' consent to participate in the study valid?

Commentary

One of the characteristics of consent is that it be free. It must be a decision rendered by a substantially autonomous agent. Both Dr. Clark, the artificial heart implant patient, and Mr. Timmons, the subject of the study to attempt to decrease encephalopathic symptoms and improve liver function, raise questions about the autonomy of their actions when they expressed consent.

Mr. Timmons' consent can be questioned on the grounds that he may not have comprehended adequately what he was being told. He was intoxicated at the time. If consent is grounded in the principle of beneficence, Mrs. Barnsworth would ask the question, "Did getting the original consent do any good?" If it did not, then presumably it serves no moral purpose. She might also ask whether the process should have been delayed until Mr. Timmons could have understood the conditions to which he was consenting. Once again she would ask whether getting the consent at that point would have done any good.

If consent is grounded in the principle of autonomy, Mrs. Barnsworth would have to ask whether getting the consent at the time it was obtained furthered Mr. Timmons' autonomy. She might also ask whether getting it at a later time would have done so.

Barney Clark's case does not pose serious problems of comprehending what is being communicated. He was a highly educated, active participant with substantial knowledge of what was being proposed. Dr. Vaughan-Cole was presumably more concerned about whether his consent was coerced because the offer was coercively attractive. There is a sense in which many offers received in life are so attractive that they cannot be resisted reasonably. A rational, autonomous person who assesses the options—the advantages and disadvantages of accepting such an offer—cannot always be described as being unacceptably coerced. The question is what makes attractive offers unacceptably coercive. One consideration is whether the one making the offer could have dealt with the problem in some other way. If Barney Clark's surgeons could have performed a simple operation to correct his heart problem, but insisted instead on offering only an artificial heart or death, then they would have been making an offer that would be seen by many as unacceptably coercive. Since they apparently had no other alternatives to offer, their offer may have been a fair one, assuming that they did not mislead him about the potential benefits and risks.

Mr. Timmons' case raises another problem. Assuming he did at some point consent with adequate autonomy to enter the study to reduce encephalopathy, does that mean he is obligated to stay in the study until it is completed or does he have a right to cancel his consent? That is a problem also raised in the next two cases.

Case 95: The Nurse Caught Between her Religious Values and a Research Protocol

Rachel Kornblatt had been employed at a nationally known cancer research institution for about a year. The opportunity to participate in cancer research was exciting to Ms. Kornblatt. She especially appreciated the opportunity to work with other nurses in designing research protocols to study nursing interventions in the care of patients with particular types of cancers. One such patient, Jacob Rosenbaum, had just consented to participate in a study of self-administered, mouth-care techniques. Mr. Rosenbaum had myeloblastic monocytic leukemia, a usually fatal disease of the blood. Like Ms. Kornblatt, he was also an Orthodox Jew. Understanding his religious tradition and its practices, Ms. Kornblatt tended to look after Mr. Rosenbaum in ways that could not be matched by the other nurses on the research unit. His presence on the unit gave all of the staff an excellent opportunity to learn about specialized needs of the Orthodox Jewish patient and the way in which religious values and traditions were observed by the religious Jew. It was the first time that the research unit had had such a patient.

Mr. Rosenbaum had already been admitted to a short-term study of the effects of a combination chemotherapy for his particular leukemia. When Ms. Kornblatt explained that he met the criteria for participation in the self-administered, mouth-care study, he eagerly agreed to consent. Ms. Kornblatt explained that he would be randomly assigned to a schedule of self-administered, mouth-care that would involve nurse examination and culturing of his oronasal surfaces. Mr. Rosenbaum was a good study participant and did not seem to mind the frequent examinations and cultures done by the nurses. The almost constant oral bleeding that he experienced was very distasteful to him. It also made it very difficult for him to maintain his daily dietary observances based on religious traditions.

Unfortunately, Mr. Rosenbaum's condition deteriorated more quickly than anyone had expected. Once he became unresponsive and unable to participate in his mouth-care routine, he was removed from the mouth-care study. He continued, however, to receive his combination chemotherapy and have frequent blood and other laboratory tests.

Ms. Kornblatt was off work for a 3-day weekend. When she returned, she was shocked to learn that the combination chemotherapy was still being administered to Mr. Rosenbaum. This had not been done in previous protocols for this type of cancer, and Ms. Kornblatt was particularly opposed to Mr. Rosenbaum's continued participation in a study with this provision. Her reasons were based on her knowledge of her religious traditions and the value that Mr. Rosenbaum also placed on the observance of orthodoxy. It was apparent that Mr. Rosenbaum was dying from the effects of his disease. He was bleeding from all orifices of his body and moaned in pain at the slightest movement of his body. His hemoglobin was very low, and he was experiencing increasing cardiac involvement. Why was the research protocol being continued on this particular patient?

When Mr. Rosenbaum's medical team made rounds, she voiced her concern about Mr. Rosenbaum and was told that the research protocol would continue until death occurred. In fact, some of the goals of the study depended on the continued administration of the combination chemotheraphy until death.

Ms. Kornblatt explained that Jewish tradition advocated full medical treatment until that point at which it was known that the individual was dying. Once this point was reached, Jewish tradition considered it a moral wrong for anything or anyone to impede the dying process of dying. Based on this tradition and her knowledge of Mr. Rosenbaum's adherence to his religious values, Ms. Kornblatt thought it was morally wrong for her or anyone else to continue the research protocol with this patient. She asked the physicians to remove Mr. Rosenbaum from the study.

The physicians refused. Mr. Rosenbaum had been informed about the policies of the research institution prior to his admittance. He had known that admittance into this particular study involved continued treatment until death. Therefore, he must have also known or realized that it would not be possible to observe his religious traditions concerning death. While the physicians would do everything to make Mr. Rosenbaum comfortable and free of pain, the combination chemotherapy would continue. Ms. Kornblatt disagreed. What would she say to Mr. Rosenbaum's already grieving family who firmly wanted the IV tubes and frequent blood tests discontinued for his final hours of life? How could she continue to maintain the IV infusion of the combination chemotherapy in opposition to her own strongly held religious values?

Case 96: The Research Subject with Rare Blood Cells: Is Consent Required for Cloning Them?*

Signe Colson was a nurse working in the leukemia research clinic of a large medical center. Mrs. Colson welcomed patients to the leukemia research clinic, checked their records, recorded their vital signs, and briefly interviewed each patient for problems and/or progress since his or her last visit. Following blood work in the laboratory, other necessary tests, and an examination by the physician, each patient again stopped by Mrs. Colson's office to sign any consent forms for the withdrawal of blood, to clarify instructions for new medications, additional testing, or research protocol requirements, and to obtain a return appointment. This was the time when many of the patients asked for further explanation of their physician's recommendations and for other information important to them.

One day, Mrs. Colson was troubled by the questions that one of her patients was asking. Mr. Johnstone was a patient enrolled in an ongoing study of

*The names in this case are fictitious, but the case is based on actual events cited in Statement of John L. Moore Before the Subcommittee on Investigations and Oversights, House Committee on Science & Technology, Hearings on the Use of Human Patient Materials in the Development of Commercial Biomedical Products, October 29, 1985

the research center. He had previously been diagnosed as having hairy-cell leukemia, a rare and potentially fatal form of leukemia. He questioned why he still needed to return to the clinic for repeated blood tests and examinations. Four years ago Mr. Johnstone had undergone a splenectomy to slow down his form of leukemia and had subsequently enjoyed an extraordinary recovery from his leukemic disorder. He visited the clinic twice a year at the request of his physician, who claimed that his blood had some unique characteristics that were of interest to him and his research staff. Mr. Johnstone was especially concerned about the consent form that Mrs. Colson had asked him to sign on this particular visit. She replied that it was a new standard form that had to be signed for the removal of blood from patients and that the tests were necessary for his continued health care. Mr. Johnstone, however, wanted to know more about the research activity involving his blood and whether there were any commercial products or potential financial interests involved in the research being performed on his blood. Mrs. Colson assured Mr. Johnstone that the form was only a formality made necessary by the procedural rules of the hospital, but Mr. Johnstone did not seem convinced by her explanation. She told Mr. Johnstone that she would have his physician telephone him to answer his specific questions. Again, she assured him that a number of the clinic's patients were involved in research studies of their blood and that the form was a standard document now being used by the clinic. Later in the day, she informed Mr. Johnstone's physician of the questions he had asked and soon forgot the matter.

Two years later, Mrs. Colson was shocked to read in the newspaper that a former patient of one of the clinic physicians was suing the medical center for use of his blood products to develop commercial biomedical products without his knowledge and consent. The patient was claiming that his blood cell properties had been used for private commercial gain and personal financial profit on the part of the physician without his knowledge, consent, and participation. As a result of his physician's negotiations concerning his blood cells, a for-profit biogenetic firm had been granted exclusive access to the patient's blood cells and their products in exchange for payment to the physician of approximately half a million dollars and other advantages, which would accrue both to the physician and his employer. The biogenetic firm had, in fact, cloned the unique genetic sequence of the patient's white blood cells responsible for producing useful substances in the treatment of leukemias. The patient was Mr. Johnstone. Had Mrs. Colson unwittingly played a role in deceiving a patient about his consent to have blood drawn for "research."

Commentary
As with Mr. Timmons, the alcoholic patient in the study attempting to reduce encephalopathy, these two research projects raise the question of the right to withdraw consent. Mr. Rosenbaum, the Orthodox Jewish patient being cared for by nurse Rachel Korn-

blatt, apparently consented without question to entering the study. Unfortunately, he then deteriorated to the point where he could neither approve or disapprove of continuing. The question, in part, is whether he can withdraw the consent once it is granted. If the basis of consent is autonomy, then normally persons are able to agree to participate and to withdraw their agreement. The DHHS regulations specifically require that any consent process include informing that "the subject may discontinue participation at any time without penalty or loss of benefits to which the subject is otherwise entitled."[2] Something seems to have gone wrong in Mr. Rosenbaum's case.

Part of the problem is that Mr. Rosenbaum himself is no longer in a state in which he can decide to withdraw even though Ms. Kornblatt has reason to believe that he would, based on his religious tradition. The question then becomes one of who should function as Mr. Rosenbaum's surrogate when he is no longer able to speak for himself. The physician seems to have assumed that authority while Ms. Kornblatt may want to claim that role as well, based, in part, on the fact that she shares the religious tradition of the patient. In the cases in the next two chapters we shall see that there are good reasons that the family, within limits, also have a claim to that role.

Ms. Kornblatt has several strategies open to her. She could try to persuade the physician that it is in Mr. Rosenbaum's interest to stop, implying that he is the appropriate decision-maker. She could step into the role of patient advocate, claiming authority herself to stop the procedure. She could press the argument that the family should be the surrogate for purposes of withdrawing approval for participation in the study (pointing out to them that they could ask in this way). Or she could ask for some outside body (an ethics committee or a court) to make the critical decision. Which should she do?

Signe Colson, the nurse working in a leukemia research clinic that has cloned a cell line derived from Mr. Johnstone's hairy-cell leukemia, in some ways faces a similar problem. In this case, however, Mr. Johnstone is alert, involved, and apparently autonomous. He is capable of withdrawing his own consent. One question is whether some consents are irrevocable. Another, in Mr. Johnstone's case, is whether he really gave an adequately informed consent.

No doubt Mr. Johnstone consented to something. He presumably consented to withdrawing the blood, apparently he consented to use of his blood for research. But he had presumably not been told that his blood would be used to develop a cell line that would have potentially significant financial implications. We shall see in the cases in the next chapter that it is debatable whether Mr. Johnstone was told enough for his consent to be called informed. It could be argued that he needs to be told the information he would want to know to make an autonomous choice. In this case would he want to know that at least hundreds of thousands of dollars could be made from the use of his cells?

Even if Mr. Johnstone did give an adequate consent, Mrs. Colson needs to face the question of whether he can withdraw his consent. Certain consents probably cannot be withdrawn, for example, those on the basis of which irreversible decisions have been made, such as performing surgery. The philosophical literature explores consents that contain within them the provision that the one giving his consent cannot change his mind. If this consent contained such a provision, would Mr. Johnstone still be able to withdraw? If it did not contain this provision, should he be able to withdraw?

Case 97: Sensitive Information in the Employee's Health Record*

Jane Sanborn was the occupational health nurse for a well-known manufacturer of parts for NASA projects. Among her responsibilities was the completion of the health status section of a form, which included both personal and health history for periodic health examinations of the company's employees. The physician completed the medical portion of the health report, recorded a decision about the employee's fitness for work, and returned the report to Ms. Sanborn who maintained a confidential file for employees' health reports and records. Employees were asked to sign a statement on the health report to the effect that information in the report relating to employee fitness for the job could be shared with the employer as necessary.

One day Ms. Sanborn received a memo directing her to send copies of 16 employees' health records to a federal agency in Washington, D.C., for participation in a study involving employee health in government-sponsored programs. The agency maintained a centralized data bank that was often used for research involving health record searches. Ms. Sanborn questioned the request and asked for more information about the particular study. No explanation was provided, and the original request was repeated. Ms. Sanborn responded that she would send the health records as soon as she obtained the consent of the employees. She then discussed the matter with the physician and the administrator of her company. Ms. Sanborn was told that she should comply with the request—it was the accepted practice to send any requested employee health records, since they were under federal contract with NASA. No consent was ever obtained from the employees. Under pressure from both the physician and the administrator, Ms. Sanborn was uncertain what she should do.

Commentary

One problem that arises in research is that of consent for the use of records. Statistical analysis of data drawn from medical records can be extremely valuable for epidemiological studies in increasing understanding of disease patterns, such as result from occupational health risks. Sometimes this can be done in a way that poses only limited problems of confidentiality. If, for example, an occupational health nurse such as Jane Sanborn were to remove all identifying information from the files before sending them to Washington, it would be difficult for individual patients to be identified. Of course, there are still risks of violating confidentiality. For example, if all 16 records were reported to have a stigmatizing medical problem, and those 16 employees could be identified as a group, then the removal of identifiers from individual records would mean nothing.

Aside from the problem of confidentiality, are there any ethical issues raised by sending employee records for inclusion in epidemiological research? In effect, these employees are subjects of a study without their consent. If beneficence is the basis for

*Adapted from Fry ST: Confidentiality in health care: A decrepit concept? Nursing Economics 2:413–418, 1984; also, Flaherty MJ: Confidentiality of patients' records. In Curtin L, Flaherty MJ: Nursing Ethics: Theories and Pragmatics, pp 315–316. Bowie, MD, Robert J Brady Co, 1982

assessing consent, the question would be answered by determining if obtaining the employees' consent would increase the net benefit. The employees in this case might be hurt by the study. They might lose their jobs if certain results are found. On the other hand, requiring the consent could harm others, if that requirement makes it significantly harder to do the study. It seems like a close call whether more good or harm would be done by requiring the consent. More important, some people believe that beneficence is not the basis on which this question should be decided. They believe that the critical issue is autonomy of the patient. Then the critical question is whether the employees (the potential subjects) would want to be asked. Some people might take the view that they would have no objections to searches of their records provided reasonable safeguards were employed. Other, however, might object. They might object in principle, or they might fear bad consequences. In either case, Ms. Sanborn might ask whether these employees have been told what they would want to know. For example, they might have been told when they were hired that their records could be used in this way. If they agreed then, they would have given a "blanket consent" to record use for research. Some hospitals are now asking for such blanket consents when patients enter hospitals. If there is no blanket consent, it might be argued that reasonable employees would want to know nothing about this use of their record so that, in effect, they have been told already "all that they wanted to know." Ms. Sanborn's task is to determine how the consent requirement applies and, if it does, whether the consent is adequate for the purpose.

In the next chapter, the consent issue is presented in cases involving clinical therapy rather than research.

References

1. Nuremburg Code, 1946. In Reich WT (ed): Encyclopedia of Bioethics, vol 4, pp 1764–1765. New York, The Free Press, 1978
2. U.S. Department of Health and Human Services: Final Regulations Amending Basic HHS Policy for the Protection of Human Research Subjects: Final Rule: 45 CFR 46. Federal Register: Rules and Regulations 46 (No. 16, January 26, 1981):8366–8392
3. National Commission for the Protection of Human Subjects of Biomedical and Behavioral Research: The Belmont Report: Ethical Principles and Guidelines for the Protection of Human Subjects of Research. Washington, DC, U.S. Government Printing Office, 1978
4. U.S. Department of Health and Human Services: Additional Protections for Children Involved as Subjects in Research: Final Rule: 45 CFR 46. Federal Register: Rules and Regulations 48 (No. 46, March 8, 1983):9814–9820.
5. President's Commission for the Study of Ethical Problems in Medicine and Biomedical and Behavioral Research: Making Health Care Decisions: A Report on the Ethical and Legal Implications of Informed Consent in the Patient–Practitioner Relationship, vol 1. Washington, DC, U.S. Government Printing Office, 1982
6. Faden R, Beauchamp TL (in collaboration wtih King NNP): A History and Theory of Informed Consent. New York, Oxford University Press, 1986
7. Veatch RM: Three theories of informed consent: Philosophical foundations and policy implications. In National Commission for the Protection of Human Subjects of Biomedical and Behavioral Research: The Belmont Report: Ethical Principles and Guidelines for the Protection of Human Subjects of Research. Washington, DC, National Commission for the Pro-

tection of Human Subjects of Biomedical and Behavioral Research, DHEW Publication No. (05)78-0014, pp 26-1 through 26-66

8. Levine RJ: The boundaries between biomedical or behavioral research and the accepted and routine practice of medicine. In National Commission for the Protection of Human Subjects of Biomedical and Behavioral Research: The Belmont Report: Ethical Principles and Guidelines for the Protection of Human Subjects of Research, Appendix I, pp 1-1 through 1-44. Washington, DC, U.S. Government Printing Office, 1978

9. Ramsey P: The Patient as Person, pp 11–58. New Haven, CT, Yale University Press, 1970

10. National Commission for the Protection of Human Subjects of Biomedical and Behavioral Research: Research Involving Children: Report and Recommendations, pp 6–8. Washington, DC, U.S. Government Printing Office, 1977

11. American Nurses' Association: Human Rights Guidelines for Nurses in Clinical and Other Research. Kansas City, American Nurses' Association, 1985

12. American Nurses' Association: Code for Nurses with Interpretive Statements, p 1. Kansas City, American Nurses' Association, 1985

13. Levine RJ: Ethics and Regulation of Clinical Research, pp 49–67. Baltimore, Urban & Schwarzenberg, 1981

14. Veatch RM: Justice and research design: The case for a semi-randomization clinical trial. Clin Res 31(Feb):12–22, 1983

Chapter 13

Consent and the Right to Refuse Treatment

The problems of consent for research on human subjects, raised in the previous chapter, set the stage for a more detailed examination of the ethics of consent for medical treatment and the right to refuse treatment. This is an important topic in nursing ethics because the nurse may be the patient's primary contact concerning consent for specific treatment or procedures performed by health personnel. Although surgery, complex medical procedures, organ donation, and even routine medical treatments may have been explained by other members of the health team, the nurse is often in the position to clarify the procedure and ensure that the consent of the patient is truly informed. In many acute care institutions, the nurse may even be a legal witness to the consent process including the adequacy of patient consent.

In this chapter, case studies will explore the ethical dimensions of consent, including the elements and standards of consent. Once those basic dimensions of consent have been explored, the cases will focus on problems of comprehension during the consent process and of voluntary decision-making by the one giving consent. Finally, the meaning of the concept of consent for incompetent patients will be explored.

Informed consent is a relatively new notion in health care ethics. It emerged in the 20th century from two different ethical concerns. First, traditional professional ethics has long been concerned with protecting the patient from harm and promoting the patient's welfare. It recognizes that the patient who is informed of potential side effects, contraindications, and so forth is often in a better position to protect his or her own interests. Such a patient becomes an active partner in his or her own health care. Thus, if guided by the traditional ethical principles of beneficence and nonmaleficence, the health professional would tend to give information necessary to make sure the patient is reasonably informed.

There are, however, significant problems in grounding an informed consent ethic in the principles of beneficence and nonmaleficence. These principles seem only to require informing the patient, not obtaining actual consent. In cases where the physician correctly believed that the treatment was in the patient's interest and the patient did not believe so, merely informing would adequately notify the patient of possible side effects for which the patient should be alert and would permit the patient to report any contraindicated conditions. It would not, however, offer the patient any real choice in the treatment.

A second principle, that of autonomy, has become an alternative foundation for the requirement of informed consent. It affirms the right of competent patients to control interventions involving their own bodies. Under the principle of autonomy, the patient is given the authority to evaluate treatment options based on his or her own beliefs and values. Treatments may be rejected even if they are believed beneficial by the health care professional. In fact they may be rejected even if they are deemed beneficial by the patient—if, for example, the patient would rather conserve resources for other family members.

In 20th century American law, the requirement of informed consent has been grounded in the principle of autonomy—or what the courts often refer to as the principle of self-determination. In the 1914 landmark case of Schloendorff v. Society of New York Hosp., Judge Cardozo articulated the principle that was to become the foundation of the consent doctrine:

> Every human being of adult years and sound mind has a right to determine what shall be done with his own body; and a surgeon who performs an operation without his patient's consent commits an assault for which he is liable for damages.[1]

Even with this acknowledgment that the patient is required to consent to treatment, many years passed before it was explicitly acknowledged that in order to consent, one had to be informed. In 1960 Justice Schroeder, in the important Kansas case of Natanson v. Kline, argued that where a physician misrepresents a procedure or fails to point out its consequences, he may be subject to a claim of unauthorized treatment (*i.e.,* treatment without consent).[2] That argument has generated the public debate over what elements of information must be transmitted for a consent to be adequately informed, one of the issues raised by the cases in the first section of this chapter.

Yet, even if we know what the elements of consent are—that alternative procedures must be explained and that purposes as well as risks must be disclosed—the issue of just how much of each element must be conveyed will still have to be confronted. If we agree that risks of the procedure must be explained, then just how *many* risks must be explained for consent to take place? Certainly, not all risks must be discussed, since the list of risks of most procedures could be infinite. Some standard of reference is needed to confront the issue.

Traditionally, it was assumed that professionals decided how much information was conveyed as decided by the consensus of their professional colleagues, but other standards are emerging based on what patients would want to know.

The movement, both in the courts and in ethical debate, has been very much in favor of these newer standards for determining how much to disclose to patients. Attempting to determine whether they apply to the nurse as well as to the physician will be one of the critical issues in the cases in this section of the chapter. We do know that the American Nurses' Association (ANA) *Code for Nurses* begins with a forceful commitment to client self-determination and says that

Clients should be as fully involved as possible in the planning and implementation of their own health care. Clients have the moral right to determine what will be done with their own person; to be given accurate information, and all the information necessary for making informed judgments; to be assisted with weighing the benefits and burdens of options in their treatment; to accept, refuse, or terminate treatment without coercion; and to be given necessary emotional support. Each nurse has an obligation to be knowledgeable about the moral and legal rights of all clients and to protect and support those rights.[3(p2)]

The problem presented in the cases that follow will be to determine whether that is an acceptable summary of the nurse's role in informed consent and, if so, whether it requires the nurse actually to do the informing in certain cases or merely to ensure that the client receives the information.

After we have looked at cases that pose problems in determining the elements of consent and the standards for determining how much information to disclose, we shall examine a case in which the ethical issue is whether the patient has comprehended what has been disclosed. This will be followed by a series of cases involving patients who, for one reason or another, may not be able to participate as voluntary, substantially autonomous decision-makers. We will first look at a case involving a client whose mental faculties can be presumed to be intact, but who is in an environment where freedom to make decisions may be constrained. Our example will be from a nursing home. Then we shall look at a client who has compromised capacity for rational planning and choice (*i.e.,* a patient who has been sedated prior to the consent process).

Finally, we shall examine three cases of patients who may not be capable of substantially autonomous decision-making, beginning first with a clearly incompetent patient, a 7-year-old girl, then moving to the psychiatric patient and finally an adolescent.

THE ELEMENTS AND STANDARDS OF CONSENT

The first problem in understanding consent is determining what information should be transmitted. This will depend, in part, on the ethical principle underlying consent. If the only objective is to make sure that the patient's welfare is promoted, then the emphasis is likely to be on risks of side effects where the patient can take action to avoid harm. If, however, the objective is to facilitate patient freedom of choice, then many other kinds of information might have to be transmitted. These might include the purpose of the intervention, the alternatives, and side effects about which the patient can do nothing.

The Department of Health and Human Services (DHHS) regulations regarding human subjects' research, which were summarized in the previous chapter, include a list of "basic elements" of informed consent.[4] Those elements were presented in Table 12-1. Whereas some of those elements apply only to research consent, many of them are appropriate for any consent, including consent to routine therapy. They were built largely on an autonomy model and, therefore, contain many elements beyond what the subject would need to know to protect himself or herself from harm. In deciding what information to disclose to the patient in each of these categories, some choices will have to be made. There is a very large amount of information that can be communicated about any medical intervention, even a simple one. No reasonable person would want to know it all. It would take too long and would include many items that are too trivial. In deciding which information is important enough to include, however, some standard is necessary for making the judgment. Nurses should be aware that different standards for making these choices lead to very different disclosures. Traditionally, a so-called *professional standard* was used. Under this standard, a practitioner had to disclose whatever his or her colleagues similarly situated would have disclosed.

The problem with this standard is that there are cases in which a professional's colleagues would uniformly not have disclosed some information and still some patients would want to know it or would find it material in deciding whether to consent to an intervention. Perhaps physicians, for example, tended not to disclose because they were guided by the Hippocratic principle of beneficence, whereas patients may have wanted the information in order to exercise autonomous choice.

The nurse may face a similar problem in areas where he or she obtains consent. There may be cases in which the nurse's colleagues would not have disclosed information and yet patients would want to know.

In order to get around this problem, those committed to the autonomy principle have supported a newer standard, referred to as the *reasonable person standard*.[5,6] According to this standard, the health care professional must disclose whatever a reasonable person in the patient's position would need to know in order to exercise self-determined choice about the intervention.

Whereas this avoids the problem created by the professional standard whenever the consensus among professionals differs from that of reasonable patients, it still leaves unresolved another problem. Obviously, not all patients are the same. In fact, not all are "reasonable." What should happen when a patient would like more or less information than would the hypothetical reasonable patient? A third standard, sometimes called the *subjective standard,* is emerging to deal with this problem. It requires disclosure of what a reasonable person would want to know modified by the unique needs and desires of the patient insofar as the practitioner knows them or ought to know them. This might require, for example, asking the patient if he or she has any special concerns. It might require the practitioner to add information based on his or her particular knowledge about the patient or on what the practitioner could reasonably be expected to know about the patient.

The following cases show how the nurse confronts problems of making sure all of the appropriate elements of consent are included and how he or she must draw upon some standard for deciding how much information to transmit.

Case 98: Intubating the Dead Patient:
Treatment Practice without Consent*

Mr. Ellsworth, who was 87 years old, was brought into the emergency room by the local rescue squad in a complete cardiac arrest. All emergency procedures

*Case supplied by Kathleen M. Stilling, M.S.N., R.N. Used with permission

were performed, including the establishment of an airway, peripheral intravenous lines, urinary catheterization, and more. After resuscitation attempts had been performed for 45 minutes, the patient was pronounced dead by the attending physician, and family members were notified. When the family arrived at the emergency room, Mary Pope, the evening staff nurse, found the attending physician teaching intubation techniques to five medical students. They were using Mr. Ellsworth's corpse for the practice. She quietly notified the attending physician that the family had arrived and wanted to talk to the physician. They also wanted to see their loved one's body. The attending physician, however, said that he would be busy teaching the medical students for another 15 to 20 minutes. When Miss Pope asked whether Mr. Ellsworth had given permission for his body to be used for teaching purposes, the attending physician ignored Miss Pope and asked her to tell the family that he would be busy with another patient for a few more minutes.

Case 99: How Much Information Did the Patient Need to Know?

Mr. Longwood was a 64-year-old single school teacher admitted to the hospital for indigestion, anorexia, and weight loss. After laboratory testing and a full gastrointestinal (GI) workup, an abdominal mass was suspected. An exploratory laparotomy was performed and extensive cancerous lesions of the GI tract were found and excised. When he arrived in the surgical intensive care unit (SICU), Mr. Longwood had a gastrostomy, jejunostomy, and chest tubes. Because of respiratory problems encountered during the surgery, he also had an endotracheal tube in place, and his breathing was maintained with a respirator. Joellen Ullman was assigned as his primary nurse.

When Mr. Longwood began to regain consciousness, Ms. Ullman explained the machinery and tubing that were maintaining and monitoring his bodily functions.Mr. Longwood was asked by the physician in Ms. Ullman's presence if he had any questions. He did not raise any. Dr. Jankowski did not explain in any detail about the post-surgery recovery period and possible complications. The patient, however, seemed very confused and alarmed and soon began to express anger and frustration at his altered condition. Communicating with a pad and pencil, he related how much he was appalled by the extensive and disfiguring surgery. He had signed a routine operative permit for an exploratory laparotomy that listed the gastrostomy and jejunostomy as "possible" surgical procedures, but he had not comprehended what those procedures involved. After communicating this to his surgeon, he wrote to Ms. Ullman that he would not have permitted the surgery that was performed if he had realized the condition in which it would leave him and that he had extensive cancer. He wrote that he would rather have lived a shorter life without the drastic alteration to his body.

Mr. Longwood never did leave the SICU. He developed infections, abdominal wound dehiscence, and several pneumothoraxes, and he became respirator dependent. He slipped in and out of consciousness. A cardiopulmonary arrest resulted in a tracheostomy. He also developed bradycardia, and his pulse rate would drop to zero when he was suctioned. When back on the ventilator, he would revive and then beg Ms. Ullman to let him die. His physicians refused to discontinue life-prolonging measures. After weeks of difficult treatments and miserable suffering, Mr. Longwood died. Yet Ms. Ullman could not forget his pleading eyes and frequent scribbled notes asking, "Why didn't someone tell me this could happen?"

Case 100: Ms. Jolene Tuma and the Leukemia Patient*

In 1976, Ms. Jolene Tuma cared for a patient with myelogenous leukemia. The patient had been told by her physician that the condition could best be treated with chemotherapy. The drugs to be used were, of course, very potent and had undesirable side effects that reduced the body's defense mechanisms and that made the patient susceptible to infection. Mechanisms to protect the patient from infection (reverse isolation) were explained to the patient, and, after discussion with her family, she consented to treatment.

On the morning chemotherapy was to begin, Ms. Tuma brought the prescribed medication to the patient's room. She sat with the patient for a while discussing her 12-year fight against leukemia. The patient related that she attributed her past success in combating leukemia to her belief in God and to the faithful practice of her religion. The patient and Ms. Tuma then discussed the use of nontraditional treatments for leukemia, including laetrile and herbal treatments. Other alternatives such as natural foods and massage treatments through reflexology were also discussed. The patient indicated to Ms. Tuma that she preferred natural treatments for her disorder rather than the chemotherapy. She felt, however, that her family wanted her to undergo the chemotherapy treatment even though she was worried about its effectiveness and its side effects. She asked Ms. Tuma to discuss some of the alternatives for cancer treatment with her family. Ms. Tuma agreed to do so and made arrangements to meet with the patient's family that night. The chemotherapy was started with the understanding that the patient could request that it be discontinued, pending the meeting with the family.

When the family learned of the the planned meeting, they immediately called the patient's physician. He did not interfere with the meeting and did not discuss the matter with the patient. He did order that the next dose of chemotherapy be held until after the planned meeting. Later, meeting with the family, Ms. Tuma discussed the prescribed treatment, its side effects, and alternatives provided by natural foods and herbs, as well as the fact that the patient would have difficulty obtaining treatment for her disorder, particularly blood transfusions, if she left the hospital without treatment. By the end of the meeting, the patient agreed to remain in the hospital and continue chemotherapy. The next

*For a full discussion of this case, see Gargaro WJ: Cancer nursing and the law. Cancer Nurs 5:131–132, 1982

dose of her chemotherapy had been delayed for 1 1/2 hours but was resumed. The patient died after 2 weeks, during which she experienced adverse side effects from the chemotherapy and was comatose much of the time.

As a result of her actions with this patient, Ms. Tuma's license was suspended. The patient's physician had complained about her actions to the hospital, the hospital lodged a complaint with the Idaho Board of Nursing claiming interference with the patient–physician relationship, and a hearing was held. As a result of the hearing, it was determined that Ms. Tuma had engaged in "unprofessional conduct," and her license was suspended. Tuma appealed to District Court and requested a trial. The request for a trial was denied, and Ms. Tuma filed an appeal with the Supreme Court of Idaho. The court ruled in her favor, and her license was restored.

Discussions of Ms. Tuma's case appeared in the nursing literature and provoked a considerable amount of comment on and interest in the role of the nurse in patient consent to treatment. What do you think Ms. Tuma's responsibilities were to this patient in this situation once she realized that the patient did not comprehend the information necessary for informed consent to chemotherapy treatment?

Case 101: The Patient Who Waived Informed Consent*

Mr. Fred Morrison, 49 years old, was admitted to the hospital for a cardiac catheterization. During the initial nursing assessment, Ms. Tricia Farraday asked Mr. Morrison why he was being admitted to the hospital. He stated that he was to have a "heart test" because his doctor thought the test was needed. When Ms. Farraday asked what kind of test his doctor wanted him to have, Mr. Morrison said he did not know but that his doctor could tell the nurse. When the assessment was finished, Ms. Farraday noted that Mr. Morrison had a knowledge deficit of his condition and of his reason for admission. She recorded this information as part of her nursing diagnosis and conveyed the information to the nurse on the next shift.

The next morning, Ms. Farraday noticed that Mr. Morrison was being taken out of his room and sent to surgery. She inquired whether his physician or anyone else had visited him and discussed his diagnosis and the impending cardiac procedure. Checking the consent form in his chart, she noticed that it had not been signed. Ms. Farraday immediately called the resident and told him that the patient could not leave the unit until his consent form had been signed. The resident quickly came to the unit and explained the need for Mr. Morrison to sign the permit but did not explain the procedure. When the resident asked the nurse to witness the consent form, Ms. Farraday refused because the resident had not given the patient adequate information for an informed consent. When she asked the patient what he would like to know about the procedure, Mr. Morrison claimed that he did not want to know very much. "I leave all that to my doc-

*Case supplied by Stephen P. Boychuck, B.S.N., R.N. Used with permission

tor,'' he stated. Ms. Farraday wondered whether a patient can avoid being informed and whether she ought to witness the consent form. Since the patient did not want to be informed, must she still abide by the requirements for informed consent?

Commentary

These four patients all raise the question of just how much information should be transmitted for the consent to be adequately informed. The first case—87-year-old Mr. Ellsworth, whose body was being used as teaching material upon which medical students could practice intubation techniques—presses us to the limits of the consent requirement. If the purpose of obtaining consent is to protect the patient from harm, it would seem to follow that if the patient cannot be harmed by an intervention, then no consent is necessary. Mr. Ellsworth is the limiting case of a patient who cannot be harmed.

Still, the nurse, Mary Pope, may have had some concern beyond protecting Mr. Ellsworth from harm. She may have been worrying about the harm that could be done to the family waiting to visit one last time with their loved one. Or she might have had in mind something beyond benefits and harms entirely. She may have been concerned about the infringement of Mr. Ellsworth's dignity or his right of self-determination.

In this particular case, the concern for self-determination or autonomy raises a problem. To what extent do the deceased have autonomy claims? To what extent could they? This is a problem arising in ethics and law regarding the treatment of the deceased. It is a philosophical question raised when wills are read or when other wishes of the deceased are considered.

At the level of law, there is a simple answer. All states have passed the Uniform Anatomical Gift Act (UAGA), which governs the use of the corpse for medical purposes.[7] It is normally thought of in cases of transplantation of organs, but it also governs the use of the body for teaching and research, as well as other therapeutic uses beyond transplant. Among other things it specifically requires that, before a body is used for any such purposes, including teaching, proper consent be obtained. This can come through the patient's permission in the form of a document signed while he or she is still competent, or, if patient consent is not available, permission can be obtained from the next of kin. This obviously did not happen in this case. Thus, practicing intubation techniques on Mr. Ellsworth's body can be described as use of the body without consent. It raises the question, however, of how much the patient or the next of kin might want to know before consenting. Obviously, if Mr. Ellsworth had happened to have filled out a UAGA card some years before his death, he would have no information at all about how his body might be used. If his family had to be asked, how much and what kind of information about the teaching use should they be told?

A similar question arises in the case of Mr. Longwood, the 64-year-old school teacher suffering the aftereffects of abdominal surgery. In Mr. Longwood's case, it is clear that he, in some sense, consented to the surgery. Yet it is doubtful that he was adequately informed. His physician, Dr. Jankowski, appeared to take a position similar to that of Mr. Ellsworth's physician. Information should be dispensed judiciously, only when it will do some good for the patient. It is obvious that information would do no good for Mr. Ellsworth. It is more controversial whether it would have done Mr. Longwood any good.

Joellen Ullman, Mr. Longwood's nurse, might have disagreed with the judgment about how much should be disclosed. She might have concluded that Mr. Longwood would have been better off if he had been told about the potential surgical complications, the respiratory problems, the tubing, the disfigurement, the infections, and all.

Rather than having each of them guess whether Mr. Longwood would have been better off with or without the surgery, they might have reasoned that he should have enough information in order to exercise a choice about whether he wanted the surgery done—that is, they might have appealed to autonomy rather than beneficence. Had they done so, they would have to consider many of the elements for consent outlined by the DHHS regulations. For example, they might have had to give a fair account of the potential risks, as well as the benefits. They would have had to specify how much good the surgery could have done, as well as the reasonably forseeable harms. They would have had to spell out the alternatives so that the patient could make a choice among them. They would have had to make sure he understood that he could refuse his surgery if he so desired. Review the elements of an informed consent as outlined in Table 12-1 to see how many of them would apply to nonresearch settings such as Mr. Longwood's surgery.

Even after agreeing on the ethical principle underlying informed consent and the elements of the consent process that need to be explained to the patient, there are still likely to be questions over how much detail needs be included. It is here that the controversy arises over the proper standard for an adequately informed consent.

If the traditional professional standard were used, it is possible that in both Mr. Ellsworth's and Mr. Longwood's case there was an adequate consent. Under the professional standard, the critical question is whether this physician's colleagues similarly situated would have disclosed anything more than their physicians did. In Mr. Ellsworth's case, absolutely nothing was disclosed, yet his attending physician might be able to demonstrate that none of his colleagues similarly situated would have said anything either. Likewise, in Mr. Longwood's case, if the physician could demonstrate that none of his colleagues would have gone into any more detail about the potential side effects and complications of the surgery, then the *pro forma* consent signed by Mr. Longwood might have been considered adequate. It is really an empirical question that could be answered by asking a number of the physician's colleagues.

The reasonable person standard for an informed consent would ask an entirely different question. It is not concerned about collegial consensus. Rather, it asks whether the patient (or the surrogate for the patient in the case of Mr. Ellsworth) has adequate information to exercise a substantially autonomous choice about his or her care. Would a reasonable patient scheduled for exploratory surgery for an abdominal mass in Mr. Longwood's condition want to know of the potential consequences and of the alternatives including not doing the surgery? If they would, then the physician would have an obligation to tell Mr. Longwood about them. That question might also be answered empirically, but not by asking the physician's colleagues. Rather, it would be answered by asking a group of reasonable people whether they would want the information.

One of the problems with the reasonable person standard is raised by the cases of the patients cared for by Jolene Tuma and Tricia Farraday. They both were caring for patients who seemed to have unusual information requirements. Ms. Tuma's patient seemed to want details about alternative treatments in which many reasonable people probably would not be interested. Ms. Farraday's patient, on the other hand, seemed to want virtually no information at all. In either case it might be concluded that reasonable people would not want to know the amount and kind of information that these patients wanted.

It is in situations like these that defenders of the subjective standard would want to modify the reasonable person standard. Ms. Tuma's patient apparently had a great interest in religious healing, unorthodox therapies, laetrile, and herbal remedies. If the professional standard were used by Ms. Tuma, there is no doubt that these alternative treatments would not be mentioned. Likewise, if Ms. Tuma had the obligation to discuss only those pieces of information that the reasonable leukemia patient would want to know about, it is likely that these treatments would not be included.

But when Ms. Tuma is assessing what the reasonable patient similarly situated would want to know, does she take into account the patient's expressed interest in these nontraditional treatments? Does she have a duty to disclose what the reasonable leukemia patient with an interest in nontraditional remedies would want to know? Or does the patient's unusual interests make her an "unreasonable patient?"

Surely, neither Ms. Tuma nor any other health care professional has an obligation to try to guess whether her patient has unusual interests such as those of her present patient. On the other hand, once those unusual interests are made known, some people would argue for the shift to the subjective standard in which the duty of the professional is to disclose those things that a reasonable person would want to know, adjusted for the unusual agenda of the present patient. Does that mean that Ms. Tuma had not only the right, but the duty to discuss with her patient nonorthodox therapies?

The same logic might be applied to Tricia Farraday's patient, Fred Morrison. He was scheduled for cardiac catheterization, which he understood only as "heart tests." He obviously had little idea of the risks, benefits, and alternatives. He seemed not to have the information that the reasonable person would want to know, such as how much good the tests might do, how dangerous they are, and so forth.

Mr. Morrison is, in effect, waiving his informed consent, expressing his confidence in his physician's judgment about the benefit–risk ratios and the wisdom of doing the tests. That may not be wise on Mr. Morrison's part. He may believe, erroneously, that deciding whether the test should be done is a medical matter, to be decided by an expert in cardiology. In fact, many subtle value judgments must be made. People with different risk-taking profiles might decide differently, especially in borderline cases. People with different life agendas might also decide differently. If Mr. Morrison desperately wants to see a daughter's graduation from college within the next week, but then is less concerned about long-term survival, he will make a different choice than if he has no crucial short-term agenda, but wants to achieve long-term survival. Those are trade-offs that are not made on the basis of cardiological expertise. When Mr. Morrison leaves the matter up to his physician, he may simply be confused about the nature of the choice, and either his physician or someone else, such as his nurse, may have to set him straight.

On the other hand, he may well understand exactly what he is doing when he waives his right to give an informed consent. When he opts instead for what could be called an uninformed consent, he may be saying that he knows his cardiologist's values well and that he knows that his cardiologist understands his own risk-taking profile and life agenda. If that is so, then perhaps it is not entirely irrational for Mr. Morrison to yield the decision-making to someone else—in this case, his cardiologist.

We are still left with the question of whether it is ethical to waive the information necessary to make a really autonomous choice in such a situation. Some people might conclude that there is a moral duty to face life's critical choices such that it is morally irresponsible to give over such choices to someone else. Maybe Ms. Farraday holds such a view.

Even if there is such a duty to make critical choices oneself, it does not follow that a nurse or a physician has a right to impose information on a patient who is conscientiously trying to refuse it. If the subjective standard is applied to Mr. Morrison, it may turn out that his information requirements are much less than what the reasonable person standard or the professional standard would require. In that case, holders of the subjective standard would accept Mr. Morrison's waiver.

COMPREHENSION AND VOLUNTARINESS

Even if all of the kinds of information (the elements of consent) are provided and even if the proper standard of consent is used, still other requirements must be met. The information must be comprehended, and the one giving the consent must be capable of making substantially autonomous, voluntary choices.

Even assuming that the person is not constrained in his or her choices by the lack of freedom or by internal limitations in capacity to choose, it is still possible that information will be presented in a form or in a manner in which the individual does not comprehend.

There are at least two ways in which a consent may be inadequately voluntary. Some potential decision-makers may have their options constrained. This is critical for those in confining institutions such as boarding schools, the military, prisons, and nursing homes. It may also apply to patients who have few choices because of lack of resources. The first case in this section involves this kind of constraint. The second way in which choices can be inadequately voluntary is when there are internal incapacities on the part of the one asked to consent. Psychiatric patients and the mentally retarded might be so constrained. So might a patient temporarily incapable of making voluntary choice because of drugs or medication affecting the ability to think clearly. The second case in this section presents such a problem.

Case 102: Giving Flu Vaccine Without Consent

Sonja Pearson was the day supervisor of a 50-bed nursing home facility. One day the facility's owner and medical director sent a directive to the staff: "All patients are to receive influenza vaccination unless specifically noted to be allergic to eggs or egg products. This is a facility policy, and no family or physician consent need be obtained." Mrs. Pearson and the other nursing staff refused to participate in the vaccine administration. The vaccine was given by the medical director and a physician assistant.

Several months later, the state director of public health visited the facility when it was discovered that the death rate for the month that the vaccine was given was triple the usual rate in those particular age-groups. He asked to see the consent forms for the vaccine signed by the nursing home residents. Was it appropriate to give the vaccinations without consent? Should Mrs. Pearson inform the state health department of the vaccine administration without patient consent?

Commentary

Mrs. Pearson needs to decide when, if ever, it is appropriate to treat patients without consent and if she should be willing to disclose to the director of public health that consent was not obtained. Several possible reasons might be given by the medical director and the facility's owner for their directive not to obtain consent before administering the immunizations. First, some of the patients in the nursing home may have been incapable of consenting because of the lack of the capacity to understand and to make voluntary choices. Perhaps they believed that the immunizations would be in their patients' interest and that in such cases they automatically have the right to treat without consent. The judgment that the patients would be better off vaccinated against influenza is a judgment involving value trade-offs. It requires comparing the risk of the immunization itself with the risk of the influenza. While that is not technically a medical choice, the judgment that these patients would be better off vaccinated is a plausible one.

It is not clear, however, that either the facility owner or the medical director have the moral or legal authority to authorize medical treatments on incompetent residents at least if it is not an emergency. If the patients are truly incompetent, someone ought to be in a guardian role. This might be a spouse, family member, or someone else designated for that role. Perhaps the facility owner or medical director has been designated guardian, but that is not clear in the case. If treatment is being rendered for the patient's own good, then guardian consent can be obtained.

It is also possible that the facility's owner and the medical director believed that they were not administering the vaccine for the individual patient's own good, but rather as a public health measure—that is, to protect other patients. It is sometimes argued that public health concerns justify compulsory treatment of potentially infectious disease without the consent of the patient. Under such circumstances it is even possible that the treatment may, on balance, not be beneficial for the individual patient, but, nevertheless, is believed to be justified because of the benefits to third parties. It is then not patient-centered beneficence, but aggregate or social beneficence that is the principle underlying the directive.

In the cases in Chapters 3 and 4, we discovered how controversial treating patients on grounds of social benefit can be. We particularly wondered whether it should be the clinician, normally committed to the patient's welfare, that made the decision to treat in such cases. It is very doubtful that either the medical director or the facility owner have the legal authority to treat patients on public health grounds without consent.

Mrs. Pearson appears to have reached the conclusion that the immunizations without consent were not justified. She might have reasoned that her patients were competent and had not consented or that they were incompetent and guardians had not consented. On the other hand, she might have reasoned that this was a public health measure, for which consent might not be necessary, but that neither person issuing the directive had the authority to issue it. In any case, once Mrs. Pearson and her colleagues refused to participate and, especially, once they have been asked for the documentation of the consent by the state director of public health, it is hard to see why they would not be obliged to disclose the lack of consent. For one reason or another, a nonvoluntary treatment had occurred. If it was a justified omission of consent, the staff members should be prepared to defend what they had done.

In some institutions, it is "standard policy" not to obtain explicit consent for certain routine procedures. Giving immunizations may be such a procedure. The nurse confronted with such an institutional policy may be placed in a very difficult situation. Mrs. Pearson is obligated to obtain an effective consent. In some cases, that consent might be implied (because the procedure is so obviously favored by the patient and so easy to understand that nothing need be said). If the patient extends an arm for drawing blood, the institution can perhaps assume that the patient understands the risks adequately and agrees to have the blood drawn. However, not all patients can always be assumed to be giving this kind of implied consent. This might be especially true for nursing home patients who may not comprehend what is being done. If the institution is administering the immunizations as a matter of policy, then it should be prepared to justify the assumption that patients are giving implied consent. The nurse is placed in the position of having to assess the legitimacy of this assumption of presumed consent.

Case 103: Consent from a Sedated Patient

Mrs. Jorczak, 54 years old, was diagnosed with carcinoma of the colon. Alert, oriented, and intelligent, she understood her diagnosis. Surgery was recommended, and she agreed to surgical excision of the tumor and whatever else could be done for her.

Following surgery, she experienced many complications and remained in the surgical intensive care unit (SICU) for 3 months. She experienced cardiac failure, temporary respiratory failure, renal failure, sepsis, and dehiscence, and required multiple surgical procedures. As her complications continued, Mrs. Jorczak began to question the wisdom of the many procedures ordered for her. Her family, however, encouraged her to do whatever the physician felt was necessary. One day, after being extubated and on low level vasopressors, she was asked to sign a permit for revision of her colostomy and removal of scar tissue from her previous surgical procedures. Mrs. Jorczak refused, stating that she could no longer tolerate any procedures and that she wanted to die a peaceful death. The nurse who was usually assigned to care for Mrs. Jorczak related the patient's wishes to the resident. He called the attending physician, who ordered a stat dose of valium, 10 mg IM, for the patient. One half hour later, the attending physician visited the patient and had her sign the permit. He then stopped by the nurses' desk and asked that the patient be prepped for surgery. The nurse asked: Is this patient's consent valid?

Commentary

Mrs. Jorczak appears to be the victim of an attending physician who is confused about what it means to obtain a consent from the patient. He may even be the kind who uses the vulgar term *"consenting" the patient,* as if getting consent means coaxing the patient to sign a sheet of paper. However, that clearly is not what consent means. It means a voluntary choice by a substantially autonomous agent. Was Mrs. Jorczak making such a choice?

It is clear that patients in principle have a right to change their minds. The mere fact that a patient originally refused the surgery for revision of her colostomy and removal of scar tissue does not foreclose forever her right to consent to the procedure. By the same token, had she originally consented to the surgery, she would retain the right to withdraw her consent at any time before the procedure actually took place.

But in Mrs. Jorczak's case the second so-called consent, the one in which she might be said to have changed her mind, is certainly a suspect consent. The first problem is that it was obtained while she was sedated. Generally, important decisions made while the mind is altered through chemical means should be viewed as suspect. If Mrs. Jorczak were permanently in a mentally compromised state (not by sedation, but by brain pathology) and that were the only communication we had from her, the case would be complicated. It might be argued that the suspect consent from the clouded mind was the best that we could do. In such a circumstance, we might argue that her approval was adequate. Alternatively, we could insist that she was incapable of substantially voluntary choice so that a guardian would have to be appointed for her.

In Mrs. Jorczak's case, however, we have additional information. We know what she said when her mind was clear. There is good reason to believe that her first decision was carefully thought out over a long period of time. There may even be reason to suspect that the sedation was given precisely to coerce her to consent. In such cases, the nurse and the attending physician may have obtained nothing more than a piece of paper with a signature. The nurse asks if the consent is valid. She might have asked whether there was any consent at all.

What steps should be taken by an attending physician or a nurse who believes that Mrs. Jorczak needs to have the surgery even though she is unwilling to consent to it? Could they try to have Mrs. Jorczak declared incompetent? If so, on what grounds?

CONSENT FOR INCOMPETENTS

One strategy suggested in the two previous cases was to attempt to have the patients declared incompetent so that treatment might be rendered without their personal consent. It is clear that incompetent patients need medical treatments and that they cannot themselves consent to treatment. Some provision must be made for them to be treated without their own consent. This raises the question of how the concept of consent has bearing on such patients.

Insofar as consent is a way of facilitating autonomous choice by persons, it makes no sense at all to have someone else, a parent, a relative, or a court, consent for the incompetent patient. If the term *consent* is used at all for incompetents, it must be based on some other ethical concern. Presumably, that concern is the best interest of the incompetent one, the principle of beneficence. A surrogate for the incompetent patient could be used to ensure that the patient's best interest is being served. This is so different from the function of consent in the case of competent patients that sometimes people prefer to speak of "permission" from the guardian or surrogate rather than "consent."

Even if the function of the surrogate is to try to do what is best for the incompetent one, sometimes this judgment is controversial. Sometimes the surrogate may sincerely try to do what is best, but choose an answer with which many people would disagree. The first case in this section deals with a young girl whose parents made a controversial judgment about her best interest.

Case 104: The Case of the Overweight Child

Tracey Waters is a 7-year-old girl who has been overweight since she was 2 years old. She has been followed by the well baby clinic and public health nurses in her community for her weight problem, but all attempts at weight reduction and family teaching have failed. A first grader, Tracey now weighs 128 pounds. Her teacher had discussed Tracey's weight problem with Jane Seymour, the school health nurse, several weeks ago. Today, however, she reports that Tracey is beginning to fall asleep during classroom activities. When she called Mrs. Waters, she learned that Tracey is a restless sleeper at home and often wakens her parents three to four times per night with irregular and noisy breathing.

Mrs. Seymour, finding Tracey's parents uncooperative in discussing their child's weight problems and classroom sleeping, has notified the school authorities. Upon recommendation by the school, the parents agree to a physical examination of Tracey by the health department physician. He recommends that Tracey be admitted to the hospital for controlled weight reduction and follow-up care. Mr. and Mrs. Waters refuse to agree to this intervention, stating that "Tracey is a lovable, chubby child, and we love her just the way she is." Mrs. Seymour is now in a dilemma. Should she cooperate and assist the school authorities in making a Protective Services referral on Tracey's behalf? Being an experienced school health nurse and having known the Waters family for many years, she wonders whether it would be morally justified to attempt to override the parents, and if overriding the family's decision in this matter is really the best action for Tracey's interests, in the long run.

Case 105: Refusing Treatment for a Delusional Parent

Rosa Green, a 60-year-old woman with symptoms of negativism and paranoia, is transferred from a medical unit to the psychiatric unit of a large medical center. The nursing staff assess her to be delusional and capable of harming herself while delusional (not suicidal). Her 38-year-old son, her only living relative, is asked to consent to the use of psychotropic medications in treating his mother. Mr. Green refuses because his mother experienced multiple side effects from similar medications several years ago. Twelve hours later, Mrs. Green is discharged without treatment. The nurses question whether or not action could have been taken to initiate treatment in Mrs. Green's case without the family's consent.

Case 106: Involuntary Sterilization of a Problem Teenager*

Sheila Myers, staff nurse on a busy surgical unit, received an admission from the emergency room. The patient, 17-year-old Lisa Duncan, had an elevated body temperature (101.6 F) and significant abdominal pain. The admitting note revealed that Lisa had been sexually active since age 13, had one living child (age 3 years), and did not consistently use birth control methods. A pregnancy test performed in the ER was negative. Lisa was accompanied by her mother.

Both surgical and gynecologic consults recommended a exploratory laparotomy. Immediate surgery was ordered, and an operative permit was placed on Lisa's chart. The permit was for "exploratory laparoscopy, laparotomy, possible appendectomy, possible bilateral salpingo-oophorectomy, possible hysterectomy." The attending physician took the chart into the room, talked with both Lisa and her mother, the daughter signed the permit, and Mrs. Myers prepared the patient for surgery. While in the patient's room inserting a Foley catheter, Ms. Myers asked the patient if she understood the nature of her impending surgery. The patient understood that she might have an appendectomy, but did not seem to realize that she might have a hysterectomy and a bilateral salpingo-oophorectomy and did not understood what these procedures entailed. When the nurse explained what these procedures were, the patient became very emotional and said that she would not permit them because she wanted to have a family in the future. Ms. Myers then discussed the matter with the patient's mother. The mother realized that a S & O and a hysterectomy were possible outcomes of the surgery and told Ms. Myers that in view of her daughter's sexual activity, "It might not be a bad thing. I don't want her to give me any more kids to raise." She then went on to relate that she had six other children in addition to Lisa's 3-year-old daughter and that it was very hard to cope with all these responsibilities.

Ms. Myers called the resident and explained that the patient did not understand her surgery and that she thought the consent for surgery was probably invalid. The resident came to the unit to talk to the patient and later asked the nurse why she had gone into detail about the surgery to be performed. Ms. Myers explained that there seemed to be some difficulty between the patient and her mother and that Lisa did not understand that she might have a hysterectomy. After talking with the mother and realizing that the patient was 17 years of age, the resident drew up another permit (same wording) and asked the mother to sign it. When she did so without question, Ms. Myers was not sure

*Case supplied by Mary Ann Turjanica, M.S.N., R.N. Used with permission

that there was anything more that she could do. Could a mother permit invol-
untary sterilization of her teenage daughter under these conditions?

Commentary

Mrs. Seymour, the school health nurse involved with the overweight first-graders, is asking the right questions. She recognizes that it will be difficult to determine whether overriding the parents will really be in Tracey's long-term interest. It will certainly be
disruptive of the family dynamics. Her parents will be treated as neglectful or abusive
toward their child. Of course, it may not be that they are malevolent. It is possible for
abuse or neglect to come from the most committed parents. It happens in many medical
situations when parents have unusual views of what is in their child's interest. Nevertheless, labeling them this way and forcing them to confront protective agency authorities will be traumatic, not only for the parents, but for Tracey.

A more complex question is whether it is morally the right thing to do. When the
parents refused to give their permission for the hospitalization of their daughter, they
were basing their judgment on some set of beliefs and values that apparently led them
to the conclusion that it was not in their daughter's interest to be treated this way. Possibly they had ulterior motives. That ought to disqualify them from the decision-making
role, but there does not seem to be any evidence that that is the reason for their choice.
Rather, they seem simply to believe that their daughter does not need this radical a treatment and that she is just a "lovable child."

Assuming that their motives are good, but that many people would disagree with
their judgment, a complex ethical issue is raised for Mrs. Seymour. Is it the role of the
Protective Services agency to ensure that the parents really do what is best or is it sufficient that they choose a course that is tolerable? It may be that both hospitalization and
the parents' alternative are choices that some persons in the parents' position would
make. It is not even clear how a social agency would go about deciding exactly which is
best.

The question is how much discretion any family should have in making these
choices for their incompetent members. If the family must do literally what is best, it
would have no discretion at all. If, on the other hand, family members have discretion,
what is its basis?

Some are now arguing that families are important units within a society and that
they need considerable freedom to function well.[8] Some courts are even recognizing parental authority to refuse medical treatments for their children on these grounds.

At the same time, the parents cannot possibly have unlimited freedom of choice
when it comes to the welfare of their children. Some decisions are simply beyond what
can be tolerated. Cases in which members of Jehovah's Witnesses refuse consent for
their children to have blood transfusions are handled by the courts in this way. Treatments are ordered in these cases even against religious objections of parents. The critical question is when the parents have gone beyond what can be tolerated. That may be
the question that Mrs. Seymour must answer before she can determine whether to seek
to have the Waters' decision about Tracey's hospitalization overturned.

The case of Rosa Green, the 60-year-old delusional woman transferred to the psychiatric ward, presents problems similar to those of Tracey Waters. The nursing staff,

whether they realize it or not, made a critical decision when they asked Mrs. Green's son to consent (or give permission) for treatment with psychotropic medications. Normally, as an adult, Mrs. Green would have the right to consent or refuse consent for treatment. The nursing staff apparently have made the decision that she is not competent to consent or refuse consent for the proposed treatment. On what basis do physicians or nurses have authority to make these determinations? Normally, if a patient is treated as incompetent, it is either because the patient falls into a category of people presumed incompetent—children like 7-year-old Tracey Waters—or because they have been declared incompetent by a court. Private citizens are on shaky ground when they take it upon themselves to treat a person as incompetent. Sometimes persons are so obviously incompetent that no question is raised such as when they are comatose. But Mrs. Green is not that obviously incompetent. Asking her son's permission is implying not only that she is obviously incompetent, but also that her son is her obvious guardian. Both assumptions could be debated.

Once the staff have decided to treat her son as her guardian, they are, in principle, committed to accept his choice. Had he agreed to the administration of the psychotropic agents, his judgment would never have been questioned. But when he gives a controversial answer, he is in a position that is very much like Tracey Waters' parents. Once again the key question is not whether he gave the best answer, but rather whether he gave a tolerable answer. Was his answer tolerable and what should be done if it was not?

The case of Lisa Duncan, the teenager causing problems for her mother, raises similar issues. If we could assume that her mother was her guardian, with the power to consent to (or give permission for) treatments—just like the Waters family and, arguably, Mrs. Green's son—then we would only need to determine whether her mother's judgment was acceptable. Lisa Duncan, however, is 17, not 7. She is not conspicuously delusional, like Mrs. Green. She is very close to the age at which her mother would have no legal role in her medical care. Should Lisa herself be expected to give consent for her surgery? That appears to be what the staff believed when they originally asked her to sign. It is questionable whether they can change tactics and ask her mother to sign once they discover that Lisa gives an answer that they do not like.

But were they correct in assuming in the first place that Lisa could consent to her own surgery? Although she is almost at the age of majority, she has not actually reached it. She is still a minor and for normal situations would probably not be capable of giving a valid consent. There are special situations in which minors can consent for medical treatment, such as when they are *emancipated*, that is, legally independent of a parent's care and responsibility. They can also be determined to be "mature minors" capable of understanding the nature of the issues at stake and, therefore, treated as adults for purposes of giving consent. That requires a judicial determination that the minor really is mature, however.

There is a third situation in which minors may approve of medical treatments without parental permission. Certain groups of treatments, including in many jurisdictions contraception, abortion, venereal disease treatment, and sterilization, can be authorized by the minor without parental approval. The reason for these laws is controversial. Some interpret them to be saying that the minor is capable of giving a real consent, that is, a substantially autonomous judgment, in these areas. It seems strange, however, that they could give a valid consent in these area, but not in others. The other possibility is that even though the minor cannot give a valid consent, he or she can be treated without parental involvement because the very process of getting parental involvement might discourage the adolescent from getting needed treatment. That would imply that there is not a real autonomous consent, but nevertheless an approval for the treatment that is legally valid even without parental permission.

Would that same logic work in Lisa's case? In her case, the parent was actually involved and made a judgment purportedly about her best interest. It might be argued that she was really more concerned about her own welfare, especially the burdens of raising Lisa's children. Should that be grounds for removing her from the decision-making role in the sterilization? Assuming that her mother was working at least in part out of a concern for Lisa's welfare and that her judgment was within reason, what should Sheila Myers make of the fact that Lisa, herself, obviously does not approve? Should a minor always have the right to veto a medical procedure approved of by the parent? If not, should 17 year olds have such a right? Should all minors have the right to veto their parents' decisions on certain critical medical issues such as sterilizations? If so, which ones?

These same questions arise in decisions made not only about overweight children, delusional adults, and sterilization procedures, but also in even more critical decisions that are literally matters of life and death. The problems of consent and treatment refusal for terminal illnesses raise many of these same issues. They will be explored in the next chapter.

References

1. Schloendorff v. Society of New York Hosp., 211 N.Y. 125, 105 N.E. 92, 95 (1914)
2. Natanson v. Kline 186 Kan. 393, 350 P. 2d 1093 (1960). In Katz J (ed with the assistance of Capron AM, Glass ES): Experimentation with Human Beings, pp 529–535. New York, Russell Sage Foundation, 1972
3. American Nurses' Association: Code for Nurses with Interpretive Statements. Kansas City, American Nurses' Association, 1985
4. U.S. Department of Health and Human Services: Final Regulations Amending Basic HHS Policy for the Protection of Human Research Subjects: Final Rule: 45 CFR 46. Federal Register: Rules and Regulations 46:8366–8392, 1981
5. President's Commission for the Study of Ethical Problems in Medicine and Biomedical and Behavioral Research: Making Health Care Decisions: A Report on the Ethical and Legal Implications of Informed Consent in the Patient–Practitioner Relationship, vol 1, pp 102–104. Washington, DC, U.S. Government Printing Office, 1982
6. Faden R, Beauchamp TL (in collaboration with King NNP): A History and Theory of Informed Consent. New York, Oxford University Press, 1986
7. Sadler AM, Sadler BL, Stason EB: The Uniform Anatomical Gift Act. JAMA 206:2501–2506, 1968
8. President's Commission for the Study of Ethical Problems in Medicine and Biomedical and Behavioral Research: Deciding to Forego Life-Sustaining Treatment: Ethical, Medical, and Legal Issues in Treatment Decisions, p 215. Washington, DC, U.S. Government Printing Office, 1983

Chapter 14

Death and Dying

The care of the terminally ill patient presents nurses with some of the most difficult and dramatic ethical problems they will have to face. The basic principles of Part II all have impact on the ethics of the care of the dying patient. Many of the arguments are carried out in terms of what will benefit the patient or protect the patient from harm, that is, in terms of the principles of beneficence and nonmaleficence. On the other hand, much of the debate over the right to refuse treatment has been argued in terms of the principle of autonomy. Patients, so it is argued, should have the right to self-determination even regarding matters of life and death. Likewise, the principles of truth-telling, and fidelity, often are applicable to situations involving dying patients. What they should be told about a terminal diagnosis and whether family members can be consulted before a terminally ill patient is told are issues related to the discussion of these principles in Chapters 6 and 7. The principle of avoiding killing, however, introduces many issues that are often seen as directly relevant to the care of the terminally ill patient. The cases in Chapter 8 explored the question of whether there was an independent moral duty to avoid killing other human beings and, if so, whether that duty prohibited omitting life-prolonging treatments or only prohibited active killing. Those cases also examined the question of whether withdrawal of treatment is to be thought of more as an omission or an action, whether a distinction can be made between direct and indirect killing, and whether some treatments (such as medical provision of nutrition and hydration) are so basic that they can never be justifiably omitted. All of these issues are important in terminal care.

The care of the terminally ill also raises some issues that are usually formulated in terms unique to these patients. The first is what role the definition of death ought to play in the care of such patients. In this chapter's first case we shall see that one of the first problems faced by the nurse may be whether to treat the patient as dead or as a still-living, though terminally ill patient. We shall see that calling a patient dead is very different legally and ethically from deciding to allow a living patient to die. There are certain procedures—organ removal for transplantation, research uses of the cadaver under the

Uniform Anatomical Gift Act (UAGA), and the use of the corpse for teaching purposes—that can be initiated only after the person is pronounced dead. Some patients who are still alive, however, may appropriately be allowed to die according to at least some ethical systems of thought.

Even if there is agreement that the nurse's client is still alive, there is reason to ask whether treatment should continue. These questions arise first in the case of the competent patient or the patient who had expressed wishes while competent. Various mechanisms, sometimes called living wills, are used by patients to express their wishes about terminal care. The nurse may face problems when he or she knows that a living will has been executed yet either the nurse or some other member of the health care team believes that the treatment should continue. Beginning in 1976, state laws have been passed giving certain terminally ill patients the right to refuse treatments. Now a substantial majority of states have passed similar legislation. Questions still arise, however, when patients do not completely comply with the law or when, even though patients do comply, some members of the health care team believe that their wishes should not be followed. The second group of cases deals with competent and formerly competent patients who have expressed their wishes about terminal care.

The most complex cases involve patients who have never been competent to express their wishes (because they are infants, children, or mentally retarded) or who, though once competent, have simply never made their wishes known. In these cases, when patients are terminally or critically ill someone must take responsibility for deciding about their care. In some states (such as New Mexico, Arkansas, and Virginia) the law makes provision for some other person, usually the next of kin, to become the surrogate decision-maker or agent for the patient. In other cases, the next of kin is presumed to be the appropriate surrogate and is asked whether treatment should continue.

We are learning about the limits of such surrogate decision-making. The range of discretion for surrogates is not as great as that of substantially autonomous competent patients. However, it appears that surrogates also should be entitled to some discretion. Proposals to deal with incompetent patients have included roles for the physician, the family, the courts, and special committees at the hospital level, as well as for instructions written by the patient while competent. The nurse's role in these decisions can be critical when he or she is the only one in a position to be aware that decisions are being made that may be contrary to the interests of the patient. It is one place where the nurse's role as advocate for the patient can be most critical. The nurse may play other roles, as well. Increasingly, nurses are being asked to serve on hospital ethics committees. The cases in the third section of this chapter explore the issues of surrogate decision-making.

Finally, there may be times when the limits on scarce resources do not permit the health care team to do all that the competent patient wants done or that the surrogate for the incompetent patient requests. These issues usually arise when the desired treatment is very expensive or time-consuming and offers little hope of benefit. Such questions are arising more and more frequently. The cases in the final section explore these problems.

THE DEFINITION OF DEATH

Medical technology has advanced to the point that it is sometimes difficult to tell whether the patient is dead or alive. This problem began to arise when mechanical ventilators and other support systems were developed to permit prolonged maintenance of patients suffering severe head trauma or prolonged periods of anoxia. Because of ventilator support, these patients could continue respiring indefinitely. With a source of oxygen, their heartbeats could often be maintained, as well. They were alive according to traditional definitions of death based on the irreversible loss of all vital functions.

This became a practical problem in the late 1960s when organ transplantation, especially heart transplantation, produced a need for organs from deceased patients whose organs were still viable. While the need for organs was the most dramatic stimulus to the definition of death debate, many other less dramatic decisions hinged on whether the patient was alive or dead. It is not normal practice to use nursing and medical services to maintain cadavers. Deciding whether the patient is dead may determine when treatment will be stopped. Critics emphasize, however, that often it will be appropriate to stop at least some medical interventions while the patient is still alive. The UAGA, which regulates the use of human tissues from newly dead individuals, authorizes use of body parts not only for transplantation, but also for research, education, and other therapeutic uses. Even if no concrete use of the newly dead body is anticipated, it is important for family members and health care personnel to know when the individual should be treated as dead and when as alive. The first case illustrates the problem.

Case 107: When Parents Refuse to Give Up*

Nine-year-old Yusef Camp began experiencing symptoms soon after eating a pickle bought from a street vendor. He felt dizzy and fell down; he could not use his legs, and he began to scream. By 10:00 PM that night he was hallucinating. He was transported by ambulance to D.C. General Hospital, where he went into convulsions. His stomach was pumped, and traces of marijuana and possibly PCP were found. He stopped breathing. By the next morning, brain scans showed no activity.

Four months later, Yusef's condition had not changed. The physicians believed his brain was not functioning and wanted to pronounce him dead based on brain criteria. Several difficulties were encountered. First, there was some disagreement among the medical personnel over whether his brain function had ceased completely. Second, at that time the District of Columbia had no law authorizing death pronouncement based on brain criteria. It was not clear that physicians could use death as a grounds for stopping treatment. Most importantly, Ronald Camp, the boy's father, protested vigorously any suggestion that treatment be stopped. A devout Muslim, he said, "I could walk up and say unplug him; but for the rest of my life I would be thinking, was I too hasty? Could he have recovered if I had given it another 6 months or a year? I'm leaving it in Almighty God's hand, to let it take whatever flow it will."

The nurses involved in Yusef's care faced several problems. Maggots were

*Weiser B: Boy, 9, may not be "brain dead," new medical examination shows. Washington Post, Sect. B, p 1, September 5, 1980; Weiser B: Second doctor finds life in "brain dead" D.C. boy. Washington Post, Sect. B, p 10, September 12, 1980; Sager M: Nine-year-old dies after four months in coma. Washington Post, Sect. B, Col. 1, p 6, September 17, 1980

found growing in Yusef's lungs and nasal passages. His right foot and ankle became gangrenous. He showed no response to noises or painful stimuli. The nurses had not only the responsibility for maintaining the respiratory track and the gangrenous limb, but also for providing the intensive nursing care needed to maintain Yusuf in debilitated condition on life support systems. Had the aggressive care been serving any purpose, they would have been willing to provide it no matter how repulsive the boy's condition and despite the presence of many other patients desperately needing their attention. However, some of the nurses caring for Yusuf were convinced that they were doing no good whatsoever for the boy. They were only consuming enormous amounts of time and hospital resources in what appeared to be a futile effort. In the process, other patients were not receiving additional care, which certainly could be of benefit to them. Could the nurses or the physicians argue that care should be stopped because Yusef was dead? Could they overrule the parents' judgment about the usefulness of the treatment even if he were not dead? Could they legitimately take into account the welfare of the other patients and the enormous costs involved in deciding whether to limit their attention to Yusuf?

Commentary

Many issues are raised by this complex case. First, the nurses and physicians need to understand the role of the definition of death in this case. Apparently, some of the physicians believed that a person should be considered dead when the brain function is irreversibly lost. That is a view that is accepted with increasing frequency.[1] Deciding whether to call a person dead when his brain stops functioning rather than when spontaneous heart and lung functions irreversibly cease is not a scientifically determined decision. No amount of scientific evidence will help one to decide whether a person should be treated as dead. Many states have now passed legislation or have had court cases that have established that brain criteria should be used for death pronouncement. Moreover, the President's Commission for the Study of Ethical Problems in Medicine and Biomedical and Behavioral Research has endorsed such a position. Still, several jurisdictions have not formally adopted brain-oriented definitions of death. The first problem faced by the nurses in this case is how they should respond if physicians attempt to pronounce death based on brain function loss in a jurisdiction that has not authorized a shift in the definition of death.

In fact, several different positions on the definition of death have emerged during the past several years. Some still hold to the notion that a person should not be considered dead until heart and lung functions cease (even if it is well-established that the person will never regain consciousness at any level). They hold that they are dealing with a still-living critically ill, comatose patient. For them, it is still possible to ask the question of whether such a patient should be allowed to die. They might use arguments, such as those discussed in Chapter 8, to conclude that the morally appropriate course is to allow the still-living patient to die by withdrawing support. If ventilator and other supports are withdrawn, the patient will die very soon. At issue for those concerned about organ procurement is the damage to organs that may result from this procedure. Defenders of this view, however, hold that whether organs can be procured should not be the basis on which a definition of death is chosen.

Others hold that whether a person should be treated as living should depend not so much on relatively trivial functions such as circulation and respiration, but on the more critical capacities to integrate bodily functions and exercise mental function. They believe that a person can appropriately be treated the way society treats dead people whenever those functions are lost even if the heart and lungs continue to function. In some institutions, the nurse may hold one of these views, while the physician may hold the other. In fact, it is likely that there will be differences between nurses or physicians over these nonscientific issues.

Within the past decade, a third distinct position has begun to emerge. It acknowledges that persons who have lost all brain function should be treated as dead, but questions whether all persons who retain any brain function should be treated as living. They have in mind a person perhaps like Yusef Camp, who still has some lower brain functions—reflex arcs or even respiratory center activity. Such a patient would not be dead based on the current legal brain-oriented definitions of death. He would be "vegetative." These people argue that personal identity is forever lost[2] or that capacity for consciousness and social interaction is lost,[3] and that, for those reasons, the individual should be treated as dead even though some "unessential" brain functions remain.

It is important for the nurse to realize that even if Yusef Camp or a similarly situated patient is considered still living, it is reasonable to ask whether it is morally appropriate to stop treatment in order to let the patient die. Cases later in this chapter will look at the limits of parental responsibility in making such choices.

COMPETENT AND FORMERLY COMPETENT PATIENTS

We have seen in the cases in Chapter 13 that mentally competent patients have the legal right to consent (or refuse consent) to medical treatments. This is based in part on the ethical principle of autonomy. Giving patients the right to consent may also tend to promote good. Patients who want to refuse a treatment will tend to be harmed, at least psychologically, if the treatment is rendered. They often know whether the benefit will exceed the harm, based on their own system of values. If, however, this right to consent is based on benefits and harms—the principle of beneficence—it could be overridden in cases where there is good reason to believe that the patient would really be better off without the consent.

The right to consent is not limited in cases where the patient is terminally ill. In fact, when the patient is inevitably dying, many would argue that the harm that could be done by the omission of treatment at the patient's request would be minimal. In any case, the right of the mentally competent patient to refuse life-prolonging treatment is now recognized widely, both as a matter of law[4] and of ethics.[5] There are certain persons who, based on religious and philosophical objections, hold that it is morally wrong to make such decisions,[6] but they are a minority, and even they tend to acknowledge the right of persons to make such choices.

The minority that remains committed to the preservation of life (even "at all costs") includes some physicians. Although it does not occur as commonly as in the past, nurses may find themselves facing a physician who insists that even a competent patient or a patient who clearly expressed his wishes while competent but is now incompetent continue to receive treatment. That is the issue in the first case in this section.

Treating Against the Wishes of the Patient

Case 108: The Patient Who Had a Cardiac Arrest in the Wrong Hospital*

Jesse Newton, a 68-year-old disabled man, has had a 14-year history of coronary artery disease. Since age 54, Mr. Newton has suffered three myocardial infarctions (MIs). He now complains of angina at rest, has ventricular arrhythmias, and (in the past 18 months) has been admitted to the hospital five times for treatment of congestive heart failure.

Mr. Newton was aware of his heart condition and had said that he did not wish to live as a "cardiac cripple" or to be placed on life support equipment. He discussed his concerns with his wife. They both agreed that should Mr. Newton suffer another MI or cardiac arrest for any reason, no heroic measures were to be carried out. Mr. Newton signed a Living Will in accordance with the legal requirements of his state and gave a copy to his cardiologist.

Several months later, while visiting a sister in a neighboring state, Mr. Newton was involved in a single-car accident. He was transported to a local hospital for treatment of closed head injuries with temporary loss of consciousness, facial lacerations, and cardiac contusion. He was admitted to a neurosurgical nursing unit and hooked up to a portable bedside EKG monitor. During the first 8 hours of his hospitalization, his EKG demonstrated frequent PVCs, and he complained of angina that was unrelieved by sublingual nitroglycerin (NG) or morphine. Mrs. Sherri Brooten, the nursing supervisor responsible for the neurosurgical nursing unit, was concerned that Mr. Newton's cardiac status could not be adequately monitored on this particular unit. She began to make arrangements to transfer him to the coronary care unit (CCU).

Before the transfer could be accomplished, Mr. Newton had a cardiac arrest. He was defibrillated, and his cardiac rhythm was quickly restored and maintained by medications while his respirations were maintained by hand ventilation. When he awakened after his arrest, Mrs. Brooten explained what had happened to him. Mr. Newton became agitated, saying that he did not want this to happen again and that the nurse should contact his wife immediately. Mrs. Newton was contacted and brought a copy of the Living Will to the hospital. Mrs. Brooten showed the Living Will to Dr. Gross, the attending physician handling Mr. Newton's case. Dr. Gross read it and then decided that the document should be ignored. It was not valid for his state, and Mr. Newton would receive all necessary treatment while a patient under his care. Did this decision release the nurses from all obligations to respect Mr. Newton's requests?

*Case supplied by Sandra K. Reed, M.S.N., R.N., C.C.R.N. Used with permission

Commentary

Mr. Newton is one of an increasing number of patients who have thought in advance about their terminal care. He had executed a document that is sometimes called a living will. One standard form of this document can be obtained from the group called Concern for Dying in New York City. Also available are other models for stating one's wishes, such as the one called the Christian Affirmation of Life distributed by the Catholic Health Association.

The first question is what the physician might mean when he states that the document is not valid for his state. Perhaps he is aware that many states have passed laws specifically authorizing patients to write in advance their wishes about terminal care. These laws vary somewhat from state to state. In California's law, for example, the advance directive is legally binding only if the patient has been certified terminally ill for 14 days before the document is signed.[7] In other states, this is not required. In some states, proxy decision-makers can be designated as part of the statute. The physician might say he believes that the statutory law in his jurisdiction does not authorize such advance directives or that such directives are not binding. A few states have, in fact, failed to pass such laws.

Even if Mr. Newton is not hospitalized in a state with such a law, however, other complex legal and ethical questions arise. Neither Mrs. Brooten nor the physician is in a good position to interpret all of them. For example, common law generally requires patients to consent to treatment. Patients may also refuse to consent. Would a so-called living will written by a competent patient constitute a refusal to consent to treatment under common law even if there is no specific statute on the matter? Alternatively, if Mr. Newton's own written statement is not valid as a treatment refusal, is Mrs. Newton the presumed surrogate with the responsibility to make what is called a "substituted judgment," that is, a judgment based on what she has reason to think are Mr. Newton's wishes? If so, can the written statement by Mr. Newton be used by his wife as evidence of his wishes? And if so, can the physician treat against Mrs. Newton's judgment?

Assuming that Sherri Brooten has doubts about the legitimacy of the physician's decision to treat, what should she do? She is in an awkward position. If she treats, she may be treating against the refusal of the patient, which could raise legal as well as ethical problems for her. If she refuses to treat, however, she at least faces practical problems of her relation with the physician. If she is wrong about her interpretation of the case, she could be seen as abandoning a patient.

Many nurses would take some initial steps to clarify the situation. They would talk with colleagues, gathering opinions on the appropriate moral and legal course. They might speak with their supervisor. They might, if they had good rapport with the physician, discuss their reservations about the situation directly with him. They might exercise their right to refuse to participate in the case on grounds of conscience. That would free them from direct involvement, but it might not absolve them of responsibility.

What additional steps might a nurse take who believes that the moral or legal rights of Mr. Newton are being violated even if she is personally free from involvement in the case? Would it be appropriate for Mrs. Brooten to speak with nursing supervisors, with hospital administrators or attorneys, with the chief of medicine? Would it be appropriate for her to suggest to Mrs. Newton that she seek legal advice, that she contact a patient advocacy group, or that she transfer her husband to another hospital where the instructions of her husband would be honored? Should Mrs. Brooten take the case to the local hospital ethics committee for further review or advise Mrs. Newton to do so? If she obtains legal advice that the physician is within his rights to treat even in the face of the declaration by Mr. Newton, would she then be free to withdraw from the case? Would it be appropriate for her then to take any of the other suggested actions?

The Patient in Conflict with the Physician and Family

Case 109: The Patient Says "Yes"; the Physician and Family Say "No"

Fifty-eight-year-old Frank Graham was admitted to the emergency room (ER), unresponsive and without spontaneous respirations. He had been found on the driveway alongside his house, having fallen from a ladder while he was cleaning the rain gutters of his house. A neighbor had started CPR, which was maintained by the rescue squad during transport to the hospital. Once in the ER, Mr. Graham was placed on a ventilator, and his blood pressure and pulse were restored. Subsequent testing ruled out CVA and MI; x-rays did show a C1, C2 fracture. His initial unresponsiveness was attributed to cerebral edema. Several days later, he began to focus his eyes on his nurse, Mrs. Cauthen; he could blink and also move his eyes to commands.

A neurological consult indicated that the patient's situation was irreversible and that the family should be consulted for discontinuation of treatment. Mr. Graham's wife wanted to see her husband before discussing his treatment. When she visited him, he did not open his eyes and did not respond to her voice. Later that evening, she called the physician and told him that she did not want her husband's life prolonged in this manner. The physician told her that another consult was ordered for the next day. After consulting with that physician, he would then talk to her again about any decisions that would be needed.

The second consulting neurosurgeon felt that the patient was capable of understanding the situation, and he explained the nature of the injuries to Mr. Graham. He told the patient that he would not be able to survive without the support of the ventilator. He asked Mr. Graham to look in a certain direction if he wanted the ventilator continued. Mr. Graham did this several times. The neurosurgeon and Mrs. Cauthen agreed that his wishes should be respected. When the attending physician read the consult report, he decided that he would not discontinue the ventilator, but that he would not treat Mr. Graham's current electrolyte imbalance (hyperkalemia), arrhythmias, hypotension, or pneumonia. A DNR order was written. Mrs. Graham was consulted and concurred in these decisions. Mr. Graham was not told of this last decision; he was simply told that his ventilator would not be removed unless he desired it to be removed.

Mrs. Cauthen was very uncomfortable with the kind of limited treatment being given Mr. Graham and the fact that he was not being consulted about his treatment. Since she was the one who spent the greatest amount of time with Mr. Graham, she felt that her nonresponse to his many developing problems was contributing to his death.

Commentary

In some ways, this case is like the previous one. Here, however, the neurosurgeon went to great lengths to involve the patient, Mr. Graham, in the ventilator decision, and the wife and attending physician agreed that his wishes about the ventilator should be respected. On what basis, then, did the attending physician and Mrs. Graham take it upon themselves to decide to omit various treatments and to write a so-called DNR order?

There is a growing body of literature on the use of the "do not resuscitate" decision.[8-10] Some of the early guidelines written by local groups held open the possibility that a decision not to resuscitate could be made by the physician and/or family without consulting the patient even though the patient was competent.[11] This is an example of the older, paternalistic thinking, sometimes referred to as "therapeutic privilege," rooted in the principle of beneficence. Almost all commentators now recognize, however, that if there is a presumption in favor of resuscitation, it is the patient who has the authority to confirm or cancel that presumption as long as the patient is competent to do so. Otherwise, a patient could have life-sustaining therapy omitted without his knowledge or approval. In fact, at least one case has led to legal action for failure to resuscitate a patient without informing her in advance that she would not be resuscitated.[12]

While no similar extended discussion of withholding treatments for other conditions such as hypotension or pneumonia has taken place, similar principles would seem to apply. In the cases in Chapter 8, treatments were deemed extraordinary if they were useless or gravely burdensome based on the patient's judgment. Were Mr. Newton to have refused these treatments, they would surely be expendable, but, given the fact that he apparently desired that the ventilator be continued, it is at least possible that he would also have desired these other treatments.

Mrs. Cauthen is thus on firm ground in feeling uncomfortable. She is in a position somewhat similar to that of Mrs. Brooten, the nurse in the previous case, and she might explore similar options.

There is one difference that might be significant. Whereas Mrs. Brooten's patient was trying unsuccessfully to refuse treatment, Mrs. Cauthen's patient may well want the treatment that is being withheld. It is the physician and family who have decided to omit CPR and several other interventions. Yet while the patient appears to have a virtually unlimited legal right to refuse treatment, he clearly would not have the right to insist on every imaginable intervention. He probably does not have the right to insist on unconventional treatments or experimental treatments, for example. Before Mrs. Cauthen protests, she should explore whether a request from her patient for treatment would be of this kind. It is conceivable that some physicians would object on moral grounds to providing antibiotics for pneumonia for a patient in Mr. Graham's situation. If antibiotics were requested, then the physician would have the right to withdraw, at least if some other physician were available to assume his role. It seems clear, however, that the treatments Mr. Graham may really want (treatments he might request if asked) are not of the sort that a health care institution could categorically refuse to provide. They are not comparable to administration of laetrile or experimental therapies. If that is the case, Mrs. Cauthen appears to be justified in objecting. Her problem will be one of determining which channel is most appropriate for making her objection. Of course, there is always the possibility that no matter how and to whom she makes her objection, the other treatments will not be given, and thus Mrs. Cauthen will remain in "moral distress."[13]

The Problem of the Ambiguous Patient

Case 110: To Resuscitate or Not?

Jessica Holmes is an experienced oncology nurse specialist caring for Mr. Sweitzer, an 61-year-old man with metastatic cancer of the bone. Admitted for an above-the-knee (AK) amputation, Mr. Sweitzer developed respiratory distress immediately after his surgery. He was resuscitated successfully, but he now suffers organic brain damage and continued confusion. This once-active patient now has limited mobility and is in considerable pain from the amputation. He also seems frightened by his confusion. At times, he cries and tells Mrs. Holmes that he would rather die than live as he is living now.

The mental change in Mr. Sweitzer worries his family. They visit him often, but believe that his confusion is a temporary condition and that he will soon recover and return home. They do not seem to be aware of the brain damage that he suffered after surgery.

Several weeks after his surgery, Mrs. Holmes observes that Mr. Sweitzer has developed an intermittent pattern of Cheyne-Stokes respirations. In discussing Mr. Sweitzer's condition with the physician, she learns that the physician wants the patient to be resuscitated if he develops cardiopulmonary arrest, despite the fact that Mr. Sweitzer indicates otherwise. Since the family does not really understand Mr. Sweitzer's condition, they also want everything done for their loved one. Yet Mrs. Holmes thinks that it would be cruel to resuscitate this particular patient. What should she do?

Commentary

This case is in some ways similar to the two previous ones. It may simply be another case of a physician refusing to follow the patient's wishes. If so, Mrs. Holmes faces a problem like those of Mrs. Brooten and Mrs. Cauthen. As in Mr. Graham's case, the family may even be siding with the physician against the patient. Mrs. Holmes' problem may be more complicated, however, because it may not be as clear exactly what the patient really wants. Mr. Sweitzer has given Mrs. Holmes a clear signal at times that he would rather not be treated, yet he has suffered brain damage and seems confused. It is not clear exactly what he wants.

There are several possibilities. He may be competent, but ambivalent. Sometimes patients are competent beyond doubt but cannot make up their minds. If that is the case, the physician and family may be on the right track. The issue may not be whether they have the authority to decide, but rather that even though the patient has the authority to decide, he is not giving a clear answer. Surely, the rule of thumb should be that when the patient is ambivalent, treatment should continue (at least until he makes up his mind).

More likely, the doubt is over whether Mr. Sweitzer really is competent. A treatment refusal by a clearly incompetent patient is not binding. Consider, for example, a small child who refuses surgery. We shall see in the next group of cases that for incompetent patients someone must be the presumed surrogate for the patient—whether it be the physician, the next of kin, or someone else. The problem here, however, is whether Mr. Sweitzer is competent to make these critical decisions.

Legally, no one involved, Mrs. Sweitzer, Mrs. Holmes, or the physician, has the authority to declare Mr. Sweitzer incompetent. If there is doubt or if there is a dispute, some adjudication will be necessary. Mrs. Holmes' task may be to raise the question of whether a patient can be treated against his consent. It may be to question whether Mr. Sweitzer is really incompetent, as the physician and the patient's wife appear to presume. She might use one of the mechanisms discussed in the previous cases or some other (such as asking for a psychiatric consult or, conceivably, if the case becomes critical, reporting the case to public authorities). In any case, if the nurse's role is to be an advocate for the patient, she will have a duty to see that Mr. Sweitzer's wishes are respected insofar as he is competent to express them and to see that his interests are served insofar as he is not competent to express his wishes. It is to the incompetent patient that we now turn.

NEVER-COMPETENT PATIENTS AND THOSE WHO HAVE NEVER EXPRESSED THEIR WISHES

While for the competent and formerly competent terminally ill patient the moral conflict is over the tension between judgments about what is in the patient's interest and what serves patient autonomy, that conflict cannot arise for patients who have never been competent or who have never expressed their desires while competent. For young patients like Yusef Camp, the opening case in this chapter, some surrogate decision-maker must be found. For these patients, the moral objective is to have someone choose what will be in the patient's best interest. While for the formerly competent patient, the surrogate decision-maker will try to do what the patient would have wanted (applying the so-called substituted judgment test), for the never-competent patient—the small child or the severely retarded patient—the surrogate will have to try to determine what is really in the patient's interest (the so-called best interest test).

Two kinds of questions arise. First, who should that surrogate be? Should it be a family member, a health care professional, or a court-appointed guardian? Second, once the surrogate has been chosen, how much discretion should that person have in assessing the best interests of the patient? Many of the most controversial cases involve the designated surrogate making a good faith choice about what he or she believes is in the incompetent one's interest, but one with which many people would not concur. Do we insist that the surrogate make the best possible choice of what is in the patient's best interest or only that the choice be within reason?

Many individuals think that parents should not have the authority to make critical treatment choices for their infants. When an infant is severely afflicted, for example, the parents may have a long-term conflict of interest. They might have obligations to other children; they also have interests of their own. The proper care of the infant may not be the result of parental choice. On the other hand, it is not clear that even if the parents are excluded from decision-making that the physician is the appropriate surrogate for the incompetent patient. Physicians clearly differ tremendously among themselves over what counts as appropriate care for infants and other incompetents. One physician might believe that the parents should be spared the agony of rearing this infant. Another physician, perhaps one who has had a marriage suffering from infertility or who stands in a religious tradition that favors sustaining the lives of such infants, might have a very different response.

Other approaches to decision-making for never-competent patients might include use of an infant care review committee.[14] This is a hospital ethics committee oriented specifically to decisions regarding critically ill infants. While some have argued that there is nothing so unique about infant care that a separate committee should be created, others have maintained that special personnel (pediatricians, specialists in institutionalization of handicapped infants, and special education experts) could be included. Such committees, however, have no legal authority to make critical decisions for infants. The most they can do is provide counsel and advice. Moreover, committees appointed at local institutions might not completely neutralize the biases of individual practitioners. A particularly conservative or liberal hospital might have a committee that reflects that orientation no matter how well-meaning the administrators who appointed the committee. The incompetent patient might still be subject to random variations in decisions.

Another alternative to the use of parents as decision-makers is to go routinely to a court or child protection agency for a publicly authorized guardian. While that may be necessary in controversial cases, most people do not think it appropriate to resort to such bureaucratic mechanisms in all cases requiring decisions on medical care for infants.

Some people object to health care professionals, infant care review committees, and public agents serving as surrogates for the infant because they believe that, in principle, the choice should belong to the parent, at least within reason. The parents or next of kin should have some discretion, according to this view, in deciding what counts as appropriate treatment, basing their choice on family beliefs and values. The notion of familial discretion is the issue in the next group of cases.

How Much Discretion Should the Family Have?

Case 111: Selective Treatment of Meningomyelocele: Two Cases of Parental Choice*

Sherri Fincham is a pediatric nurse specialist who has worked on a pediatric neurosurgical unit for more than 10 years. She is especially well-qualified to care

*Adapted from Homer MB: Selective treatment. Am J Nurs 84:309–312, 1984

for children born with spina bifida and meningomyelocele. She is well-versed in the problems that nurses often encounter in decision-making concerning these children and their deformities. Two cases represent the diverse choices that might be made by parents in the care and treatment of their children.

(1) Michael Adams was born with a lumbar meningomyelocele. His parents were told that there was no hope, that they should "let him go." Mr. and Mrs. Adams were aware that Michael would have some residual handicap, but they were eager to do all they could do to save his life. After 5 days, the parents took Michael home and sought other medical treatment. Admitted to another institution, Michael was leaking cerebrospinal fluid (CSF) but had good movement at his hips and toe movement on the right foot. He was alert and responsive, and had good reflexes. Because Michael's back had been open for 5 days, his physicians decided not to close the wound until they had seen three consecutive negative wound cultures. Unfortunately, the wound cultures remained positive for *Pseudomonas,* and the infant develop ventriculitis. He was treated with bilateral external ventricular drainage systems (EVDs) and ventricular irrigations with antibiotics. The meningomyelocele was closed, and administration of antibiotics was continued. After 10 days of negative CSF cultures, the EVDs were removed. When Michael later developed increased intracranial pressure, a ventriculoperitoneal (VP) shunt was inserted. His parents did not give up, and neither did Michael. Three months and 2 days after his birth, Michael was able to return home with his parents.

(2) John Brody was also born with a large lumbar meningomyelocele, kyphosis, bilateral club feet, and bilateral dislocated hips. His meningomyelocele was closed, and a partial kyphectomy was performed hours after his birth. John's parents were optimistic and eager for additional information about their child's condition. As in Michael's case, complications soon developed. John's back began to leak CSF, and an EVD was inserted. Several days later, he developed fever and spells of apnea. His CSF cultures were positive for *Staphylococcus aureus,* and ventriculitis was diagnosed. After treatment with antibiotics, John recovered, was alert and responsive, and began feeding well.

John's parents, however, had become discouraged and sought another medical opinion. They then decided against further treatment for John. When the physicians wanted to initiate further treatment, the Brody's transferred John to another hospital. They stated that they were more concerned for the quality of John's life than whether it would be possible to keep him alive. They became very angry when Ms. Fincham and the other nurses expressed displeasure with their choices for John. The parents said that they did not feel guilty about their decision but resented being made to feel guilty by the nursing staff.

(Postscript) By the age of 4 years, Michael was walking with braces and crutches. He is moderately retarded, but talkative and friendly. He has not been able to develop bladder and bowel control, and so he wears diapers all the time.

John was discharged from the hospital without a VP shunt at his parents request. He died at home about 6 months later.

Commentary

The pair of cases of meningomyelocele involving nurse Sherri Fincham are typical of the cases of critically ill newborns that generate great controversy today. Other cases involve infants born with Down's syndrome and gastrointestinal atresias, as well as low-birth-weight infants. Common to all of these cases is the patient's obvious lack of ability to decide for himself or herself. Moreover, without treatment the patient will almost certainly die. With treatment the patient will live but with handicap of varying degrees of seriousness.

In the cases in Chapter 8, we saw that the most straightforward approach to these cases begins with the assumption that the surrogate decision-maker should try to serve the best interests of the patient. The President's Commission and the Catholic Church are among groups that have supported the notion that treatments are expendable when they are disproportionally burdensome for the patient. We also saw that two criteria are now frequently used for deciding when treatments are disproportionately burdensome. When the treatment is useless, it will offer no benefit and is surely expendable. Likewise, if there is grave burden with relatively modest expectation of benefit, the treatment is likely to be disproportional. Some parents, such as Mr. and Mrs. Brody, made the decision that the benefits of aggressive treatment of the meningomyelocele do not justify the burdens of the treatment. It is not clear whether the Brodys were considering the burdens of the treatments themselves, the burdens of the handicapped life that would result, or the burdens resulting from the institutional care that might be necessary. All three factors have been considered by some parents. There is some controversy over which of these burdens are legitimate considerations.

The Brodys may also have taken into account burdens to other persons, themselves or other children in the family, for example. It is also not clear what role these considerations ought to play. From the case report, however, we have no evidence that the Brodys were malicious or that they were considering anything other than John's welfare.

The Adams, facing essentially a similar situation, came to a very different conclusion. They thought it was in Michael's interest to be treated aggressively. Ms. Fincham seems to agree more with the Adams than with the Brodys. There is evidence that many in our contemporary society side with Ms. Fincham and the Adams even if substantial numbers concur with the Brodys and would make the same decision they did.

The problem for Ms. Fincham is what difference it makes whether she and a purported majority of the population agree with the Adams and disagree with the Brodys. It hardly seems the kind of issue that should be decided by majority vote. If, for example, the majority of the population believed that such infants would be better of having treatment stopped, it would hardly be a justifiable conclusion that the Adams should be forced to stop against their will. Ms. Fincham has a number of avenues available to her to intervene, including reporting the case to child abuse authorities. In fact, such a step may be required by current federal regulations governing the care of handicapped newborns.[15] They require that states have mechanisms available for reporting cases of "medical neglect including instances of withholding of medically indicated treatment from disabled infants with life-threatening conditions."[15] The only cases excluded are those in which

1. The infant is chronically and irreversibly comatose;

2. The provision of such treatment would merely prolong dying, not be effective in ameliorating or correcting all of the infant's life-threatening conditions, or otherwise be futile in terms of the survival of the infant; or

3. The provision of such treatment would be virtually futile in terms of the survival of the infant, and the treatment itself under such circumstances would be inhumane.

Even in these cases, appropriate nutrition, hydration, and medication must be provided. The infants with meningomyelocele (as well as those with Down's syndrome and atresias, and those with low birth weight) would appear not to fit any of these exceptions.

By contrast, the President's Commission for the Study of Ethical Problems in Medicine and Biomedical and Behavioral Research appears somewhat more open to the conclusion that parents could justifiably find some treatments unreasonably burdensome even if these conditions are not met. The Commission speaks of cases in which benefits are ambiguous or uncertain, and accepts foregoing treatment in such circumstances.[5(p218)]

If it is true that decisions about what is useless and what is a disproportional burden are inherently evaluative judgments, then it is likely that there will continue to be disagreement. The question faced by Ms. Fincham and others assessing surrogate decisions is how much discretion the parents or other surrogates should have in making the evaluations.

One approach is to insist that the guardians make the most reasonable judgments about what is in the incompetent one's best interest. That would give the incompetent patient the best chance of having his or her interest served, but it would require some routine reassessment of every surrogate decision. The alternative is to give the surrogate some latitude, at least in ambiguous cases.

It is not clear why parents and other surrogates should have such latitude. Some argue that it is because the family is a fundamental unit in our society. Society expects the parents to draw on family beliefs and values in making many choices for their children: in choosing school systems, in socializing children in religious and other values, and so on. Some people hold that families therefore deserve some discretion beyond that given to a judge or some other decision-maker. The President's Commission, for example, says that

> There is a presumption, strong but rebuttable, that parents are the appropriate decision makers for their infants. Traditional law concerning the family, buttressed by the emerging constitutional right of privacy, protects a substantial range of discretion for parents.... Americans have traditionally been reluctant to intrude upon the functioning of families, both because doing so would be difficult and because it would destroy some of the value of the family, which seems to need privacy and discretion to maintain its significance.[5(pp212,215)]

This suggests some range of discretion for parents in their decisions. The next question is just how much discretion should be allowed. Surely, parental variation cannot be unlimited. The parents must at least be within reason when they judge what is in their ward's interest. Drawing that line will be a judgment call. It is slightly different, however, from the judgment call made by those who insist that the parents must choose what is really best.

What does this mean for Ms. Fincham? If she believes that the parents in these meningomyelocele cases have the duty to make what is really the best choice, then it appears that in at least one of the cases they have not done so, and she must intervene—she must ask for ethics committee review, report to the child welfare agency, or seek judicial intervention. If, however, she accepts the notion of a range of parental discretion, she will have to decide not what is best in each case, but rather whether either of these pairs of parents has exceeded the reasonable limits of parental discretion.

Nonfamily Surrogates

Case 112: Who Decides for the Dying Patient?*

Mr. Burntree, 67 years old, was admitted by his internist to the medical–surgical unit with the diagnosis of probable bowel obstruction. Mr. Burntree had a history of two myocardial infarctions, chronic obstructive pulmonary disease (COPD), and arteriosclerotic heart disease (ASHD). A surgeon was consulted, and Mr. Burntree underwent surgery in the late afternoon. A cancerous growth was removed from his colon, and a permanent colostomy was performed. He returned to the unit several days later (a Friday afternoon), alert, oriented, and aware of his condition. He was receiving IV fluids at the rate of 125 ml/hr and had a Foley catheter in place. His urinary output for the previous 8 hours had been only 200 cc. Both the internist and surgeon were aware of this fact.

During visiting hours, Mr. Burntree was visited by Ms. Scanlon, a friend with whom he had made his home for the past 10 years, after having been divorced for about 6 years. Ms. Scanlon was very attentive to Mr. Burntree and appeared quite concerned about him. Later in the afternoon, Mr. Burntree's daughters from his previous marriage called the nurse's station. They talked with Liz Holden, the evening charge nurse. The daughters were from out of town and were requesting information about their father's condition. Both seemed unaware of their father's postoperative diagnosis. Miss Holden advised the daughters that his condition was stable and that they could talk with their father on his room telephone.

By the end of the 3 to 11 shift, Mr. Burntree's urinary output was a total of 85 cc. Miss Holden contacted the surgeon on call (both internist and surgeon were signed out to their respective partners for the weekend) and received orders to give Mr. Burntree Lasix IV and to increase his IV fluids to 166 ml/hr.

By the next afternoon, Mr. Burntree's condition had deteriorated significantly. His urinary output had failed to increase during the night. The surgeon on call was notified during the day, and he ordered Lasix IV, as well as blood albumin, O_2 per NP, and the insertion of a NG tube to low suction. Given the patient's diagnosis and condition, the day nurse requested a DNR order. The physician on call refused, citing his unfamiliarity with the patient and his family. By early evening, Mr. Burntree was extremely restless and confused. He was pulling

*Case supplied by Dawn G. Snyder, M.S.N., R.N. Used with permission

off his O₂ cannula and tried to climb out of bed, necessitating the use of a Posey restraint. Within an hour, the patient was diaphoretic and extremely lethargic with Cheyne-Stokes respirations. The surgeon on call was notified, but no additional orders were given, and he did not come to visit Mr. Burntree. At this time, Mr. Burntree's daughters called again for a report on their father's condition. They were informed of his deteriorating condition. The daughters were adamant that they wanted everything done for their father and that they would arrive at the hospital within 3 to 4 hours.

Mr. Burntree's friend, Miss Scanlon, who had been visiting him all afternoon and evening, talked to Miss Holden and stated that she just wanted Mr. Burntree kept comfortable. She did not want any heroic measures taken. Mr. Burntree had apparently shared his diagnosis with her, and since he had COPD, he had asked that he not be kept alive "hooked up to any machines" in order to live. Miss Holden assured Miss Scanlon that she would record this information and notify the physician on call.

Before she could reach the physician by telephone, Mr. Burntree suffered a cardiac arrest. Whose directions, the daughters' or the friend's, if any, should Miss Holden follow?

Commentary

Mr. Burntree's case is all too typical of many terminally ill patients. He apparently had views about terminal care, but no one took the responsibility for documenting them. There are suggestions that a record of the patient's wishes be part of every routine hospital intake interview and that the patient be asked if he has an advance directive or would like to prepare one. Had that been done in this case, much of the confusion would have been avoided.

The first nursing intervention is a puzzling one. The day nurse apparently asked for an "order" opposing resuscitation. There is no evidence that she based the request on the patient's wishes or even those of Ms. Scanlon. Should a nurse (or a physician) contemplate nonresuscitation without some confirmation that it is the patient's or surrogate's wishes?

Liz Holden, the charge nurse, was then left in an awkward situation. If Mr. Burntree's wishes are known, they presumably should be followed, but the evidence of his wishes is very indirect. On the other hand, there is substantial circumstantial evidence that Mr. Burntree might have preferred to have Ms. Scanlon as his agent for transmitting his decision or making a decision on her own if his wishes could not be discerned. However, can a health care professional (physician or nurse) take it upon himself or herself to designate a friend, even an apparently close and devoted one, as the patient's surrogate? Can she do so especially when there are natural relatives standing by ready to assume the role of surrogate?

While in this particular case the legitimacy of Ms. Scanlon may be obvious, that will not always be the case. In other cases, apparent friends may step into the decision-making role when there is no clear evidence how well they know the patient's wishes or how devoted they are to the patient. Can health care professionals decide by themselves which apparent friends are the appropriate agents for their patients?

Even if Mr. Burntree had chosen not to write a substantive advance directive expressing his wishes about terminal care, he might have executed a "proxy directive." Sometimes referred to as a durable power of attorney, it designates the person who should serve as the decision-maker in the event that the patient can no longer speak for himself. That would have easily clarified Liz Holden's dilemma.

Since no one took the initiative to get either a substantive directive or a proxy directive, Liz Holden is now in a difficult situation. Would it not have been prudent for her (or anyone else sensitive to the potential for confusion) to have insisted in advance that some responsible decision-maker be designated, by court action if necessary. The next of kin is the presumed surrogate when one has not been designated in advance by the patient. This is true by statute is a few states, but also presumed in common law and in clinical practice. The next of kin has the responsibility first to determine what the patient would have wanted based on the patient's values (substituted judgment) and then to use his or her own judgment about what would be in the patient's best interest if the patient's own wishes cannot be surmised.

If the next of kin is the presumed guardian, that would appear to give the daughters the edge in authority. Ms. Scanlon then would have two possible ways of intervening. She could argue, based on the evidence she has available, that the substituted judgment based on Mr. Burntree's values should be that treatment cease. If necessary, she could have the daughters removed from decision-making authority if they continued to make choices contrary to Mr. Burntree's wishes. Second, Ms. Scanlon could try something even more radical. She could try to argue that she is, *de facto,* Mr. Burntree's next of kin. Whether that strategy would be successful is debatable.

Where does that leave Liz Holden as Mr. Burntree arrests before all of this is worked out? She has several options:

1. She could take it upon herself to replace the daughters with Ms. Scanlon as surrogate.
2. She could accept the rule that the next of kin is the presumed surrogate until someone else is designated.
3. She could, as the day nurse may have done, simply use her own judgment and do what she thinks is best.
4. She could "err on the side of life," resuscitating this time but then insisting that the decision-making authority be clarified so that if another crisis occurs, the proper course is well worked out.

Which course would you follow if you were Ms. Holden?

Divisions within the Family

Closely related to the problems raised in the last case is the situation occurring when two or more family members are all willing to step into the surrogate role. Whereas the friend might be eliminated as an authoritative decision-maker until some official sanction is given for her agency, that would not be the case when the disagreeing significant others are both family members. The following case is illustrative.

Case 113: When Parents Disagree on Death*

Celia Alinger, a 6-year-old girl with a closed head injury as a result of a recent automobile accident, was a very sick pediatric patient. Her respirations were maintained by a ventilator, and she received nutrition by a central hyperalimentation line. She had several bone fractures (left clavicle, several ribs) and had not regained consciousness 5 weeks after the accident. There was a general concern that Celia had suffered permanent brain damage from the accident, but testing to date was not diagnostic. Celia also suffered from Down's syndrome. Prior to the accident, Celia attended a day school for the mentally retarded and was progressing well in self-care activities.

Celia's parents both worked and usually visited her separately. Mrs. Alinger was an office worker, and Mr. Alinger worked as a janitor for the city school system. They spaced their visits around the care of their two other children, ages 8 and 3, and their work schedules.

When additional testing did not rule out the possibility of permanent brain damage, Mrs. Alinger confided to Celia's nurse, Trish Kendrick, that she was very concerned about the quality of Celia's life. She said, "The children have a hard time understanding and accepting Celia now—what will it be like if Celia has permanent brain damage? Perhaps we should let her die without all this effort to keep her alive." At Ms. Kendrick's urging, she expressed her views to the attending physician.

When Mr. Alinger arrived during the late afternoon, it was apparent that he had not spoken to his wife about Celia's condition and the results of the additional testing. When the guarded prognosis was explained to Mr. Alinger, he asked the nurses if they could do more for his daughter. He wanted no treatment spared and rejected the idea that Celia might remain in a vegetative state.

At a staff–family conference several days later, it became apparent that the parents were deeply divided in their wishes for Celia's continued care. Mr. Alinger expressed deep feelings of guilt for driving the day of the accident and for fathering a mentally impaired child. Mrs. Alinger expressed resentment and bitterness concerning the day-to-day social interactions and psychological burdens of having a retarded child. She did not want to prolong Celia's life when it had such a bleak outlook. She was also questioning how she could cope with the long-term management of Celia as a severely mentally and physically impaired child. The staff members were also divided in their opinions about Celia. Ms. Kendrick and the attending physician wanted to do whatever the parents wished, but since the parents could not agree, they felt caught in a double bind.

Commentary

The first critical decision made by nurse Kendrick and the physician was an acknowledgment that they were willing to accept whatever decision the parents reached. That separates this case from many of the others in this section, in which nurses were strug-

---

*Case supplied by Susan Ford, B.S.N., R.N. Used with permission

gling with the question of whether they ought to be willing to go along with the parental decision. To say that they were willing to go along with either a protreatment or anti-treatment decision is to say either that they are exactly at the indifference point between benefits and harms or that they have accepted the idea that parents should have a range of discretion in deciding about care for critically ill children. It is also to say that they believe that either option would be within reason, and so the nontreatment decision would be acceptable or at least tolerable as the protreatment one would be.

If this child were an infant, could this child have treatment omitted without violating the federal regulations summarized earlier in the chapter? Is there some reason that treatments cannot be omitted on infants, but older children similarly situated are not given similar ''protections'' under the regulations?

Once Ms. Kendrick has accepted the idea that either decision would be acceptable, then her problem (and the problem of the physician) is to reach some resolution. It seems clear that the Alingers need some help beyond what either Ms. Kendrick or the physician can provide. They need some counseling to explore the community resources available for the care and support of their daughter. If Mrs. Alinger's decision is based on her concern that she cannot cope with the long-term management of Celia, perhaps her fears can be ameliorated if she knows what social supports are available. Mr. Alinger has expressed guilt feelings over his involvement in the accident. He may also feel some unexpressed (and inappropriate) guilt over fathering a daughter with Down's syndrome. He may well need psychological support in helping work through this critical decision.

This appears to be the kind of case in which the counsel of a local ethics committee would be of great help. Such a committee should have among its members or consultants not only people who can help the family work through the ethical choice, but also resources for psychological counseling and authorities on the social support networks available in the community. Ms. Kendrick may have other resources available to assist the parents in working through their decision. If that final decision is one that Ms. Kendrick finds morally or legally unacceptable, then she will have to consider the alternatives examined in the previous cases in this section.

LIMITS BASED ON THE INTERESTS OF OTHER PARTIES

Thus far the cases in this chapter have focused on the principle of autonomy and its conflict with the patient's welfare (beneficence). This problem arose first with competent and formerly competent patients and then with patients who have never expressed their wishes about terminal care while competent. Even then we saw that some degree of familial autonomy is being advocated by many participating in the current debate. At the same time, the principle of beneficence seems to place some limits on the range of familial and other surrogate choices. Sometimes the welfare of these noncompetent patients seems to require overruling parents and other surrogates.

There are other cases where it is the welfare of other parties that may be in conflict with the decision rendered by the patient or surrogate. This may arise where the patient is permanently comatose and, by many people's judgment, has no further possibility of benefit from treatment. It may also arise when the patient might benefit, but the benefits are extremely small in comparison with the potential social or economic costs to others. These become what are essentially problems in the ethics of allocation of scarce resources. The principles of beneficence (now interpreted broadly to include welfare of all affected parties) is in potential conflict with the principles of autonomy and justice. Increasingly, as a society, we are having to ask whether there are cases in which patients or their surrogates should be prohibited from having care they desire because of the burdens that result to other parties. In the 1950s, Pope Pius XII, in clarifying the concept of extraordinary means, stated that means may be expendable if they involve grave burden to oneself *or another*.[16] In the future, nurses will be facing these social conflicts more and more. They will arise particularly in the care of the terminally ill.

Case 114: Treatment at What Cost?

Suzanne Grimes, RN, was assigned to care for Mr. Desmond, a 67-year-old man with chronic obstructive lung disease and cor pulmonale. During his 6 weeks in the hospital, Mr. Desmond had developed tracheal necrosis and paratracheal abcesses from prolonged mechanical ventilation. Several days ago, his physicians had decided that his trachea could not be repaired, and it was now discovered that he was also suffering from sepsis. After discussing Mr. Desmond's prognosis with his physician, Mr. Desmond's family had agreed to discontinue treatment. Mr. Desmond was now totally incommunicative and incapable of participating in this critical decision. The plan was to make Mr. Desmond as comfortable as possible until his inevitable death from sepsis and respiratory failure.

During the morning, Mr. Desmond was visited by his oldest daughter, who lived thousands of miles away and who had not seen her father for several years. She was visably alarmed by Mr. Desmond's condition and by the fact that no treatment was being given for his declining physical condition. After conferring with the rest of the family, she announced that the family would like to try an alternative treatment for Mr. Desmond. They called the physician and requested that massive doses of vitamins be given to Mr. Desmond. The physician agreed to their request. He then called Miss Grimes and asked her to begin instituting massive intravenous vitamin therapy.

Miss Grimes protested the use of this form of therapy in the care of an inevitably dying patient. She consulted her supervisor. The supervisor agreed with the physician and the family. "I don't understand why you are protesting the vitamins," she said. "It won't take much of your time to administer them; it won't cost the family a lot of money; and it might help them cope with their father's imminent death," she told Miss Grimes. "Besides, vitamins won't hurt Mr. Desmond. He won't notice them, since he is dying anyway. So why the fuss?"

Miss Grimes still disagreed with the plan. She argued, "We are giving the family false hopes; we are setting a precedent for family requests for any treatment on dying patients." According to Miss Grimes, it was not so much the cost of the requested therapy as the fact that a family could make requests of nursing staff that were of no proven benefit to the dying patient. Was it fair that families could make such requests? Miss Grimes did not think so.

Case 115: The Economic Side of Prolonging Life

Leon Davies, age 16, has Duchenne muscular dystrophy. Despite his relatively young age, his disease is at an advanced stage. He has already lost functional use of all extremities, is dependent for all activities of daily living and suffers frequent sleeplessness and headaches because of breathing difficulties. Leon's father died when Leon was an infant. His mother is disabled and lives on a fixed income in a small rural community in another state. Because of his mother's inability to care for him, Leon has been in the custody of the Department of Social Services for the past 7 years. He has been placed in a private institution for children with physical disabilities, where he is supported by a combination of federal and state funds. He sees his mother about twice a year and considers the staff of the institution his "real family." As his physical condition has deteriorated, staff have noted that Leon is becoming uncooperative and distant from staff and peers. They are often unsure what to do to relieve his headaches and sleeplessness.

Recently, Leon's physician has talked with him about the possibility of being placed on a respirator to prolong his life. It has been made clear that such a decision would probably improve his sleeping and decrease his headaches but that Leon should not expect improvement in any of his other functions.

Simone Gauthier, a nurse and the director of the institution where Leon lives, has discussed Leon's care with his physician and has concluded that it is unlikely that Leon will be able to stay at her facility if he is placed on a respirator. The institution does not maintain 24-hour nursing care, and staff would be unable to provide the level of nursing care that he would need on a respirator. She also wonders whether the state could really afford the approximately $200,000 extra a year that would be required to provide respirator care for Leon. Mrs. Gauthier has tried to talk with Leon about his own wishes with respect to a respirator, but Leon has been vague. He finally said that he did not know what decision to make. Neither Mrs. Gauthier's institution nor the physicians have discussed what they plan to do for Leon when his inevitable respiratory failure occurs.

Commentary

The first issue raised by these cases is whether the nurses are motivated out of concern for burdens to others or for what is best for the patient. This is particularly unclear in the case of Suzanne Grimes, responsible for the care of Mr. Desmond, the patient with chronic obstructive lung disease. She perceives that the family has opted for a totally useless therapy. She might object purely out of concern for the patient. On the other hand, her supervisor pointed out that the vitamin therapy will not burden the patient. If

Miss Grimes were motivated purely out of concern for her patient, she might well be indifferent to the proposed treatment.

On the other hand, Miss Grimes clearly felt uncomfortable. Partly, she seemed concerned that family members not be able to ask for utterly useless interventions and get them (even if they do make the family comfortable). The most sensible reason for her to object would be that providing intravenous megavitamin therapy would involve some costs and would require nursing time. Other patients' interests would be compromised by the time devoted to a useless intervention. Moreover, if the treatment is utterly useless, why should a nurse have to devote her energy to such a procedure just because a family member believes that it might help?

It seems reasonable to concede that it is very unlikely that the vitamins will help. In the previous section, however, we discussed the emerging theory that family members should be given some discretion, provided it is within reason.

This leaves Miss Grimes with three possible objections to family decision. First, she could argue that the daughter had exercised undue influence and that, therefore, the decision should not be honored. She might hold that the wife, as next of kin, should be the real decision-maker assuming that Mr. Desmond could not participate. If the wife had, in fact, accepted the treatment proposal after persuasion from her daughter, however, on what basis could Miss Grimes reject the decision?

Second, she could argue that the family decision about what will serve Mr. Desmond's interests is so grossly in error that it should be overturned. Just as hospital attorneys go to court to overturn unreasonable treatment-refusal decisions made by parents, so they could seek to have overturned a familial decision that is so implausible that it would constitute abuse of the patient. That action, however, also creates problems. First, it would require a court action to have the family removed from the decision-making process. Second, it is highly debatable whether the family's decision is so contrary to Mr. Desmond's interests that a court should intervene. After all, he is not likely to be hurt by the treatment.

That leaves one other possibility: that even though the family decision is a tolerable one in terms of Mr. Desmond's interest, it still violates the principles of justice and beneficence to the extent that the family judgment can be overridden. Could Miss Grimes sustain such an argument here?

A similar analysis could be applied to the case of Yusef Camp, the boy who suffered severe, possibly total brain function loss after eating a pickle laced with a hallucinogen. The parents could be opposed in their request for continued support of their son on the grounds that they are beyond reason in their decision that it might benefit the boy. In their case, as in Mr. Desmond's, that would be a hard argument to make, since Yusef is not likely to be affected one way or the other. The alternative is to argue that the nurses' burden (having to clean maggots from the respiratory track, debride the gangrene, and provide intensive support) or the economic burden on society justifies overriding the parents.

In the case of Leon Davies, Simone Gauthier has clearly shifted her focus from the welfare of the individual patient to consider a more social perspective. Is there doubt in Ms. Gauthier's mind that the expensive institutional care would be in Leon's interest? Mrs. Gauthier reasonably observes, however, that a price of $200,000 for an extra year of institutionalization on a respirator is a great deal of money. At some point, a limit must be set.

In all three cases, the question must be raised of whether these are issues appropriate to the clinical nurse's agenda. If a decision is made that Yusef Camp's or Mr. Desmond's care should be limited in order to protect the welfare of others, should these issues be raised by the nurse or by someone else—that is, should an administrator, the board of trustees, or health insurance planners be setting these limits?

Whoever makes these choices will face the alternatives for allocating scarce resources discussed in the cases in Chapters 3 and 4. They might give the resources to those who are most willing to pay for them; they might use them where they will do the most good; or they might distribute them to those in greatest need. Should the nurses in these cases make these choices themselves, or should they turn to someone else for the decisions?

References

1. President's Commission for the Study of Ethical Problems in Medicine and Biomedical and Behavioral Research: Defining Death: Medical, Legal and Ethical Issues in the Definition of Death. Washington, DC, U.S. Government Printing Office, 1981
2. Green MB, Wikler D: Brain death and personal identity. Philosophy and Public Affairs 9(2):105–133, 1980
3. Veatch RM: Death, Dying, and the Biological Revolution. New Haven, Connecticut, Yale University Press, 1976
4. In re Quinlan. 70 N.J. 10, 355 A. 2d 647 (1976)
5. President's Commission for the Study of Ethical Problems in Medicine and Biomedical and Behavioral Research: Deciding to Forego Life-Sustaining Treatment: Ethical, Medical, and Legal Issues in Treatment Decisions. Washington, D.C., U.S. Government Printing Office, 1983
6. Bleich JD: The obligation to heal in the Judaic tradition: A comparative analysis. Rosner F, Bleich JD (eds): Jewish Bioethics, pp 1–44. New York, Sanhedrin Press, 1979
7. California "Natural Death" Act. 1976 Cal. Stat., Chapter 1439, Code, Health and Safety, sections 7185–7195
8. Miles SH, Cranford R, Schultz AL: The do-not-resuscitate order in a teaching hospital. Ann Intern Med 96:660–664, 1982
9. Minnesota Medical Association: Do Not Resuscitate (DNR) Guidelines. January 24, 1981
10. Youngner SJ, Lewandowski W, McClish DK, Juknialis BW, Coulton C, Bartlett ET: "Do not resuscitate" orders. JAMA 285:54–57, 1985
11. Beth Israel Hospital: Guidelines: Orders not to resuscitate. In President's Commission for the Study of Ethical Problems in Medicine and Biomedical and Behavioral Research: Deciding to Forego Life-Sustaining Treatment: Ethical, Medical, and Legal Issues in Treatment Decisions, p 503. Washington, DC, U.S. Government Printing Office, 1983
12. Frances Okun v. The Society of New York Hospital. Supreme Court of the State of New York. County of New York. Summons. Index Number 13167/84, June 1, 1984
13. Jameton A: Nursing Practice: The Ethical Issues. Englewood, NJ, Prentice-Hall, 1984

14. U.S. Department of Health and Human Services: Infant care review committees—Model guidelines. Federal Register: Notices 50(72):14893–14901, April 15, 1985

15. U.S. Department of Health and Human Services: Child Abuse and Neglect Prevention and Treatment Program: Final rule: 45 CFR 1340. Federal Register: Rules and Regulations 50(72):14878–14892, April 15, 1985

16. Pope Pius XII: The Prolongation of Life: An Address of Pope Pius XII to an International Congress of Anesthesiologists. The Pope Speaks 4:393–398, 1958

Index

Abortion, 2, 9, 10, 276
  avoiding killing *vs*, 155
  confidentiality and, 145, 147–148
  cultural differences related to, 185–186, 188–189
  genetic counseling and, 199–207
  moral rules and, 30–33
  personal values of nurse and, 31–33
  sex of fetus and, 187–188, 190–191
  in surrogate mothers, 210
  in unmarried teenager, 187, 189–190
Absolutism
  empirical, 5
  theological, 5
Acute care center, 127
Acute myelocytic leukemia, 98
Adenosine adaminase (ADA) deficiency, 211–212
Adoption, 87, 143, 145, 146, 148, 209
Advocate for the patient, 69, 70, 72, 94, 108, 280, 289
Alcoholism, 118, 126, 127, 227, 250, 254
Allocation of health resources. *See* Justice
Ambulatory health clinic, 145
American Nurses' Association (ANA) *Code for Nurses*
  interpretation of, 31, 55
  issues addressed by
    benefit to patient *vs* benefit to others, 24–26
    confidentiality, 141–144, 147, 150, 242
    employment conditions, 76
    incompetent practice, 46–47
    indirect killing, 169
    obligations to client, 3, 57–59, 61
    obligations to community, 69
    obligations to self, 31, 78–79

patient right to information, 124, 133, 260–261
  as source of moral authority, 37–38, 40
Amniocentesis, 188, 191, 199–201, 204
Anencephalic infant, 158
Annas, G., 178, 214
Aquinas, Thomas, 6, 12, 178
Artificial insemination, 198, 207–211
Authority. *See* Moral authority
Autonomy of patient, 101–115
  abortion and, 190
  avoiding killing and, 155, 163–164, 172
  conflicts involving, 18–19, 23, 24, 27, 29–30, 40, 197
  in death and dying, 279, 283, 289, 299
  diminished capacity to claim, 102–105
  ethical principles related to, 56, 57, 69
  external constraints on, 105–109
  fidelity and, 147
  in human experimentation, 234–248, 251, 225, 257
  justice and, 82–84, 91, 98
  normative ethics and, 8
  overriding, 109–114
  in psychiatric nursing, 215–216, 219–221, 224
  and right to refuse treatment, 260–262, 266, 267
  veracity and, 129, 132
Autosomal dominant condition, 203
Avoiding harm. *See* Maleficence
Avoiding killing, 155–178. *See also* Killing
  abortion and, 184–191
  actions and omissions in, 156–159
  autonomy and, 101
  conflicts related to, 9, 27, 30–31

305